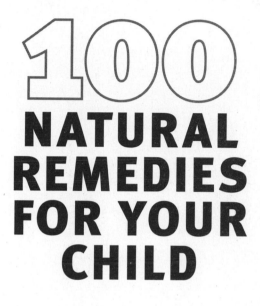

# 100
# NATURAL
# REMEDIES
# FOR YOUR
# CHILD

# 100
# NATURAL REMEDIES FOR YOUR CHILD

THE **COMPLETE GUIDE TO**
Safe, Effective Treatments
for Childhood's Most Common Ailments,
from ALLERGIES to WEIGHT LOSS

## Dr. Jared M. Skowron

RODALE.

© 2011 by Jared M. Skowron

Rodale books may be purchased for business or promotional use or for special sales. For information, please write to:
Special Markets Department, Rodale Inc., 733 Third Avenue, New York, NY 10017

Printed in the United States of America
Rodale Inc. makes every effort to use acid-free ♾, recycled paper ♻.

Book design by Kara Plikaitis

**Library of Congress Cataloging-in-Publication Data**

Skowron, Jared M.
    100 natural remedies for your child : the complete guide to safe, effective treatments for childhood's most common ailments, from allergies to weight loss / Jared M. Skowron.
        p.      cm.
    Includes index.
    ISBN 978-1-60961-115-6 paperback
    1. Pediatrics—Popular works.    2. Children—Health and hygiene—Popular works.    3. Children—Diseases—Alternative treatment—Popular works.    4. Naturopathy—Popular works.    I. Title.    II. Title: One hundred natural remedies for your child.
    RJ61.S335   2011
    618.92—dc23                                                                2011016621

**Distributed to the trade by Macmillan**
2   4   6   8   10   9   7   5   3   1   paperback

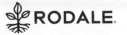

We inspire and enable people to improve their lives and the world around them.
www.rodalebooks.com

*For my parents,*
*And all parents who do the very best for their children.*

# — CONTENTS —

## Neurological

## Endocrine

## Exanthems (Viral Rashes)

## PART III: BODY SYSTEM REMEDIES

## APPENDIX

# — ACKNOWLEDGMENTS —

**A LONG LINE OF DOMINOES LED** to this book. It starts with my parents and my teachers, building my background of interest to search for a real solution to a problem and to never be satisfied with adequate. I need to thank Dr. Peter D'Adamo, who put me in touch with my fantastic agent, Janis Vallely, who connected me with the wonderful Lynn Lauber, who made my stories sing. More thanks goes to Julie Will, Marie Crousillat, Gena Smith, Marilyn Hauptly, Nancy Elgin, David Kiefer, and all the enthusiastic sales, marketing, editing, and publicity folks at Rodale. Huge thanks to my wife, Nicole, who is beside me every step of the way, and thanks to my patients, who prove to me that natural therapies are real and sometimes, miraculous. Last, but not least, is thanks to you: the parent, the grandparent, the teacher. It is the love you have for your children that fuels a search for the very best for them. I thank you for your limitless pursuit for their great potential.

# — INTRODUCTION —

## Why Natural Medicine, Why Now?

**IF YOU HAD THE CHOICE,** would you rather give your depressed son fluoxetine (Prozac)—a strong prescription drug with possible side effects that include abdominal pain and suicide—or fish oil and vitamin B complex supplements?

Would you rather see your daughter's acne treated with isotretinoin (Accutane)—a medication for which the FDA requires prescribers, pharmacies, and patients to follow a strict risk management program because it causes birth defects and may be linked to inflammatory bowel disease—or eliminate fat-free milk and other dairy items from her diet?

If you're like most parents, you'd probably feel more comfortable trying natural remedies first, using safe, effective options and ultimately wanting your child to be healthy and happy. In the 21st century, parents understand that a greener, cleaner environment includes their children's bodies.

Yet many parents don't have quick access to reliable natural, science-based remedies. That's why I've written this book: to help parents who want to prevent their children from having to take unnecessary medications or having to undergo unneeded surgeries or other invasive treatments. I also want to share the rewarding results of my clinical experience treating children who suffer from a variety of medical conditions with natural remedies. Why go to such extreme lengths when there are natural options that are safer, less costly, more effective, and readily available?

Many childhood disorders can be gently and safely treated with naturopathic medicine. That's why so many parents visit my Connecticut office in search of cures for their children's attention deficit disorder, asthma, colic, autism, and other health conditions that don't require a heavy dose of medication.

Two years ago, Marie drove 3 hours in order to carry her gravely ill daughter, Emily, into my office. She knew I am a top pediatric expert in natural health, and she had already been to countless doctors in some of the most prestigious pediatric groups in the country, from Harvard to Johns Hopkins to the Cleveland Clinic. Along the way, she'd met many experts, but she'd found no answers to the illness that had mysteriously attacked her young daughter.

Emily suffered from mitochondrial disease, a potentially fatal disorder. The mitochondria, the energy-producing cells in her body, had simply stopped working. Her visits to the top hospitals in the country had provided her with a diagnosis, but they didn't give her the answer to her real question, "How do I feel better?" Once a vibrant 10-year-old who trained her Afghan hound for competitions, Emily now was bedridden and listless, plagued by migraines and chronic fatigue.

Marie was frantic; her daughter's life seemed to be slipping away, and no MRI or CT scan had been able to locate the source of the problem. I often meet parents like Marie who are desperate for answers, whose children are suffering from complex, often serious disorders. Many of these chronic conditions—from obesity to diabetes to asthma—aren't caused by bacteria or viruses, but by something more far-reaching: what they are eating and the way they are living their lives.

Through rigorous testing and examination, I was able to discover the root cause of Emily's illness: She not only had a severe vitamin deficiency, but also serious food sensitivities. As a result, her muscles had atrophied and her gastrointestinal system had begun to shut down.

One of the things I love most about naturopathic medicine is that we spend time with patients to discover the root cause of illness. We get a full sense of the patient as a person, not a disease, run scientific tests that are often overlooked by mainstream physicians, and discover a safe, natural therapy that helps the patient at the deepest level. While the physical exam remains the same regardless of who performs it, lab work and other testing methods are extremely varied. The laboratories that naturopathic physicians use for standard blood work also perform nutrient analysis, heavy metal toxicity screens, and other tests to see how you are functioning.

Many sick children have a genetic intolerance to specific foods, and their bodies react to these foods as if they are fighting off an infection. Emily was no exception. When we tested her, we found that she had a serious sensitivity to cow's milk. We eliminated it from her diet; substituted goat, rice, and soy milks; and then began making plans to rebuild her health, including instituting a regimen of vitamins, herbal remedies, and nutritional supplements. These included:

1. Vitamins and supplements: High doses of the B vitamins; coenzyme Q10 (CoQ10); Seacure protein supplement

2. B vitamins and CoQ10 are essential for the production of energy. Our cells need these nutrients so their energy factories (the mitochondria) can create adenosine triphosphate (ATP), which the cells then use to power their work. Seacure is a fish protein supplement (not a fish oil) that heals the intestines.

3. Herbs: *Rhodiola*
   The herb *Rhodiola rosea* is known for boosting energy levels in people with fatigue.

4. Homeopathics: UNDA 3, UNDA 6
   Used in drainage homeopathy for the cells, these two compounds contain herbs and metals that support digestion and the liver.

In my practice, I detoxify many of my patients with safe, effective homeopathic drainage remedies. They are specific combinations of diluted herbs and metals. The principle behind their use is one you probably remember from high school chemistry, "like dissolves like": The diluted metals in the remedies grab onto toxins in the body and remove them.

Emily had never felt a treatment work before. Her other physicians had tried a multitude of drugs that didn't make her feel better or more energetic.

Natural medicine strives to include a person's total environment in the healing process. Emily's beloved dog Hank had always been an important part of her life. In fact, her family relied on Hank to alert them when Emily experienced painful muscle spasms. Now we included Hank in Emily's treatment plan, utilizing him to help her walk again, rebuild her muscle mass, and regain her strength. When Emily was reluctant to get out of bed, Hank inspired her to get outside and take daily walks again. This dog made an enormous difference in Emily's mental state and provided her with the motivation to take an active part in her own recovery.

Observing Emily's progress was incredible. When I first met her, she was confined to a wheelchair, barely able to open her eyes or to speak. Yet within 2 months of complying with the regimen I'd prescribed for her, she was back in school, playing outside, and showing her dog competitively again. I've seen thousands of kids like Emily who don't fit into cookie-cutter diagnoses and whose parents are frustrated and scared about the lack of options to treat their sick children. My job as a pediatric naturopath is to show them that proper nutrition and vitamin and mineral supplementation are the keys to good health. There is a time and place for conventional (Western) medicine, but natural solutions, especially things as simple as a change in diet, can be seemingly miraculous cures for many of our children's most alarming and misdiagnosed ailments.

# An Epidemic of Sick Children

Ever since I was young I wanted to be a pediatrician. But as I grew older, I started to see the fragmented nature of conventional medicine. Patients were shuttled from one specialist to another, where their bodies were divvied up and treatments were prescribed that merely masked their symptoms. The main role of a pediatrician increasingly revolved around well-baby visits, prescribing antibiotics, and keeping a watch out for serious illness rather than supporting health. I didn't want to work like that; I wanted to help children live healthy lives without the chemical crutch.

Many of us believe the myth that the United States has the world's greatest health care system. After all, we spend more money than any other country on health care. In 2003, we accounted for 45 percent of the world's pharmaceutical sales. We must have the healthiest population, right?

Wrong. In fact, the health statistics of our country are downright dismal.

Consider that:

According to the Central Intelligence Agency's *World Factbook,* the United States ranks 49th in the world in life expectancy and 177th in infant mortality.

We have the unfortunate distinction of having the world's highest autism rate. In fact, a study published in 2009 in *Pediatrics* revealed that 2 percent of all American boys (that's 1 in 58) fall somewhere on the autism spectrum, while among all children the ratio is 1 in 91.

Obesity is increasingly a problem as well, with 16.9 percent of children between the ages of 2 and 19 and 18.1 percent between the ages of 12 and 19 being clinically obese. Childhood obesity substantially raises the risks for type 2 diabetes, high cholesterol, high blood pressure, heart disease, and gallstones.

Asthma affects 9.6 percent—7.1 million—American children; it is the third-leading cause of hospitalization for children under the age of 15. These and other now common illnesses—from type 2 diabetes to autism, ADHD to high cholesterol—are not caused by exotic bacteria or viruses, but by poor lifestyle habits. We're nourishing our children with fake foods. We're enabling obesity by using computers, television, and video games as babysitters. We're subjecting our kids to environmental toxins on a daily basis. And it needs to stop.

# Why Natural Medicine, Why Now?

In much of Europe, integrative medicine—which combines conventional and scientifically proven alternative medical treatments—is practiced routinely and conventional medical interventions are reserved for more serious conditions and emergencies. Natural medicine, which focuses primarily on wellness and disease prevention, generally provides the first course of treatment.

Naturopathic, or "natural," medicine is built upon the idea that the body possesses an innate ability to heal itself. When you cut your finger or are exposed to a virus, your immune system kicks in to stop the invading germs or fight the infection. Natural medicine works in tandem with this organic healing mechanism by supporting it with nutritious foods, vitamins, minerals, herbs, and homeopathic solutions composed of these elements. Naturopathic physicians base their practice on a simple yet powerful concept: putting good stuff in and taking bad stuff out.

Conventional medicine tends to overlook this idea. If you have asthma, you are given an inhaler; if you have inflammation, you're prescribed a steroid. There's little interest in discovering the underlying cause of the illness or creating a preventive strategy to keep it from recurring; even when the interest is there, conventional health care providers have little time to explore it. When physicians are tied to appointment schedules that require them to see patients every 15 to 20 minutes, it's not easy to fully assess patients' lifestyles and the factors that may play a part in their problems. But there is a new movement in conventional medical schools to train physicians in integrative medicine. As evidence of natural medicine's value accumulates, conventional medical practices change—for example, fish oil was once discounted as ineffective, but now it is scientifically proven and available as a prescription medication. Hopefully, such changes will continue so that a healthier kind of medicine, integrative medicine, will be the future for our children.

The pharmaceutical industry seems to have devised a drug for every condition of modern life, from allergies to weight loss. But these drugs come with hidden costs that are often more severe than the conditions they are intended to cure. Many of these very powerful medications are used to treat conditions that don't require such potency. There's no need to treat every bug, allergy, and sniffle with a wallop of medicine.

The public is becoming increasingly aware of the many side effects, mishaps, and recalls associated with prescription drugs. In fact, prescription drugs, even when they are used correctly (at the right doses and for the right conditions), regularly appear among the top five leading causes of death in the United States. That's probably one of the reasons why Americans are currently spending $34 billion annually on alternative medicine.

In this book, it is my goal to help you heal your children's health conditions naturally. I'm not advocating for the exchange of one health care system for another; I simply believe that we should add another layer of protection to the conventional model and integrate natural medications and treatments that can positively impact a child's developing mind and body.

Keep your pediatrician. Keep your child's prescriptions, if they are necessary to his or her health. But I urge you to try using safe, natural medicines as a first course of action, or in conjunction with your child's current treatment plan. Your children will thank you for it.

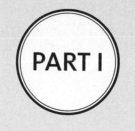

**PART I**

# NATURAL SOLUTIONS
# FOR YOUR KIDS

# THE POWER
# OF REAL FOOD

**1**

**JOAN, A MOTHER OF TWO,** called one day to tell me that her son Hal, 10, was listless, losing weight, and doing poorly in school. He had been variously diagnosed with depression, attention deficit hyperactivity disorder (ADHD), and irritable bowel syndrome (IBS) and was being medicated by three different specialists. Joan was worried that her son was being overmedicated by his doctors and wanted my opinion as a naturopathic physician.

She arrived at my office looking distressed and accompanied by Hal, who was reserved and sullen. After they sat down, Joan said, "I'm recently divorced, and I also got laid off 6 months ago. I'm working two part-time jobs now, so Hal has to fend for himself most of the day."

Hal avoided my eyes as his mother talked, as if he was embarrassed.

Joan continued, "The other morning I looked down and realized that my 10-year-old son was on more medications than my mother was at 75, and I just freaked out. Plus, he doesn't seem to be getting any better, just worse."

Hal was suffering from a list of diagnoses that many American kids currently face: ADD, depression, and IBS. He was being treated with a powerful drug cocktail that included methylphenidate (Ritalin) for his ADHD and paroxetine (Paxil), a selective serotonin reuptake inhibitor, or SSRI, for depression. Both are strong medications; in combination, they could have effects on not just his mood and behavior, but also on his appetite, energy level, and mental skills.

I asked Joan about her son's lifestyle—what was his diet like?

"I buy him healthy food, but I can't make him eat it," she responded. "I work all day and he's at school."

When I asked Hal what a typical day's food intake looked like, he listed the following:

- Breakfast: A toaster pastry and a sweetened orange drink
- Lunch: One or two slices of pizza, two cookies, and a can of soda
- Dinner: A microwaveable frozen meal followed by a bowl of ice cream and another soda

Immediately I could see that the lack of nutrients in Hal's diet, along with the hefty doses of added sugars and fats, was certainly problematic. Hal didn't consume a single serving of fruit on most days. And the food he ate was loaded with synthetic additives and colorants that may be linked to ADD, among other disorders.

But when it came to Hal's overall quality of life, the IBS was his most troubling illness. It often sidelined him from many social events and school functions, particularly sports. From Hal's somber mood, it was clear that he missed participating in such activities with his peers—and that being involved in physical activity would have a positive impact on his health.

I decided we would first try a food elimination diet (see "Elimination Diet," opposite), which removes the foods suspected of triggering an illness (in this case, IBS) from the diet and then adds them back in, one at a time, to see which ones are triggers. To facilitate this process, patients keep a daily food and symptom journal, tracking what they eat and how they feel after eating. Once several weeks' worth of information has been recorded, the patients and I sit down together to analyze the journals, and it usually becomes apparent which foods are precipitating or contributing to their illnesses.

In the weeks that followed, it became apparent that Hal's trigger was wheat gluten, which was present in virtually every meal he ate. I helped Joan create a gluten-free diet (see "Gluten or Another Wheat Protein," later in this chapter) that eliminated wheat breads and all other products made with grains that have gluten and substituted brown rice and spelt. Since Joan suspected that she had the same food allergy, she decided to follow the same eating plan.

When you start your own elimination diet, it may take time for your symptoms to decrease or disappear. Because of this, you might not associate stopping a food with feeling better 2 weeks later. Consult your naturopathic physician, who will make the connections for you.

## ELIMINATION DIET

An elimination diet removes foods from a child's diet that are suspected of being symptom triggers, then adds them back in one at a time to see whether the child feels well or ill. Common triggers are cow's milk and gluten.

While it's easy to follow this procedure, ongoing compliance with the findings can be challenging for both parent and child. No one likes giving up favorite foods— even if it makes him or her feel better.

Follow these instructions for the elimination diet. If children are old enough, they may be able to follow the procedure themselves, with your help.

1.  Keep a 7-day food diary of the foods your child eats most commonly.

2.  Keep a parallel record of gastrointestinal symptoms or mood changes and try to connect them to the foods listed in the food diary.

3.  See if the foods that match your child's symptoms have similarities, such as dairy, gluten, egg, soy, legume, or corn ingredients.

4.  If possible, avoid the foods that match the symptoms for a minimum of 1 week, preferably for 1 month.

5.  After the elimination period, reintroduce a suspect food for 2 days.

6.  If this food is causing the problem, then the symptoms may return, sometimes even worse than before.

7.  If the symptoms do return, eliminate this food from your child's diet altogether.

8.  If the symptoms do not return within 3 days of reintroduction, then you can assume that the food is not causing the problem.

9.  Continue eliminating and reintroducing a food every 5 to 7 days until you discover the offending items.

10. After avoiding an offending food for 6 to 12 months, your child's immune system may have further developed, allowing him or her to tolerate a food that used to cause a problem. Try reintroducing it. It doesn't always work, though; some foods will always have to be avoided.

While food allergies are usually present for life, food sensitivities can change for no apparent reason. The immune system is in constant flux, especially in children.

I have seen sensitivities to a food disappear as a child's immune system begins to tolerate it.

This change in their diet turned out to have a number of benefits for both Hal and his mother. Joan changed her work schedule so they could sit down and eat dinner together for the first time in years. They ate healthy, wholesome foods, and they saved money by eating at home. This junk-free diet also rid Hal's body of the additives and food colorings that may be linked to ADHD.

Surprisingly, Hal enjoyed his new diet and even agreed to take the healthy lunches his mother packed to school. Why?

I saw the answer for myself when Hal arrived for his 2-month follow-up appointment. After spending 8 weeks on a healthy diet, he was almost unrecognizable. His pallor was gone, his face and body had filled out, and he had also stopped taking Ritalin.

"Why's that?" I asked him.

"I don't feel like I need it anymore. I can pay attention pretty well now. I told my other doctor—he was surprised, but he didn't argue about it."

Joan, on the other hand, looked as if a sublayer of fat had melted off her body. She also seemed more vital and alive. "Hal is playing soccer!" she shared. "And it was his idea."

As I listened to her talk, I thought, *This is the power of food*. It is not simply our body's fuel, without which we could not survive. Food also possesses great power to affect our physical and mental well-being.

As the French gastronomist Jean Anthelme Brillat-Savarin said, "Tell me what you eat, and I will tell you what you are."

Dietary change is the core lifestyle modification in naturopathic medical practice. The easiest, least expensive, and most effective intervention you as a parent can make to improve your children's health is to feed them "real" foods, which are often the miracle cures for numerous childhood disorders. This is an area of everyday life that you can act on right now—without a prescription or special expertise, but with just a little guidance.

# What Are Your Children Really Eating?

At the end of each day, if your child's food intake were displayed on the dining room table, you might be surprised—or even shocked—by the quality and the quantity of what he consumed.

Did he really empty that bag of corn chips and half a jar of processed cheese dip? Did his lunch actually consist of two slices of pepperoni pizza, a can of soda, and a pile of vending machine candy? You might be surprised to see that your child's only "fruit" serving for the day came in the form of a "roll-up" or that the only green item in his diet was artificially colored.

My rule for children is simple: Feed them a whole food diet. If it grows from the earth, swims in the ocean, or grazes in a pasture, they can have it. There are no cookie bushes, bagel trees, or potato chip canyons anywhere that I know of.

As parents, you are a child's first role model in the world of food. Whether you're a health nut or a couch potato, your child is likely to mimic your behavior. And the habits that children form during their first 7 years will likely last a lifetime. Once your child develops a taste for unhealthy, processed foods, it can be very difficult for him or her to overcome cravings for foods that are full of sugar, fat, and salt. Your best strategy is to keep those foods to a minimum in your child's diet in the first place.

Parents should also be careful not to use food—especially sweets and junk foods—as incentives for good behavior, rewards for accomplishments, or positive reinforcement. These associations can become long lasting and contribute to disordered eating habits.

One way for parents to get a clear idea of just what their children are eating is to ask them to keep a 7-day food journal in which they record the amount of each item in every meal, snack, and dessert as well as every beverage they consume every day for a week. (This can be the same food and symptom journal they used for the elimination diet.) Older kids should be able to fill it out on their own, and you should encourage them to record their entries throughout the day so they don't forget about any candy bars or toaster pastries they might have eaten. Ask them to be specific about portions, too; instead of simply writing "ice cream," they should specify "ice cream cone" or "1 pint of ice cream." With younger kids, sit down together at the end of the day and help them try to remember the foods they ate. You should also have them note any symptoms that arose around the time they ate. Did they have a headache shortly after their snack? A tummy ache after dinner?

Linking physical symptoms with food is also a way for children to understand how their diet makes them feel and why. For example, as a child works through an elimination diet, you can explain how cow's milk and gluten products may have adverse effects on the immune system and draw connections between symptom relief and food removal.

Eventually, children will learn which foods create unpleasant symptoms, and you can help them choose whether to eliminate them from their diet entirely or simply cut down on the amounts they eat. If they have some say in that choice, they are more likely to follow through on the ultimate decision.

My 12-year-old patient Heather had lived for most of her life with undiagnosed celiac disease. She often felt ill and bloated after eating wheat or other starches. After she was diagnosed, she was happy to stick to a gluten-free diet because she realized how much better she felt.

"I don't even have to worry about compliance," her father told me. "When she's confronted with something she's not supposed to eat, she says, 'No, thanks, that will make me feel sick.'"

## Whole versus Processed Foods

A peach plucked from a tree and a sugar snap pea snipped off a vine—these are real, whole foods that many of our children rarely eat. Delivered straight from nature, they contain nutrients and vitamins that are impossible to duplicate in any pill or supplement.

Processed foods, on the other hand, are ubiquitous and often make up the majority of our children's diets, from their first bite of high-sugar cereal in the morning to their evening snack of salty, fried potato chips.

There is no good reason to feed your children manufactured meals. It may seem like packaged meals—breakfast sandwiches, pizza bagels, frozen dinners—are more convenient than preparing whole foods, but consider this: An apple and a handful of almonds is one of the most nutritious ways you can start your child's day. No microwaving or toasting involved!

In addition, junk foods such as sugary snacks and sodas may be linked to hyperactivity in children. And it has been shown that children who eat a diet rich in nutritious, wholesome foods (high in fresh fruits, vegetables, whole grains, and fish) have half the risk of being diagnosed with ADHD as do children who eat a "Western" diet (emphasizing processed, sugary, fried, and refined foods).

In fact, in a Dutch study, 25 children with ADHD whose parents fed them an oligoantigenic diet—one comprising only a few hypoallergenic foods, such as rice, turkey, pears, and lettuce—were judged by the parents to have at least a 50 percent improvement in their behavior. While this diet may seem strict, it's a wonderful example of how food can affect our cognitive function and mood.

Shop at farmer's markets and on the perimeters of grocery stores, where fresh foods are located, as opposed to at the center, where preservative-laden foods are displayed. Eating this way will help your health!

# Artificial Colors and Preservatives

Did you know that farm-raised salmon—which are gray and have lower healthy essential fatty acid content than wild salmon—are dyed deep pink to mimic the color of wild salmon? Artificial food colors and preservatives, so common in packaged products, may be graced with lyrical names—from Sunset Yellow to Allura Red—but their effects are far from poetic. They are simply additional unnecessary toxic burdens for our children to bear.

A 12-year-old girl who was in serious trouble came in to see me recently. Her skin was covered with hives and she was experiencing difficulty breathing. When I asked the mother if her daughter had any allergies, she answered, "Not that I know of."

The girl was pale and wheezing. There was no time to waste. As I began to administer steroids and an antihistamine, I noticed that she had something in her mouth.

"What's that?" I asked.

"Oh, nothing," she said, and spit out a wad of cinnamon chewing gum.

She and her mother remained in the office for an hour until her symptoms stabilized and she felt strong enough to go home.

To my surprise, mother and daughter were back in my office the next day with the same symptoms, which had grown even more severe. Once again the girl had a wad of the same gum in her mouth.

I asked the mother if she had monitored what her daughter had ingested since the day before.

"Since last night, she's only had water."

"What about the gum?"

"Oh, the gum—I wasn't counting that. She lives on that stuff."

That mouthful of chemicals my patient was chewing turned out to be the culprit. She was having a severe allergic reaction to it. It contained aspartame, a common ingredient in sugarless gum, which is thought to be a neurotoxin—a substance that affects the functioning of neurons. But that wasn't the only chemical with the potential to be responsible for her severe allergic reaction.

What else was in the chewing gum that could have killed this child had she not gotten to a doctor in time? Here's a look at the ingredients:

Sorbitol, gum base, glycerol, mannitol, acesulfame, malic acid, aspartame, citric acid, colors (Blue 2 Lake, Yellow 6 Lake, Red 40 Lake), soy lecithin, and BHT (to maintain freshness)

It's hard to know which of these chemicals caused such severe symptoms in my patient. The truth is that most of the packaged foods our children eat are like laboratories stocked with arcane chemicals that even a chemist would have trouble discerning.

Just a cursory glance at the ingredients of a frozen chicken dish reveals sodium tripolyphosphate, natamycin, calcium propionate, sulfites, modified cornstarch. How about Lunchables, a favorite meal kit for children's brown-bag lunches? A typical one contains a deep-dish pepperoni pizza, cheese crackers, chocolate chip cookies, and fruit punch—an artificially flavored smorgasbord with high-fructose corn syrup cookies for dessert. Even worse, one Lunchables variety that, thankfully, is no longer made included chocolate chips that were coated with shellac to make them shinier. That's right, shellac, more commonly used to produce a sheen on furniture and a substance secreted by a particular kind of bug.

What are the effects of these substances on our children? As a parent, you don't want to wait and find out. Once parents recognize the toxicity of these additives in their children's foods and snacks, most want to avoid them—especially those who know that research has suggested that artificial food colorings may cause neurotoxicity—damage to the brain and nervous system.

The good news is that changing to a wholesome diet of fresh foods free of these chemical additives is remarkably easy. Think of the kinds of lunches our great-grandparents might have taken with them to school—an egg, cheese, or meat sandwich on whole grain bread, nuts, and a piece of fruit. This is the way nature intended for us to fuel our bodies.

# Feeding Your Child for Health

The nutritional needs of children are much greater than those of adults because of their rapid development and growth. They need a diet rich in nutrients in order to build a physical foundation that will be long-lasting.

Children aren't just little adults. They possess unique nutritional needs at different times of their lives. In the first few years, they need high levels of healthy fats to grow smart brains. As they get bigger, they need healthy proteins, vitamins, and minerals to support growth spurts in bone and muscle. Once they enter school, immune system-supporting nutrients will help them fight off colds and infections.

So, which food choices are the best for your child? Every time you turn on the news or look on the Internet, there's a new diet or research finding that is supposed to help your child achieve the best health. The important point is to begin somewhere

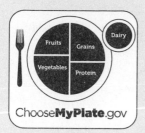

# CHOOSE MY PLATE
## 10 TIPS TO A GREAT PLATE

### MAKING FOOD CHOICES FOR A HEALTHY LIFESTYLE CAN BE AS SIMPLE AS USING THESE 10 TIPS.

Use the ideas in this list to *balance your calories*, to choose foods to *eat more often*, and to cut back on foods to *eat less often*.

• In 2011, the USDA updated the dietary guidelines for Americans and replaced the pyramid icon, long used to help parents make healthy food choices, with a plate (above).

### 1. Balance calories
Find out how many calories YOU need for a day as a first step in managing your weight. Go to www.ChooseMyPlate.gov to find your calorie level. Being physically active also helps you balance calories.

### 2. Enjoy your food, but eat less
Take the time to fully enjoy your food as you eat it. Eating too fast or when your attention is elsewhere may lead to eating too many calories. Pay attention to hunger and fullness cues before, during, and after meals. Use them to recognize when to eat and when you've had enough.

### 3. Avoid oversized portions
Use a smaller plate, bowl, and glass. Portion out foods before you eat. When eating out, choose a smaller size option, share a dish, or take home part of your meal.

### 4. Foods to eat more often
Eat more vegetables, fruits, whole grains, and fat-free or 1% milk and dairy products. These foods have the nutrients you need for health—including potassium, calcium, vitamin D, and fiber. Make them the basis for meals and snacks.

### 5. Make half your plate fruits and vegetables
Choose red, orange, and dark-green vegetables like tomatoes, sweet potatoes, and broccoli, along with other vegetables for your meals. Add fruit to meals as part of main or side dishes or as dessert.

### 6. Switch to fat-free or low-fat (1%) milk
They have the same amount of calcium and other essential nutrients as whole milk but fewer calories and less saturated fat.

### 7. Make half your grains whole grains
To eat more whole grains, substitute a whole grain product for a refined product—such as eating whole wheat bread instead of white bread or brown rice instead of white rice.

### 8. Foods to eat less often
Cut back on foods high in solid fats, added sugars, and salt. They include cakes, cookies, ice cream, candies, sweetened drinks, pizza, and fatty meats like ribs, sausages, bacon, and hot dogs. Use these foods as occasional treats, not everyday foods.

### 9. Compare sodium in foods
Use the Nutrition Facts label to choose lower sodium versions of foods like soup, bread, and frozen meals. Select canned foods labeled low sodium, reduced sodium, or no salt added.

### 10. Drink water instead of sugary drinks
Cut calories by drinking water or unsweetened beverages. Soda, energy drinks, and sports drinks are a major source of added sugar, and calories, in American diets.

**Go to www.ChooseMyPlate.gov for more information.**

Source: USDA Center for Nutrition Policy and Promotion

healthy. Start by keeping track of what your child eats and then, step by step, change his or her diet to match the recommendations for children of the same age. Remember to keep track of not only the calories and servings, but also the different types of foods.

Some additional tips for feeding your kids nutritious foods:

- When cooking, choose preparation methods that don't rely on a lot of added fat, such as baking, grilling, and broiling. Olive oil can be safely used in modest amounts for children.

- Replace packaged chips and cookies with fresh fruits, yogurt, and air-popped popcorn.

- Choose whole grain breads, pasta, and crackers over white-flour items.

- Always keep fresh fruits and vegetables on hand for easy snacks and to add to meals. If you don't want to spend time preparing them, buy them precut.

- Replace juices, sodas, and sports drinks with water.

- Avoid purchasing water bottles made of soft plastics that can leach into the water, especially when they are exposed to heat, such as in the back of a car on a hot summer day. Instead, filter water at home and fill a glass container to take with you.

- Replace high-fat dairy products with lower-fat, organic versions.

# Macronutrients and Kids

## Three Basic Macronutrients

"Nutrients" include the macronutrients—carbohydrates, proteins, and fats—which your body needs in large amounts, and the micronutrients, which are the vitamins, minerals, and other substances the body requires in small amounts. The table on page 13 indicates how much of each of these macronutrients your child needs. The ranges of the recommendations are wide because different children should get different proportions of the nutrients based on their health, weight, and other factors. Consult your naturopathic physician for specific nutritional suggestions and guidelines.

## Macronutrient Proportion by Age

| AGE | CARBOHYDRATES | PROTEIN | FATS |
|---|---|---|---|
| 1–3 years | 45–65% | 5–20% | 30–40% |
| 4–18 years | 45–65% | 10–30% | 25–35% |

Source: Institute of Medicine. Dietary Reference Intakes: Macronutrients. n.d. www.iom.edu/~/media/Files/Activity%20Files/Nutrition/DRIs/DRI_Macronutrients.pdf.

**PROTEINS.** Proteins are essential for growth. There's no life without them; next to water, they are the most plentiful substances in the body. It's important to eat protein every day. A lack of protein can result in growth failure, loss of muscle mass, a less robust immune system, and a weakened heart and respiratory system, among other health problems.

Proteins don't have to come from meats. While animal foods such as beef, chicken, turkey, fish, milk, and eggs are all good sources of protein, nuts, seeds, beans, and tofu are also protein-rich foods.

Proteins are composed of amino acids, with different amino acids being combined to make different kinds of proteins. Most proteins are similar, and there are no "good" or "bad" proteins although there are healthy and unhealthy protein sources.

## 5 Sources of Healthy Animal Proteins

Wild fish, especially wild salmon
Organic chicken
Turkey
Lean pork
Eggs from cage-free, organically raised hens

## 5 Sources of Unhealthy Animal Proteins

Hot dogs
Bacon
High-fat beef
Conventionally raised chicken
Farmed fish

# 5 Sources of Healthy Vegetarian Proteins

Beans

Hummus

Nuts

Seeds

Soy products, lightly processed (tofu, tempeh, miso, and soy milk)

**CARBOHYDRATES:** Every machine needs fuel, and the body is no exception. Carbohydrates are our major sources of quick fuel and provide us with energy. They come in many different forms, from breads and pastas to vegetables, from white flour to whole grains.

## Glycemic Indexes (GI) of Sample Foods

| HIGH GI FOODS (70 OR HIGHER) | LOW GI FOODS (55 OR LOWER) |
|---|---|
| Cornflakes 81 | Kidney beans 24 |
| Instant mashed potatoes 87 | Soy milk 34 |
| White bread 75 | Barley 28 |
| Watermelon 76 | Apple 36 |
| White rice 73 | Carrots (boiled) 39 |
| Rice milk 86 | Fat-free milk 37 |

## Glycemic Loads (GL) of Sample Foods

| HIGH GL FOODS (20 OR HIGHER) | LOW GL FOODS (10 OR LOWER) |
|---|---|
| 1 bagel 25 | 1 whole wheat tortilla 8 |
| 1 cup white rice 23 | 1 cup whole milk 3 |
| 1 cup raisins 28 | 1 grapefruit 3 |
| 35 grams macaroni and cheese 32 | 1 cup peanuts 1 |
| 1 baked potato 26 | 1 carrot 3 |

Two things to consider when choosing carbohydrates for your child are their gly-cemic index (GI) and glycemic load (GL). These are ways to understand the effects that different amounts of carbohydrates in different foods will have on your blood sugar. The GI sets out the "quality" of these carbohydrates by ranking foods accord-ing to how much and for how long they raise blood sugar after the body converts them from carbs. The higher and longer a food raises the blood sugar level, the higher the GI number. Stick with foods that have GIs of 55 or less, especially if your child has diabe-tes or is overweight or obese. White bread and cornflakes are high-GI foods, so the low-GI high-fiber whole grain bread and bran cereal are better choices. I tell my patients to eat low-GI foods like grapefruits and carrots.

While the glycemic index reflects only the *quality* of the carbohydrates in a food, the glycemic load lets you take into account the *quantity* of the food and how it and the other foods you want to eat at the same time will affect your blood sugar on the whole. A food's GL is calculated by multiplying the food's GI value by how many grams of carbohydrates your portion contains and then dividing that by 100. You can use it to compare foods to each other based on how much of them you will eat. Choose foods with a GL of 10 or lower.

Foods with high GIs and GLs often aren't very filling and are easily overeaten, sending your blood sugar soaring. This can be dangerous because it puts people who eat too much of them at risk for diabetes. Choosing the right carbohydrates is impor-tant, because the glycemic index isn't a "perfect food choice" number. Even though some candy bars and potato chips have low GIs, they are not healthy foods for your child. Common sense will steer you to the right choices.

# 7 Sources of Healthy Carbohydrates

Beans

Brown rice

Fruits

Sweet potatoes

Vegetables

Whole grain bread

Whole grain pasta cooked al dente

## 5 Sources of Unhealthy Carbohydrates

Bread snacks (bagels, muffins, doughnuts, cookies)

Corn syrup (regular and high fructose)

Cracker snacks (Goldfish, corn chips)

Sugar

White bread

**FATS:** Children need healthy fats in their diets to support growth, organ development, and brain health. Each and every nerve in our body is actually wrapped in a blanket of healthy fat. Without this fat blanket, the brain can't grow or work properly. Choose natural, heart-healthy fats (see the healthy sources list, opposite), and be cautious about eating processed foods like cookies and chips that are advertised as low fat. These foods may have a reduced fat content, but they're often filled with a laundry list of chemicals that improve the taste once the fat has been removed.

Different types of fat have different structures and affect the body differently. Monounsaturated and some types of polyunsaturated fats are healthy, beneficial fats. They help balance your cholesterol levels and are essential to the foundation of every cell. These fats are found in nuts, avocados, olive oil, salmon, etc.

Saturated fats and trans fats are bad fats that raise the "bad" (LDL) cholesterol level and prevent cells from working correctly. These bad fats are found in many foods, including fried foods, margarine, microwave popcorn, vegetable shortening, and meats. Some animal products, such as beef, have more bad fats, whereas others, such as wild salmon, have a higher level of good fats. Contrary to what you may think, not all saturated fats are bad for your heart. Stearic acid, one form of saturated fat, has no effect on cholesterol. Palmitic acid and lauric acid, two other kinds, raise both "good" (HDL) and LDL cholesterol, but they may lower heart disease risk because the HDL increase is greater than the LDL rise. The Women's Health Initiative, a comprehensive study on diet's impact on health, showed that low total and saturated fat intake had no impact on heart disease and stroke rates, even among women who had restricted them for years.

Recent medical studies suggest that trans fats are worse for our long-term health than saturated fats because although both types raise the LDL cholesterol level, trans fats also lower the level of HDL. In the past, oils containing trans fats could be commonly found in the deep fryers at many chain restaurants, but today they are, thankfully, less prevalent. But trans fats are still used in many processed foods, especially baked goods.

Fats contain fatty acids, a term we're familiar with from today's over-the-counter nutritional supplements. One type, the omega-3 fatty acids, includes the eicosapentaenoic acid (EPA) and docosahexaenoic acid (DHA) that are found in cold-water fish and are the beneficial components in fish oil supplements. Walnuts and flaxseeds contain a precursor to omega-3 fatty acids, alpha-linolenic acid, that the body must convert. Omega-6 fatty acids are found in other nuts and seeds and their oils, including soybean oil, which is used in most processed foods and fast foods. Omega-6s increase inflammation, whereas omega-3s decrease it, so properly balancing the two is important for good health.

Fats are added to many of our processed foods for a simple reason: They taste good, and make us feel full and satisfied. I remember when I was a short-order cook in high school, standing next to a fryer filled with gallons of fat we used over and over for weeks on end. Periodically, I'd fish out a french fry that had gotten lost at the bottom and was destroyed beyond belief—a shriveled strip. I remember thinking, *I wonder what all that fat does to our bodies?*

## 4 Sources of Healthy Fats

Avocados
Fish
Nuts
Soy spreads

## 5 Sources of Unhealthy Fats

High-fat dairy products such as cream
Margarine and other foods made with partially hydrogenated oils
Red meat from grain-fed animals
Shortening and solid animal and vegetable fats
Soybean oil (common in fast and processed foods)

# Portion Distortion

It's easy to confuse portion size and serving size. A serving size is a standardized unit of measurement—say, a cup or an ounce—used for reference in dietary guidelines. A portion size is the amount of food served in a single situation, like a meal or a snack.

A problem arises when the portion size you're accustomed to eating is larger than the standard serving size on the food package. This is so common that most of us aren't even aware of what a serving size looks like. We assume that the 24-ounce bottle of soda we're drinking is one serving, when in fact it's two. A 12-ounce can of Coke has 140 calories and 39 grams (almost 10 teaspoons) of sugar. A 24-ounce bottle—three servings—has 300 calories and 81 grams (over 20 teaspoons) of sugar.

Our portion sizes have increased dramatically over the past few decades, especially in restaurants. Individual portions are now so generous that they may contain two, three, or four servings of food. And these supersize servings are clearly linked to the obesity epidemic. As I tell my patients, "If you want to be large, order the large; if you want to be small, order the small."

Portion size wouldn't matter so much if people chose to eat only an appropriate amount. But few of us look at the plate of food we've been served and eat only a single serving. We tend to eat whatever is placed in front of us. As a parent, being aware of serving sizes is crucial to helping your child eat the appropriate, healthy amount. Your child may think he's pouring one serving of cereal into his breakfast bowl when, in fact, he's pouring—and eating—three or four times that amount. Help your child become aware of what a healthy portion looks like and why it's important to be mindful of how much you eat.

So what is a serving size? Here are some helpful guidelines.

1 cup (8 ounces) of vegetables = 1 baseball

½ cup (4 ounces) of ice cream = ½ baseball

3 ounces of meat = a deck of cards

# Sugars

We all know that sugars—simple carbohydrates—contribute to weight gain and are underlying culprits in our nation's obesity crisis. But sugar also plays a role in a number of other health conditions, including high cholesterol, type 2 diabetes (in combination with high fat intake), mood swings, hyperactivity, and tooth decay. And, as we all know, eating too much sugar can also affect a child's behavior, sometimes causing him to act "wired" or "hyper" and stimulating out-of-control behavior. Eating too much sugary candy causes a rapid rise and then dip in blood sugar, setting off a chain reaction of metabolic and hormonal changes that affect appetite and behavior for hours. Remember to choose foods that have a low glycemic index and a low glycemic load.

Lisa, a patient of mine who is overweight, recently came to see me with her father, who is also overweight. Lisa had recently been diagnosed with high cholesterol and prediabetes, and her father was livid.

"She's a kid; how could she possibly have high cholesterol?" he asked me.

I told him that there is now an epidemic of formerly adult-onset disorders showing up in our children. Worse, evidence shows that a child with high cholesterol will likely have the condition in adulthood. I suggested that we make some changes to Lisa's diet, but her father was convinced that she ate healthfully. So we all sat down together and I asked Lisa to write down everything she had consumed that day.

She had started her day with high-sugar cereal and a doughnut; for lunch she had one of the Oscar Mayer Lunchables along with candy and a Snapple. For dinner she had chicken fingers and fries and more Snapple.

In addition to all the fat and calories, this tallied up to nearly a half pound of sugar, which meant Lisa was consuming about 10 to 15 pounds of sugar a month. A fruit drink (Snapple or otherwise) can have more than 12 teaspoons of sugar per bottle. Was it any wonder that Lisa was obese and fighting prediabetes and high cholesterol?

# SUGAR RULE OF 4

To measure your child's intake of added sugars (not the natural sugars found in fruits and vegetables), find the number of grams of sugars on a product's label. Then divide the number of grams by 4 to arrive at how many teaspoons he or she consumed.

Example: 12 grams of sugar ÷ 4 = 3 teaspoons of sugar

A typical day's sugar intake for your child might look something like this:

**BREAKFAST**

Muffin: 8 grams of sugar = 2 teaspoons

Orange juice: 32 grams of sugar = 8 teaspoons

**LUNCH**

Chicken with honey mustard dip: 28 grams of sugar = 7 teaspoons

Soda: 52 grams of sugar = 13 teaspoons

Total sugar intake: 120 grams = 30 teaspoons

Sugar calories per teaspoon: 15 calories

120 grams of sugar = 450 calories

A child's recommended calorie intake should be between 900 and 1,400 calories per day, depending on age and gender. The example above illustrates how easy it is for up to one-half of a child's recommended daily calories to come from sugar.

# Liquid Calories

Sugary drinks, including fruit juices, are prime culprits in childhood obesity. In fact, one study showed that 2- and 5-year-old children who drank more than 12 ounces of fruit juice a day were more likely to be overweight and of short stature than children who drank less. Many parents think that fruit juice is a healthy beverage and allow their kids to drink gallons of the stuff—but juices are full of natural sugars that digest quickly because they lack the fiber of whole fruits, and they offer little nutritional benefit.

Whole fruits are healthier options. In addition to their belly-filling fiber and greater amounts of water-soluble vitamins, whole fruits are digested more slowly, so the sugar they contain is released slowly into the bloodstream. When your child drinks juice, he receives an instant sugar rush in a few big gulps.

Sodas are even worse than juices because their high acid content causes tooth decay and often stomach distress. When our children begin drinking sodas and juices at a young age, they become habituated to the taste of sweet drinks, setting them up for a lifetime of choosing sugary beverages.

If your child doesn't like drinking plain water, try adding a little bit of fruit juice to the water to give it some flavor while still diluting the juice's sugar content. It's a healthier choice, and the less-sweet taste won't cause him or her to crave sodas or other sweet beverages.

# Special Diets and Food Sensitivities

When you have a bacterial infection, your immune system creates antibodies to fight the invading bacterium that's making you sick, and you develop symptoms of fatigue, malaise, pain, and inflammation. This same reaction occurs when you eat foods that your body can't tolerate: You create antibodies that can cause symptoms such as headaches, migraines, IBS, diarrhea, constipation, hyperactivity, mood changes, joint pain, muscle pain, and more.

Every child is unique, so kids who have food allergies and sensitivities react to different foods. Symptoms of an immune reaction to a food usually appear in at least one of four parts of the body: the respiratory system, the skin, the intestines, and the brain. Common symptoms include wheezing, hives, bloating, and headaches. If you suspect that your child has food allergies or sensitivities, see your doctor.

Correctly diagnosing and treating a food allergy or sensitivity can make a remarkable difference in a child's quality of life. Such was the case for Cara, a spunky 4-year-old girl who came to see me with her mother. She was vivacious and obviously intelligent, but it seemed to me that something was amiss. By the end of the appointment I had realized what it was—she was having trouble hearing.

"Why didn't you mention her hearing?" I asked Cara's mother.

The mother blushed. "I'm always hoping that someone will find something else that's wrong that will help her hearing. It happened out of the blue 2 years ago. I've taken her to every ENT doctor in the county and they've given her every test they could think of. But they never can find the cause."

"Does Cara drink a lot of milk?" I asked her.

"Sure, with every meal. Especially this year. Our new pediatrician said it was important."

"I'm going to do a few new tests on her genetic food intolerances. Can you come back next week?"

I was not surprised to find that Cara had a severe sensitivity to cow's milk, which she was not only drinking daily, but also consuming in yogurt, cheese, ice cream, and other dairy products.

Milk was the basis of so much of Cara's daily diet. I told Cara's mother to immediately remove dairy products from her daughter's diet. Initially this was very difficult, she later told me, because those were Cara's favorite foods. But after only 3 weeks, something miraculous happened.

One day when I was in the office, the phone rang. I picked it up and said, "Hello?" There was silence on the other end, and a kind of snuffling in the background. "Hello," I repeated, "who's this?"

"It's Cara," the voice said.

"Cara! No kidding."

It took me a minute to realize what this meant. "You can hear me!"

"Yes, I can hear now. Mom said I should call you."

"Does your mom want to talk to me?"

"Just a minute," Cara said.

I realized then that the snuffling I'd heard in the background was her mother crying.

"Mom said that's okay, she just wanted to thank you."

The answers can be so easy with children once you realize what's at the root of the problem.

# Specific Food Allergies

Food allergies can be serious, even life threatening, especially those to nuts and shellfish. The trachea—windpipe—may begin to spasm or the cardiovascular system may go into shock (called anaphylactic shock) within minutes after a child eats a particular food. If your child has had a serious reaction to a food, even severe hives or wheezing, talk with your doctor about keeping an epinephrine-filled syringe with you for emergencies. This can be a lifesaver if you are not within minutes of an emergency room. However, if your child accidentally eats a food that has caused a severe reaction before, you should immediately call 911 or go to the nearest emergency room as a precaution. If the reaction is not severe enough to merit emergency treatment, closely monitor the child at home after calling your physician for guidance.

It is possible to be allergic to just about any food, but the majority of food allergies, especially in young children, are caused by:

Dairy products      Shellfish

Eggs               Wheat

Peanuts

For children who are allergic to dairy products, cow's milk is the food that most commonly must be avoided. Having a dairy allergy means that the child possesses antibodies to one or more of the protein types in dairy products, which are found in either the curds or the whey. An allergic reaction can begin immediately or several hours after the ingestion of moderate to large amounts of cow's milk products. The most common symptoms are nausea, vomiting, diarrhea, and abdominal cramps.

A milder problem children can have with cow's milk products is lactose intolerance. With this condition, the gastrointestinal tract has too little or none of the enzyme that is required to metabolize lactose, the sugar in milk. The most common symptoms of lactose intolerance are nausea and gas.

It can be difficult to ascertain whether a child has an allergy to dairy or lactose intolerance, although the latter usually doesn't occur until after the age of 5. Lactose-free products and supplements that assist in digesting regular dairy products can be used by those with lactose intolerance, but those with a dairy allergy should strictly avoid cow's milk.

When your child has a dairy allergy, make sure the dairy alternative you choose provides adequate calcium to support the needs of your growing child. (See page 28 for a list of the calcium requirements of children at different ages.)

These are the options I recommend:

## FOR INFANTS

Goat's milk          Soy formula

Hypoallergic formula

## FOR OLDER CHILDREN

| | |
|---|---|
| Coconut milk | Enriched soy milk |
| Enriched almond milk | Goat's milk |
| Enriched rice milk | |

# Shellfish

If your child has a shellfish allergy, he or she may have an allergic reaction to only certain kinds of shellfish, such as shrimp, or to all of them. Shellfish are all marine animals with shells, such as clams, mussels, crabs, lobsters, and shrimp, as well as octopus and squid.

A shellfish allergy can cause mild symptoms, such as hives or nasal congestion, or more severe and even life-threatening symptoms such as anaphylaxis and closing of the airway. For some children with this allergy, even a tiny amount of shellfish can cause a serious reaction.

# Gluten or Another Wheat Protein

Your immune system may perceive one of the four wheat proteins, such as gluten, as an enemy and attack it every time you eat it. This causes allergic symptoms such as hives and wheezing.

A wheat or gluten intolerance is different from the genetically caused celiac disease, in which the immune system attacks the small intestines and sometimes causes symptoms such as abdominal pain and bloating, diarrhea, poor appetite, and weight loss. A blood test for the antibody to tissue transglutaminase (anti-tTG) will show whether celiac disease is likely. The only treatment for this disease is avoidance of all gluten-containing foods. Untreated celiac disease increases the risk of developing colon cancer in the future.

Gluten is found in many grains, including barley, rye, and others. Children who have a problem with the gluten protein can't eat any of these grains. Children who are intolerant to another of the wheat proteins—albumin, globulin, and gliadin—only have to avoid foods made with wheat, including the wheat flour used to make crackers, cookies, pasta, pizza crusts, etc. These kids can eat other grains, such as rye. (Read your ingredients lists, though. Many oat and rye products are mostly wheat with a sprinkle of oats or rye for flavor.)

Here are some alternatives to wheat for those who have found that they need to remove gluten from their diets:

| | |
|---|---|
| Brown rice | Quinoa |
| Gluten-free breads | Rice cakes |
| Millet | Rice pasta |
| Organic popcorn | |

## Peanuts

Nut allergies are often among the most severe food allergies. Peanut allergy can cause life-threatening reactions, particularly in children with asthma. Only about 20 percent of children outgrow a peanut allergy, making it the most common food allergy in adults.

Accidental exposure to peanut-containing foods is a common problem, so it is important for children with this allergy to follow a strict peanut-free diet, wear a medical alert bracelet, and always have injectable epinephrine available.

## Eggs

Eggs, especially the proteins in egg whites, are a common cause of food allergies in children. Egg white, especially when it is raw or poorly cooked, causes a more severe allergic reaction than egg yolk does. Egg allergy usually begins in infancy, and children who have it will often refuse egg when it is given to them. The allergy usually disappears by ages 5 through 7, but it can be lifelong.

Foods to avoid include, but are not limited to, foods that are derived from or prepared with eggs, including egg substitutes, foods that contain egg albumin, and possibly French toast, cakes, cookies, pancakes, breads, ice cream, pasta, and puddings.

# 2

# THE FOUR BASICS OF NATUROPATHIC PEDIATRICS

## *Vitamins, Minerals, Herbs, and Homeopathic Remedies*

**OPTIMAL NUTRITION IS CRUCIAL FOR GROWING CHILDREN.** Poor nutrition can deprive a child of vitamins and minerals that are essential for growth. Children with iron-deficiency anemia may have difficulty learning; a deficit of vitamin D can make kids more prone to broken bones. If children are not properly nourished, the consequences for their developing minds and bodies can be profound.

It might be hard to believe that the quality of your child's diet today will affect his or her health as an adult, but the truth is, eating nutrient-rich and, if necessary, allergen-free foods will build the foundation for a lifetime of good health.

When I was in elementary school, I had a friend who ate only bologna sandwiches, chocolate pudding, and Twinkies. He was so devoted to this narrow diet that he brought these three foods to school and also insisted on eating this meal anytime he came over to my house to play. Over the years, his food preferences changed somewhat, but he still chose processed, nutritionally bereft snack foods for most of his meals. He grew increasingly obese and eventually developed type 2 diabetes and heart disease as an adult. His childhood of poor nutrition, mixed with genetic influences, led him on the path to a lifetime of poor health. And, sadly, his kids are following their father's example and have picked up many of his poor nutritional habits.

In an ideal world, we'd receive all the nutrients we need from foods, but the diets of most of us are far from perfect. And even many of the healthful foods we eat today have been stripped of much of their nutritional value thanks to processing and less than optimal agricultural and livestock-raising practices.

In my practice, I don't see patients with the nutritional deficiencies that were common a century ago, like beriberi, a disease caused by a deficiency of vitamin $B_1$ (thiamine), and scurvy, a vitamin C deficiency that affected sailors who were at sea for long periods without fresh fruits and vegetables. But I do see iron-deficiency anemia, and I've certainly treated rickets due to deficits of calcium and vitamin D. This is why the children I see in my practice receive not only a nutritional evaluation but also a review of the foods they're eating, their vitamin and mineral statuses, and a nutrient-deficiency screening.

Robby, a quarrelsome 12-year-old with brown eyes, had been diagnosed with ADHD. He found it difficult to focus in school, a problem that had worsened over time. His grades were low, which made him angry. He was smart and understood the lessons, but he couldn't take tests, sit still in his chair, or pay attention to the teacher. ADHD had been an integral part of his identity since he was in first grade.

In fact, he is part of a whole generation of young American children with this diagnosis. Given what our children are often fed, the high rate of ADHD in our country does not surprise me; studies suggest that there's an association between the two. Some studies have shown that in a subgroup of children with ADHD, artificial food colorings can worsen symptoms. Others show that simplified diets can reduce symptoms.

"Every other doctor wants me to give him Adderall"—a combination of two kinds of amphetamine—his mother, a school administrator, told me. "It's their only suggestion. And when I don't agree, they refuse to deal with me anymore. But I know there must be something else going on."

Robby's mom wanted to get to the bottom of his symptoms, not mask and suppress them. We did a thorough vitamin and mineral analysis and discovered that he was very low in magnesium, a nutrient essential for proper brain function.

Magnesium is an often-ignored but vital nutrient.

As far back as 1951, Adelle Davis wrote in her famous book *Let's Have Healthy Children*, "Magnesium is a must. The diets of all Americans are likely to be deficient. . . . Even a mild deficiency causes sensitiveness to noise, nervousness, irritability, mental depression, confusion, twitching, trembling, apprehension, insomnia, muscle weakness and cramps in the toes, feet, legs, or fingers."

She could have been describing Robby.

I gave his mother a list of magnesium-rich foods, which included buckwheat flour, oat bran, halibut, wheat flour, and spinach.

His mother stared at it in disbelief. "So this is it? You just want him to eat fish and spinach?"

"How often has he eaten these foods?"

"Probably never."

"So give it a try. I think you might be surprised," I assured her. I also gave her a list of supplements I wanted him to take.

Robby began a regimen of eating magnesium-rich foods and taking a fatty acid called docosahexaenoic acid (DHA) and a nutrient called inositol. Initially he grumbled about the loss of his cheeseburgers and fries, but his mother persevered. Very gradually, something profound occurred: A calmer and less fidgety boy began to emerge.

By the time they came back to see me 2 months later, Robby's grades were way up, and he was calmer and more focused. His mother was overjoyed.

"I can't believe nutrition could make such a difference," she admitted.

But nutrition can make all the difference.

# Micronutrients and Minerals

Micronutrients are essential for our bodies to function. They are called "*micro*nutrients" because we need a tiny amount of each every day, as opposed to the large daily servings we require of proteins, fats, and carbohydrates—the *macro*nutrients.

Vitamins, which are micronutrients, are biological molecules that help our bodies to function. Vitamin C helps the immune system; vitamin D increases bone strength; the B vitamins help change food into energy and the brain function, to name a few. Vitamins are either water soluble or fat soluble, meaning that they dissolve in one of those fluids before they are absorbed by the body. Extra fat-soluble vitamins are stored in the liver and fat tissue, whereas what the body doesn't use of water-soluble vitamins in the diet is lost in the urine. If your child takes vitamin A, D, E or K, it should be taken with a meal that contains fat because these are the fat-soluble vitamins.

Minerals, which are also micronutrients, are nonbiological substances from the earth. Among the macrominerals—those we need larger amounts of, as opposed to trace minerals—are calcium, which is necessary for strong bones and teeth; magnesium, needed by muscles; and potassium, which works the nervous system. Even though we need only tiny amounts of minerals, our bodies require all of them regularly to function optimally. Eating a healthy diet should give us all of the nutrients—both vitamins and minerals—we need, but if we don't get enough through our food, supplements are available. But don't fall into the trap of believing that your child can receive all of his or her nutrients in pills. Eating healthy foods is the best way to obtain these important substances.

# Recommended Dietary Allowance

You're probably familiar with the term % Daily Value, also known as the Recommended Dietary Allowance (RDA), from looking at the nutrition labels on packaged foods. There are many reasons to read food labels carefully, and one of them is to check whether you're meeting 100 percent of your daily vitamin and mineral recommendations. By law, food manufacturers only have to list the amounts of vitamin A, vitamin C, calcium, and iron in one serving of the food on their Nutrition Facts labels. How do you know how much of other vitamins and minerals your children are getting?

When we see 100% listed below % Daily Value on a label, we may believe that the amount of that vitamin or mineral in a serving of that product is all we need for the day. In actuality, it's the minimum amount that most of us need to prevent disease. For example, when your child gets 100 percent of his or her RDA of vitamin D, it's not the amount of vitamin D needed for optimal health, but rather the amount needed to prevent the onset of rickets.

Let's explore the optimal ranges of nutrients for a child to get. These values represent the total intake from foods, water, and supplements. Note that you can take a longer view of your child's diet than just 1 day. It's important for them to eat nutritiously, but if you don't quite meet the daily requirement today, the difference can be made up tomorrow. It is a diet that consistently lacks any of the nutrients that creates symptoms, diseases, or conditions.

| NUTRIENT | AGE (YEARS) | MINIMUM | MAXIMUM |
|----------|-------------|---------|---------|
| Calcium | 1–3 | 700 mg | 2,500 mg |
| | 4–8 | 1,000 mg | 2,500 mg |
| | 9–13 | 1,300 mg | 3,000 mg |

| NUTRIENT | AGE (YEARS) | MINIMUM | MAXIMUM |
|---|---|---|---|
| Copper | 1–3 | 340 mcg | 1,000 mcg |
| | 4–8 | 440 mcg | 3,000 mcg |
| | 9–13 | 700 mcg | 5,000 mcg |
| Iodine | 1–3 | 90 mcg | 200 mcg |
| | 4–8 | 90 mcg | 300 mcg |
| | 9–13 | 120 mcg | 600 mcg |
| Iron | 1–3 | 7 mg | 40 mg |
| | 4–8 | 10 mg | 40 mg |
| | 9–13 | 8 mg | 40 mg |
| Magnesium | 1–3 | 80 mg | 65 mg* |
| | 4–8 | 130 mg | 110 mg* |
| | 9–13 | 240 mg | 350 mg* |
| Phosphorus | 1–3 | 460 mg | 3,000 mg |
| | 4–8 | 500 mg | 3,000 mg |
| | 9–13 | 1,250 mg | 4,000 mg |
| Potassium | 1–3 | 3,000 mg | Not determined |
| | 4–8 | 3,800 mg | Not determined |
| | 9–13 | 4,500 mg | Not determined |
| Selenium | 1–3 | 20 mcg | 90 mcg |
| | 4–8 | 30 mcg | 150 mcg |
| | 9–13 | 40 mcg | 280 mcg |
| Vitamin A (retinol) | 1–3 | 1,000 IU | 2,000 IU |
| | 4–8 | 1,320 IU | 3,000 IU |
| | 9–13 | 2,000 IU | 5,610 IU |

*Amount from only supplemental magnesium; no adverse effects with any amount from food sources

(Continued)

| NUTRIENT | AGE (YEARS) | MINIMUM | MAXIMUM |
|---|---|---|---|
| Vitamin B$_1$ (thiamine) | 1–3 | 0.5 mg | Not determined |
| | 4–8 | 0.6 mg | Not determined |
| | 9–13 | 0.9 mg | Not determined |
| Vitamin B$_2$ (riboflavin) | 1–3 | 0.5 mg | Not determined |
| | 4–8 | 0.6 mg | Not determined |
| | 9–13 | 0.9 mg | Not determined |
| Vitamin B$_3$ (niacin) | 1–3 | 6 mg | 10 mg |
| | 4–8 | 8 mg | 15 mg |
| | 9–13 | 12 mg | 20 mg |
| Vitamin B$_5$ (pantothenic acid) | 1–3 | 2 mg | Not determined |
| | 4–8 | 3 mg | Not determined |
| | 9–13 | 4 mg | Not determined |
| Vitamin B$_6$ (pyridoxine) | 1–3 | 0.5 mg | 30 mg |
| | 4–8 | 0.6 mg | 40 mg |
| | 9–13 | 1 mg | 60 mg |
| Vitamin B$_9$ (folate/folic acid) | 1–3 | 150 mcg | 300 mcg |
| | 4–8 | 200 mcg | 400 mcg |
| | 9–13 | 300 mcg | 600 mcg |
| Vitamin B$_{12}$ (cobalamin) | 1–3 | 0.9 mcg | Not determined |
| | 4–8 | 1.2 mcg | Not determined |
| | 9–13 | 1.8 mcg | Not determined |
| Vitamin C (ascorbic acid) | 1–3 | 15 mg | 400 mg |
| | 4–8 | 25 mg | 650 mg |
| | 9–13 | 45 mg | 1,200 mg |

| NUTRIENT | AGE (YEARS) | MINIMUM | MAXIMUM |
|---|---|---|---|
| Vitamin D | 1–3 | 600 IU | 2,500 IU |
| | 4–8 | 600 IU | 3,000 IU |
| | 9–13 | 600 IU | 4,000 IU |
| Vitamin E | 1–3 | 9 IU | 300 IU |
| | 4–8 | 10.4 IU | 450 IU |
| | 9–13 | 16.4 IU | 900 IU |
| Zinc | 1–3 | 3 mg | 7 mg |
| | 4–8 | 5 mg | 12 mg |
| | 9–13 | 8 mg | 23 mg |

# Vitamins

## Vitamin A (Retinol)

Antioxidant (a dietary substance that may prevent or repair cell damage caused by free radicals, which are molecules that may cause some diseases and be responsible for aging; cells produce free radicals naturally, but exposure to pollutants such as tobacco smoke and asbestos can also cause them); fat soluble; promotes healthy vision and skin; helps form strong bones and teeth

**Where It's Found** Meats, liver, kidney, milk, eggs, grapefruits, carrots, sweet potatoes, pumpkins, broccoli, many dark green leafy vegetables

**If You Don't Get Enough** Impaired immunity, rash, vision problems such as xerophthalmia (dry eye syndrome) and night blindness

**Used to Treat** Chicken pox, bronchitis, eczema, gastroenteritis, herpes simplex, hypothyroidism, leukemia, measles, mumps, ear infection, pneumonia, psoriasis, urinary tract infection, vision problems, acne, psoriasis, rosacea

**If You Have Too Much** Headache that won't go away, fatigue, muscle pain, joint pain, dry skin, dry lips, irritated eyes, nausea, diarrhea, hair loss, birth defects, liver failure

## top 5 Dietary Sources of Vitamin A (Retinol)

| | | |
|---|---|---|
| Carrot juice | 1 cup | 45,000 IU |
| Canned pumpkin | 1 cup | 38,000 IU |
| Sweet potato | 1 potato | 28,000 IU |
| Cooked carrots | 1 cup | 26,500 IU |
| Spinach | 1 cup | 23,000 IU |

## B Vitamins

These were once was thought to be a single vitamin, but now eight distinct B vitamins are known; they are called "B complex" when grouped together in a supplement.

**B$_1$ (Thiamine).** Assists the body in converting food into energy; water soluble
    **Where It's Found** Lean meats; fish; beans; fortified grain products like wheat flour, breads, and cereals; white rice; oat bran; orange juice
    **If You Don't Get Enough** Beriberi, Wernicke-Korsakoff syndrome
    **Used to Treat** Numbness and tingling, cataract, heart failure, fatigue, confusion, neuropathy
    **If You Have Too Much** Stomach upset, imbalance of other B vitamins

## top 5 Dietary Sources of Vitamin B$_1$ (Thiamine)

| | | |
|---|---|---|
| White rice | 1 cup | 1.3 mg |
| Wheat flour | 1 cup | 1.2 mg |
| Oat bran | 1 cup | 1.1 mg |
| Pork | 3 oz | 1.05 mg |
| Orange juice | 6 oz | 0.6 mg |

**B$_2$ (Riboflavin).** Converts food into energy; metabolizes fats and proteins; water soluble
    **Where It's Found** Nuts, eggs, lean meats, duck, shrimp, legumes (especially soybeans), milk, yeast, mushrooms, spinach

**If You Don't Get Enough** Chapped and torn lips; sore, red tongue; oily, scaly rashes in the groin. Usually accompanied by other nutrient deficiencies; may lead to deficiencies of vitamins $B_6$ (pyridoxine) and $B_3$ (niacin)

**Used to Treat** Migraine, rheumatoid arthritis, acne, cataract, eczema, anemia

**If You Have Too Much** Itching, numbness, burning, or prickling sensations; sensitivity to light; eye damage from the sun; imbalance of other B vitamins

## *top* 5 Dietary Sources of Vitamin $B_2$ (Riboflavin)

| | | |
|---|---|---|
| Duck | ½ duck | 1.0 mg |
| Shrimp | 6–8 | 0.9 mg |
| Soybeans | 1 cup | 0.5 mg |
| Mushrooms | 1 cup | 0.5 mg |
| Spinach | 1 cup | 0.4 mg |

**$B_3$ (Niacin).** Antioxidant; water soluble; essential for converting carbohydrates into energy; helps rid the body of toxins; reduces blood cholesterol level

**Where It's Found** Brewer's yeast, broccoli, carrots, cheeses, eggs, meats, chicken, fish, milk, nuts

**If You Don't Get Enough** Pellagra

**Used to Treat** Acne, migraine, high cholesterol, hypertension, diarrhea, canker sores, fatigue, depression, scaly skin, atherosclerosis, type 2 diabetes, osteoarthritis

**If You Have Too Much** Flushed face and chest with burning and tingling, ulcers, liver damage, gastric ulcers, imbalance of other B vitamins

## *top* 5 Dietary Sources of Vitamin $B_3$ (Niacin)

| | | |
|---|---|---|
| Chicken | ½ breast | 14.7 mg |
| Tuna | 1 cup | 13.7 mg |
| Swordfish | 3 oz | 12.5 mg |
| Halibut | ½ fillet | 11.3 mg |
| Salmon | ½ fillet | 10.3 mg |

**B₅ (Pantothenic Acid).** Antioxidant; water soluble; essential for growth and the metabolism of nutrients; necessary for the production of stress hormones by the adrenal glands

**Where It's Found** Cheeses, corn, eggs, liver, meats, salmon, peanuts, seeds, vegetables, white and shiitake mushrooms, couscous, white rice, wheat germ

**If You Don't Get Enough** Depression, fatigue

**Used to Treat** Stress, heartburn, high cholesterol, fatigue, insomnia, depression, bronchitis, neuropathy, wounds, juvenile rheumatoid arthritis

**If You Have Too Much** Diarrhea, bleeding, imbalance of other B vitamins

## *top* 5 Dietary Sources of Vitamin B₅ (Pantothenic Acid)

| | | |
|---|---|---|
| Shiitake mushrooms | 1 cup | 5.2 mg |
| White mushrooms | 1 cup | 3.4 mg |
| Sunflower seeds | ¼ cup | 2.3 mg |
| Couscous | 1 cup | 2.2 mg |
| White rice | 1 cup | 2.1 mg |

**B₆ (Pyridoxine).** Used to manufacture red blood cells; assists in protein metabolism; boosts the immune system; creates neurotransmitters; water soluble

**Where It's Found** Fortified cereals, meats, beans, poultry (especially turkey), vegetables, seeds, hummus, tuna, white rice, chestnuts

**If You Don't Get Enough** Dermatitis, depression, muscle weakness, memory loss

**Used to Treat** Anemia, dermatitis, ADHD, PMS, autism, heart disease, nausea during pregnancy, depression, carpal tunnel syndrome, rheumatoid arthritis

**If You Have Too Much** Neurological problems such as loss of sensation in the legs and imbalance, sensitivity to sunlight, abdominal pain, nausea, imbalance of other B vitamins

# *top* 5 Dietary Sources of Vitamin B$_6$ (Pyridoxine)

| | | |
|---|---|---|
| Hummus | 1 cup | 1.1 mg |
| Tuna | 3 oz | 0.9 mg |
| White rice | 1 cup | 0.8 mg |
| Chestnuts | 1 cup | 0.7 mg |
| Turkey | 3 oz | 0.6 mg |

**B$_9$ (Folic Acid/Folate).** Folic acid is the synthetic form found in supplements and fortified foods; folate is the natural form found in foods; both promote proper brain function and neurotransmitter formation; water soluble

**Where It's Found** Fortified cereals, wheat flour, white rice, lentils, beans, dark green leafy vegetables, root vegetables, avocados, fortified orange juice, liver, salmon

**If You Don't Get Enough** Heart disease, depression, gingivitis, shortness of breath, diarrhea, irritability, hiatal hernia, spina bifida (fetus), cleft lip (fetus), cleft palate (fetus), heart malformation (fetus)

**Used to Treat** Heart disease, age-related hearing loss, depression, megaloblastic anemia

**If You Have Too Much** Sleep problems, stomach problems, seizures, skin reactions, imbalance of other B vitamins

# *top* 5 Dietary Sources of Vitamin B$_9$ (Folate)

| | | |
|---|---|---|
| White rice | 1 cup | 797 mcg |
| Wheat flour | 1 cup | 395 mcg |
| Lentils | 1 cup | 358 mcg |
| Black-eyed peas | 1 cup | 356 mcg |
| Orange juice | 6 oz | 330 mcg |

**B$_{12}$ (Cobalamin).** Essential to form red blood cells and maintain a healthy nervous system; aids in the production of DNA and RNA; water soluble

Note: Vegans must take this as a supplement because it is the only vitamin that you cannot get in a strictly plant-based diet. However, because vitamin B$_{12}$, unlike the other water-soluble vitamins, is stored in the liver for years, humans very rarely have B$_{12}$ deficiency.

**Where It's Found** Fish, shellfish, meats, poultry, eggs, yogurt

**If You Don't Get Enough** Anemia, fatigue, neuropathy

**Used to Treat** Pernicious anemia, heart disease, fatigue, male infertility, asthma, cognitive impairment, autism, ADHD, depression

**If You Have Too Much** Imbalance of other B vitamins

## *top* 5 Dietary Sources of Vitamin B$_{12}$ (Cobalamin)

| | | |
|---|---|---|
| Clams | 3 oz | 84 mcg |
| Oysters | 6 | 16 mcg |
| Crab | 3 oz | 10 mcg |
| Salmon | ½ fillet | 9 mcg |
| Sardines | 3 oz | 8 mcg |

**Biotin (a B vitamin).** Metabolizes carbohydrates, fats, and proteins; important for hair and nail growth; water soluble

**Where It's Found** Eggs, sardines, nuts, beans, whole grains, cauliflower, bananas

**If You Don't Get Enough** Hair loss; dry skin; red rash around the mouth, nose, eyes, and groin; fatigue; insomnia; depression; brittle nails

**Used to Treat** Hair and nail problems, cradle cap, type 1 and type 2 diabetes, neuropathy

**If You Have Too Much** No effects

## Vitamin C (Ascorbic Acid)

Antioxidant; water soluble; important for immunity; crucial for wound healing; promotes healthy skin, connective tissues, and bones; supplements should be avoided by people who have a corn sensitivity or hemochromatosis

**Where It's Found** Bell and hot peppers, broccoli, leafy green vegetables, tomatoes, citrus fruits, peaches, papaya, strawberries

**If You Don't Get Enough** Scurvy (rare), impaired wound healing, connective tissue defects (such as rash and gingivitis). Vitamin C deficiency starts with fatigue, malaise, and gum inflammation.

**Used to Treat** Asthma, herpes simplex, influenza, rhinitis, scoliosis, scurvy, colds, stress and anxiety, heart disease, hypertension, osteoarthritis, preeclampsia; also given to children to reduce complications after surgical repair of cardiac malformations

**If You Have Too Much** Diarrhea, gas, stomach upset, dehydration

## top 5 Dietary Sources of Vitamin C (Ascorbic Acid)

| | | |
|---|---|---|
| Peaches | 1 cup | 235 mg |
| Red bell peppers | 1 cup | 233 mg |
| Papaya | 1 | 188 mg |
| Strawberries | 1 cup | 106 mg |
| Broccoli | 1 cup | 101 mg |

## Vitamin D

Called the sunlight vitamin; fat soluble; deficiency is more prevalent in winter because of less exposure to sun; the only vitamin the body manufactures naturally, from exposure to sunlight; crucial for a strong immune system and bones; increases calcium absorption for bone health

In today's video game society, many children aren't spending enough time outside to produce sufficient vitamin D. Have your child's vitamin D level tested before supplementing; it is necessary for a growing child's bone health, but too much can cause side effects.

**Where It's Found** Fish, salmon, swordfish, trout, halibut, pork, fortified milk, eggs

**If You Don't Get Enough** Rickets in children (rare, but on the rise in the United States), osteoporosis in adults, depression, seasonal affective disorder, pain, fatigue, multiple sclerosis, some cancers

**Used to Treat** Asthma, Crohn's disease, depression, type 1 diabetes, eczema, influenza, earache, psoriasis, rickets, scoliosis, warts, osteoporosis, seasonal affective disorder, heart disease, multiple sclerosis

**If You Have Too Much** Kidney stones, thirst, itchy skin, change in bowel habits

## Vitamin E

Antioxidant; fat soluble; stops the production of dangerous reactive oxygen molecules when fat breaks down; enhances immune function; protects against heart disease and cancer; promotes healthy skin

**Where It's Found** Nuts, sunflower seeds, wheat germ, leafy green vegetables, tomato paste, vegetable oils, eggs, avocados

**If You Don't Get Enough** Muscle weakness, vision damage, impairment of balance and coordination

**Used to Treat** Skin problems, type 2 diabetes, PMS, herpes simplex, influenza, muscular dystrophy, eczema, vision problems, preeclampsia, rheumatoid arthritis

**If You Have Too Much** Increased risk of bleeding, especially if your child is taking a blood thinner such as warfarin (Coumadin), clopidogrel (Plavix), or aspirin

## top 5 Dietary Sources of Vitamin E

| | | |
|---|---|---|
| Tomato paste | 1 cup | 16.4 IU |
| Sunflower seeds | 1 oz | 11 IU |
| Spinach | 1 cup | 10 IU |
| Turnip greens | 1 cup | 6.4 IU |
| Hazelnuts | 1 oz | 6.4 IU |

## Vitamin K

Makes proteins that clot blood and form and maintain healthy tissues and bones; newborns have little of this vitamin, so they're given a shot; fat soluble

**Where It's Found** Berries, leafy green vegetables

**If You Don't Get Enough** Excessive bleeding (very rare)

**Used to Treat** Bleeding in people taking blood thinners, osteoporosis

**If You Have Too Much** Should be avoided by children with G6PD deficiency

# Omega-3 Fatty Acids

Three main types: eicosapentaenoic acid (EPA), docosahexaenoic acid (DHA), and alpha-linolenic acid (ALA); have cardioprotective effects; assist in fetal brain development

**Where It's Found** Fatty fish and fish oil (EPA, DHA), some algae, ground flaxseeds and flaxseed oil (ALA), walnuts and some nut oils (ALA)

**If You Don't Get Enough** Depression, ADHD (in infants of mothers who are deficient in it), worsening of inflammatory conditions such as arthritis, worsening of blood lipid (fat) levels

**Used to Treat** Depression, arthritis, asthma, type 2 diabetes, ADHD, hypertension, high triglycerides, autism, rheumatoid arthritis, lupus, osteoporosis, bipolar disorder, eczema, inflammatory bowel disease (IBD), PMS, memory problems

**If You Have Too Much** Bleeding, abdominal pain, loose stools

# Minerals

Minerals are crucial components of your child's diet because they support virtually every body system. Iron forms red blood cells, zinc enhances the immune system, iodine creates thyroid hormones, copper supports the nervous system, calcium builds the bones, magnesium relaxes the muscles, and so on.

Many children are deficient in minerals because of poor diets. Mineral deficiency problems can arise quickly, mask other issues, and remain undiagnosed for years.

## Calcium

Most abundant mineral in the body; essential for teeth and bones; prevents progressive bone loss; lowers blood pressure

**Where It's Found** Dairy products, dark green leafy vegetables, sardines, nuts, salmon

**If You Don't Get Enough** Numbness and tingling, seizures, mood changes, rickets in children (rare, but on the rise in the United States), hypertension, muscle spasms, osteopenia and osteoporosis in adults

**Used to Treat** Osteoporosis, rickets, PMS, hypertension, obesity, high cholesterol, gastritis, gastroesophageal reflux disease (GERD), muscle spasms

**If You Have Too Much** Heart problems, constipation, stomach pain, nausea, kidney damage, confusion

## top 6 Dietary Sources of Calcium

| Collards | 1 cup | 357 mg |
|---|---|---|
| Rhubarb | 1 cup | 348 mg |
| Sardines | 3 oz | 325 mg |
| 1% milk | 1 cup | 305 mg |
| Spinach | 1 cup | 291 mg |
| Whole milk | 1 cup | 276 mg |

## Copper

Helps form red blood cells, nerve cells, connective tissues, and skin pigment

**Where It's Found** Oysters, lobster, crab, meats, whole grains, vegetables, beans, shiitake mushrooms

**If You Don't Get Enough (very rare)** Low body temperature, bone fractures, low white blood cell count, thyroid problems

**Used to Treat** Anemia, arthritis, burns, IBS, wounds

**If You Have Too Much** Stomach pain, nausea, headache, dizziness, diarrhea, metallic taste in mouth, heart problems

## top 5 Dietary Sources of Copper

| Oysters | 6 medium | 4 mg |
|---|---|---|
| Lobster | 3 oz | 1.5 mg |
| Shiitake mushrooms | 1 cup | 1.3 mg |
| Crab | 3 oz | 1.0 mg |
| Barley | 1 cup | 0.8 mg |

## Iodine

Essential for the production of thyroid hormones; extra bromide (from bread products) or chloride (from city tap water or swimming pools) in the body counteracts iodine to make thyroid hormones ineffective

**Where It's Found** Iodized salt, seaweed, dark green leafy vegetables

**If You Don't Get Enough** Hypothyroidism, goiter

**Used to Treat** Hypothyroidism, goiter, fibrocystic breasts, vaginitis, wounds

**If You Have Too Much** Thyroid disease

## Iron

Present in red blood cells' hemoglobin, which delivers oxygen throughout the body

**Where It's Found** Liver, meats, canned clams, beans, white rice, seeds, soybeans, dark green leafy vegetables

**If You Don't Get Enough** Anemia, difficulty learning

**Used to Treat** Anemia, ADHD

**If You Have Too Much** Constipation, stomach upset, hemochromatosis, skin discoloration, liver damage, heart disease

## top 5 Dietary Sources of Iron

| | | |
|---|---|---|
| Canned clams | 3 oz | 24 mg |
| White rice (enriched) | 1 cup | 10 mg |
| Soybeans | 1 cup | 9 mg |
| Baked beans | 1 cup | 8 mg |
| Lentils | 1 cup | 6.5 mg |

## Magnesium

Essential for energy production and muscle contraction and relaxation; protects against heart disease, cancer, and complications of type 2 diabetes

**Where It's Found** Soybeans, beans, green leafy vegetables (especially spinach), whole grains, buckwheat flour, oat bran, wheat flour, nuts, halibut

**If You Don't Get Enough** Anxiety, agitation, restless legs syndrome, insomnia, confusion, muscle spasms

**Used to Treat** Asthma, fibromyalgia, ADHD, autism, heart failure, hypertension, migraine, osteoporosis, PMS, restless legs syndrome; note that some of these conditions are treated with low-dose magnesium supplements over the long term, whereas others respond to a high dose usually given intravenously. Consult your physician to find out which is appropriate for your child.

**If You Have Too Much** Diarrhea, very low blood pressure, slow heart rate, stomach pain, confusion

## top 5 Dietary Sources of Magnesium

| | | |
|---|---|---|
| Halibut | 1 fillet | 340 mg |
| Buckwheat flour | 1 cup | 301 mg |
| Oat bran | 1 cup | 221 mg |
| Wheat flour | 1 cup | 166 mg |
| Spinach | 1 cup | 163 mg |

## Phosphorus

Second most abundant mineral in the body; involved in bone and tooth formation; helps release energy from nutrients

**Where It's Found** Almonds, beans, calf's liver, cheeses, eggs, fish, legumes, milk

**If You Don't Get Enough (uncommon)** Anxiety, bone pain, stiff joints, fatigue, irritability, weakness

**Used to Treat** Bone pain, loss of appetite

**If You Have Too Much** Diarrhea; hardening of the organs and some tissues; impaired metabolism of calcium, magnesium, zinc, and iron

## Potassium

Needs to be replenished after strenuous activity; helps maintain blood pressure; stimulates the kidneys to remove toxins from the body; works the nervous system; protects against heart disease and cancer

It's best to get potassium from the foods you eat. Consult your physician before taking potassium supplements, because too much of the mineral can also cause health issues.

**Where It's Found** Avocados, bananas, dates, citrus fruits, cantaloupes, honeydew melons, tomato paste, carrots, chard, beet greens, legumes, milk, molasses, nuts

**If You Don't Get Enough** Weakness, muscle cramps, irregular heartbeat

**Used to Treat** Hypertension, constipation, stroke, IBD, muscle cramps

**If You Have Too Much** Diarrhea, stomach pain, muscle weakness, abnormal heart rhythm

## top 5 Dietary Sources of Potassium

| Tomato paste | 1 cup | 2,657 mg |
|---|---|---|
| Beet greens | 1 cup | 1,309 mg |
| White beans | 1 cup | 1,189 mg |
| Dates | 1 cup | 1,168 mg |
| Banana | 1 cup | 537 mg |

## Sodium

Regulates blood pressure; little chance of a deficiency because the American diet is high in table salt

**Where It's Found** Cured meats, clams, most processed foods, seaweed

**If You Don't Get Enough** Nausea, malaise, decreased consciousness

**Used to Treat** Certain types of dehydration (by infusing a saline solution)

**If You Have Too Much** High blood pressure, bloating

## Sulfur

Essential for healthy joints, skin, hair, nails, and connective tissue; critical to protein metabolism; in supplements as dimethyl sulfoxide (DMSO) and methylsulfonylmethane (MSM)

**Where It's Found** Garlic, onions, whole grains, legumes, coconut, eggs, red meats

**If You Don't Get Enough** Sulfur deficiency is extremely rare

**Used to Treat** Acne, hair loss, arthritis, psoriasis, eczema, dandruff, warts, shingles, interstitial cystitis

**If You Have Too Much** Headache, nausea, vomiting, changes in bowel habits, skin irritation if used topically

## Zinc

Antioxidant; important for immune system health, enzyme function, and hormone function; helps with vision, taste, smell, and wound healing

**Where It's Found** Oysters, crab, beef, lamb, seeds, beans, milk, whole grains

**If You Don't Get Enough** Poor growth, weight loss, impaired taste or smell; poor wound healing; hair loss; depression

**Used to Treat** Acne, colds, sickle cell anemia, skin ulcers, ADHD, herpes simplex, Wilson's disease, hair loss, impotence

**If You Have Too Much** Stomach upset, metallic taste in mouth, nausea, vomiting, headache, hallucinations, poor muscle coordination

## *top* **5** Dietary Sources of Zinc

| | | |
|---|---|---|
| Oysters | 6 medium | 76 mg |
| Baked beans | 1 cup | 14 mg |
| Beef | 3 oz | 9 mg |
| Lamb | 3 oz | 6 mg |
| Crab | 1 cup | 5 mg |

# Naturopathic Remedies

Many modern pharmaceuticals have their origins in plants. For example, the now-synthetic active ingredient in aspirin, acetyl salicylic acid, was first derived from the salicin in willow bark, and the drug digitalis comes from the leaves of the herb foxglove.

Treating illnesses with botanical remedies is an age-old practice. With their ability to gently soothe, heal, and provide relief, they are often effective therapies for children with acute and chronic conditions.

## *Echinacea Purpurea*

A wildflower with daisylike purple blossoms, echinacea is also known as purple or prairie coneflower. A natural antibiotic, echinacea stimulates the immune system and helps the body fight bacterial and viral infections. The herb also boosts the cells' production of a virus-fighting substance called interferon. It is often used to shorten the duration of colds and flus, but scientific research has not proven that it works in children.

## Lemon Balm

Lemon balm is an herb that relaxes, lessens stress and anxiety, helps sleep and appetite, and relieves indigestion. It's thought that chemicals called terpenes may be behind the herb's relaxing effects. A substance called rosmarinic acid may be the cause of its antiviral activities, and another, eugenol, relaxes muscles, numbs tissues, and is an antibacterial.

## Calendula

The petals of calendula are used medicinally to calm inflamed tissues. Calendula contains large amounts of flavonoids, plant-based antioxidants that protect the body against cell-damaging free radicals and are used to make soothing topical anti-inflammatory formulations. Calendula also has weak antimicrobial activity. It is most often used topically for lacerations, abrasions, and skin infections.

## Garlic

Related to the onion, shallot, and other plants in the genus *Allium,* the power of garlic resides in its bulb. When its cloves are crushed, it produces allicin, one of the chemicals responsible for its medicinal effects. Garlic may prevent heart disease by making platelets less likely to clump and lowering both blood pressure and cholesterol levels slightly. It is also effective against infectious organisms (viruses, bacteria, and fungi) because allicin can block the enzymes that give them the ability to invade and damage tissues.

## Peppermint

The leaves and stem of this aromatic herb contain menthol, which soothes an upset stomach and aids in digestion. Its calming and numbing properties relax the muscles that prevent the release of intestinal gas, and its antispasmodic effect soothes irritable bowel syndrome (IBS). Menthol aids digestion by stimulating the flow of digestive juices. Peppermint is also an ingredient in topical solutions that treat symptoms of the common cold, soothe muscle aches, and ease congestion.

## Chamomile

Chamomile is a daisylike herb that gently calms frayed nerves and possesses anti-inflammatory, antispasmodic, and infection-fighting properties. The healing power of this herb is related to its volatile oil, one component of which is a substance called apigenin. It also relieves muscle spasms and treats a range of skin conditions and mild infections, including mouth sores and gum disease.

## Tea Tree Oil

Tea tree oil comes from the leaves of the tea tree, a species native to Australia but now cultivated in many countries. The oil disinfects the skin with its powerful antibacterial and antifungal agent, terpinen.

## Valerian

The roots of this perennial plant approved as a sleep aid in many European countries contain compounds that relax the mind and promote sleep. These compounds—valepotriates, valeric acid, and volatile oils—combine to make valerian a calming agent for treating anxiety disorders, diverticulosis, stomach cramps, and IBS.

## BOTANICAL MEDICINES NOT TO BE USED FOR INFANTS AND TODDLERS

Certain botanicals can be harmful to young children. These herbs—in leaf, oil, and any other form and for all methods of administration—should be avoided in children.

> *Aloe vera* (under 10 years of age)
> Buckthorn (*Cascara sagrada*) bark
> Cajeput oil
> Camphor
> Eucalyptus
> Fennel oil
> Horseradish
> Mint and peppermint oils (external application)
> *Nasturtium*
> Rhubarb root
> Senna
> Watercress

# Homeopathic Remedies

Homeopathy is based on the principle that "like cures like." In other words, a natural substance that may cause a disease or condition when given to a healthy person can cure the same condition when given in a lower strength to a sick person. Similar to allergy shots, which are tiny amounts of allergens injected over time to help the immune system build tolerance to substances, homeopathy also gives patients small amounts of offending substances to change the immune system so the body can heal itself.

Samuel Hahnemann, a German doctor, invented homeopathy in the late 1700s. It's so successful that it is used all over the world as an affordable, effective treatment option. Hospitals in which only homeopathy is practiced exist in Europe and Asia.

Homeopathy arrived in the United States in the 1800s and homeopathic schools opened across the country. However, in the United States, its use gradually declined with the growing popularity of pharmaceutical medications until the 1970s, when consumers began looking for natural preventives and treatments.

Homeopathic treatment is an excellent choice for children, and one of my personal favorites. In fact, these remedies work more effectively in children than adults and pose extremely low risks of side effects and toxicity. Most people do not know that homeopathic remedies are regulated by the FDA under the *Homoeopathic Pharmacopoeia of the United States.*

## COMMONLY USED HOMEOPATHIC REMEDIES FOR CHILDHOOD AILMENTS

Homeopathic remedies are commonly found in health food stores with the designations 30C, 12C, 6C, and others after the name—for example, Arnica 30C. This is the strength of the remedy. Your naturopathic physician may give you a different strength of a medicine, such as 12C or 200C. These homeopathic remedies are dilutions of the herbs or minerals put on lactose pellets. Typically, five pellets are dissolved under the tongue a few times a day during illness. Some remedies are given more often or less often; your naturopathic physician will tell you exactly how to give them to your child. Children with milk allergies should take liquid forms of homeopathic medicines.

Aconite: Fear of the dark

Allium: Allergies

Arnica: Bumps and bruises

Belladonna: Fever

Calcarea Carbonica (Calc Carb): Constipation

Chamomilla: Irritability

Lycopodium: Irritable bowel syndrome

Nux Vomica: Vomiting

Rhus Toxicodendron (Rhus tox): Poison ivy

Sulphur: Diarrhea, eczema

As a naturopathic pediatrician, I know that most childhood infections run their course and children's bodies heal themselves. When we recommend "watching and waiting," we wait to see if the body will heal, or worsen and require intervention, and we monitor for warning signs of severe disease. In addition to being responsible for making this decision, our role is to encourage inflammation. We believe that it's beneficial to allow fevers to run their course rather than suppress them, and we encourage parents to save antibiotics and other strong drugs for emergencies. If a child younger than 3 months of age has a fever of more than 100.5°F or a child 3 months or older has a fever higher than 105°F, take him or her to your pediatrician. We are currently seeing some strains of bacteria that are resistant to antibiotics as a result of these drugs' over-use. Saving antibiotics for emergencies will help prevent more types of bacteria from becoming resistant. Antibiotics can also cause other problems, including diarrhea and hearing loss. Natural remedies are effective treatments for mild colds and flus and should be used before antibiotics.

A powerful example of the dangers of overusing antibiotics and the benefits of natural medicine can be found in the story of 6-year-old Brandon and his 8-year-old sister. Brandon arrived at my office with right ear pain. He wasn't eating, was fatigued, and had a fever of 100°F. All signs indicated that his body was actively fighting an infection. His sister had also had chronic ear infections.

"She grew up on antibiotics," the mother told me. "Our pediatrician gave them to her five or six times a year. By the time she was older, we had to search for another antibiotic to treat her pneumonia because the one she'd been on for years didn't work anymore."

In our culture, watching and waiting are the last things parents want to do. In fact, physicians sometimes provide antibiotics for illnesses that don't even respond to them—such as the common cold—in order to make parents happy. While some physicians are changing their mind-set and prescribing antibiotics less often, others have not followed suit.

Luckily, Brandon's mother was open to naturopathic methods.

I asked her to let her son's fever run its course, monitor his temperature closely, and use fever reducers such as Children's Tylenol only if his temperature exceeded 104°F.

In the meantime, I prescribed one dose of the homeopathic remedy Belladonna 200C, which increases the strength of the immune system and lowers fever.

By the next day, the fever had broken and Brandon began sweating, a good sign. The fever had done its job and his body was successfully fighting off the offending organism. During the next several days, Brandon's appetite and vitality improved.

# **3**

# TOXIC KIDS

**OUR WORLD IS INCREASINGLY TOXIC.** Traces of pharmaceuticals can be found in our drinking water, plastics litter our oceans, and carbon monoxide and other pollutants choke the air we breathe.

In our delicate ecosystem, every action has an impact. DDT sprayed on a farm in other parts of the world eventually enters the air when it evaporates. It can be carried in the atmosphere over long distances, and possibly settle in your yard. Fertilizers from local farms end up in streams, rivers, and oceans. Deadly fumes from manufacturing plants migrate far across state lines.

There may be nothing that makes parents feel more anxious than the sense that the very environment their children live in—the air they breathe, their playgrounds, the foods they eat—contains poisons.

Luckily, toxic exposure is often preventable. And when it's not, detoxification and elimination procedures, fundamental naturopathic therapies, are available. There is plenty that parents can do to protect their children.

I see "toxic" children in my office every day. They don't come in saying that they were contaminated by a broken mercury thermometer or were exposed to pesticides at the dinner table. Instead, they come in with ADHD, autism, asthma, and eczema. Exposure to toxins is the last thing on their—and their parents'—minds.

Joanie was a solemn, underweight girl who, at age 7, had eczema and arthritis. With her knobby joints and skinny limbs, she looked decades older than her young age.

Her father, tanned and muscular, had two other children, and both were healthy. He was clearly both worried and somewhat annoyed by his daughter's unyielding problems that no mainstream doctor had been able to solve.

"Joanie's the only one of us who has any health problems," he said as I examined the girl. "We've taken her everywhere and no one can find the answer."

Joanie had arrived fresh from the conventional medical world, where her body had been viewed as a collection of disparate parts, with a different specialist managing each one. She'd visited neurological, psychiatric, and gastrointestinal doctors, each with unique expertise, tests, and conclusions.

These encounters had produced a thick pile of imaging and test results that would take me hours to read, yet no one had discovered what was wrong with her.

No one had stopped to really look at the totality of Joanie. But naturopathy does just that: We look at a patient's whole self—how she lives, eats, and feels.

I rifled through her paperwork, then put it aside.

"What are Joan's other symptoms?"

Her father counted them off. "She's sluggish, she has abdominal pains and little interest in eating. She's underweight. She often vomits. And she has had trouble concentrating and learning."

Listening to him, a bell went off in my head.

"I'm going to do some tests, one of them for toxins."

"Toxins?" the father said with a frown. "What kind of toxins? We don't live in a Superfund site [a hazardous waste site slated for cleanup] or anything. In fact, we're in a historic section—our house was built in 1910."

"This is something I do with all my patients," I told him. I continued my exam, then stopped for a moment to take notes. While I was writing, Joanie opened a bag she'd brought with her and began to play. Out came a rag doll and a miniature metal teacup.

"Who's this?"

"Mona. This is what she drinks from."

I picked up the teacup and looked at the bottom.

"Mr. Fuller," I asked, "your house, does it still have original period details—woodwork and so on?" I asked.

"Yes."

"How about windows?"

"Well, we've replaced some, but mostly we've tried to keep the originals."

When Joanie's test results came back, it was just as I'd suspected. "Your daughter has excess lead in her system, along with cadmium and arsenic," I told her father. "Her lead reading is 20 micrograms per deciliter, which is quite high, so I'd like to start chelation [a method for removing metals from the bloodstream] right away."

Her father was surprised. "Lead? Are you serious? How could this happen?"

"Well, I'm not positive, but it could be your antique windows, for one thing—I'll bet their frames are still covered in lead-based paint. That means they produce toxic dust every time they're opened and closed. This little tea set could be another culprit; it's made from lead. There are many other possibilities. All of us are harboring toxic chemicals. The good news is that there's something we can do about it here."

From the stain guard that protects our carpets to the pine freshener we use in our bathrooms, we're under constant assault by toxic chemicals. The ingredients in pesticides, cleaning products, and plastics often end up in our bodies, as well. And these toxins are present in places you'd never imagine.

Consider the McDonald's recall of more than 12 million collectible Shrek glasses because cadmium was discovered in the designs painted on them. Cadmium is a known carcinogen that research shows can also cause bone softening and severe kidney problems.

In a 2010 Learning and Developmental Disabilities Initiative biomonitoring project called Mind, Disrupted: How Toxic Chemicals May Change How We Think and Who We Are, 12 volunteers were tested for 89 chemicals known or suspected to be neurodevelopmental toxicants or endocrine disruptors. Neurodevelopmental toxicants are environmental chemicals that affect the brain, nervous system, and childhood development; endocrine disruptors alter the body's glands and the hormones they produce and adversely affect development, reproduction, and the neurological and immune systems.

All total, the 12 volunteers tested positive for 61 chemicals. Individually, the number of chemicals detected ranged from 26 to 38, and 16 of them were found in every participant. These chemicals are commonly encountered in everyday life, and most Americans are exposed to and may be unwittingly contaminated by them.

The risks posed by these potentially harmful chemicals are especially serious for fetuses. A 2004 report on the findings of the Mothers and Children Study in New York City stated that in utero exposure to polycyclic aromatic hydrocarbons (combustion products from cars, heating systems, and tobacco smoke) in polluted air are linked to preterm birth, lower birth weight and smaller head circumference, and respiratory problems and developmental delay in childhood. Other studies looking at people in the general population have found associations between pesticides and cancer, ADHD, and nervous system disorders.

Natural medicine provides safe, proven methods for removing the poisons that our children take on from the environment. I use vitamins and herbs to remove harmful toxins from the body with a natural process called chelation, in which other substances bind with the toxins to form larger molecules that are easier for the body to eliminate. These methods are safe and without side effects, and they often significantly improve health.

# Four Exits for Toxins

Naturopathic medicine identifies four major "routes" in the body through which toxins pass: liver, kidneys, lungs, and skin.

## Liver

The liver eliminates most fat-soluble toxins in the stool. Constipation and insufficient dietary fiber allow reabsorption of toxins into the bloodstream.

**Supplement Support** When the liver removes toxins from the body, it produces damaging free radicals in the process. Antioxidants help combat the cellular damage caused by free radicals. One of the most important antioxidants is glutathione. Other beneficial antioxidants include vitamins C and E, selenium, coenzyme Q10, alpha-lipoic acid, S-adenosylmethionine, methylcobalamin (methyl $B_{12}$), magnesium, and glycine. Some of these substances interact with certain pharmaceuticals, so be sure to have a naturopathic physician or pharmacist review your medications and any supplement you want to take before you start a treatment.

**Dietary Support** Broccoli, cauliflower, cabbage, and brussels sprouts help to support liver detoxification. Other beneficial foods for liver health and maintenance include beets, dandelion greens, burdock, and citrus fruits.

**Botanical Support** Milk thistle taken orally protects the liver from damage and may help liver cells recover from damage, while castor oil packs stimulate the liver.

## Kidneys

Your kidneys function as the major excretory route for water-soluble toxins. When your body expels something it doesn't want, the substance usually exits in the urine or, if fat soluble, in the stool.

Drinking adequate amounts of water is the most important thing you can do to help your kidneys eliminate toxins. As children get bigger, they need more water. Take your child's weight in pounds and divide by 2. This is the number of ounces of water he or she should drink daily. For example, if your child weighs 48 pounds, he or she should drink 24 ounces of water daily.

**Homeopathics** Staphysagria improves the kidneys' removal of toxins in the urine.

**Botanical Support** Althea, alfalfa, equisetum, sambucus, essential oils of juniper and sandalwood (in very small amounts)

## Lungs

Exhalation excretes carbon dioxide and other gas-soluble toxins.

Exercise is an easy way to move air through all parts of the lungs. Have your child play outdoors and breathe the fresh air. If the area you live in has a high level of air pollution, it is important to take time on a weekly basis to go to a park or another cleaner area for exercise.

If it's cold or rainy, put on appropriate clothing and go outside! In fact, air quality is usually better on rainy days. Or, if you can't go out for some reason, sit down with your child for a daily breathing exercise. Sit quietly for 2 minutes, taking deep breaths. Inhale for 5 full seconds, exhale for 5 full seconds. Have your child count to 5 aloud while inhaling and exhaling. Two minutes may seem short at first, but when consciously breathing, it seems like a long time. As you practice, extend it to 5 and then 10 minutes daily.

**Botanical Support** Grindelia, glycyrrhiza (licorice) in small amounts, for short periods of time

## Skin

The skin is a secondary route for ridding the body of toxins that can't be excreted in the stool or urine. This process often manifests as a rash or chronic eczema.

The best way to improve the skin is to improve internal detoxification; daily movement and exercise help clear the lymphatic system, which acts as a drainage system for fluid left over after your tissues use the other components of blood for nourishment.

Your lymphatic system has no pump like your heart for your circulatory system; instead, breathing and muscle movement keep lymph moving. Therefore, it is important to exercise to move the lymph so it can eliminate toxins. Manual lymphatic drainage helps clean your lymphatic system and will also help you shed dead cells and keep your skin glowing.

## MANUAL LYMPHATIC DRAINAGE

At bedtime, take a dry loofah or facecloth and gently rub up the extremities toward the heart. Starting with your legs, wipe from your feet to your thighs. Then move to your arms and gently wipe from your hands to your heart. Finally, wipe up the abdomen and chest to your heart. The most important word to remember is "gently." This is not a massage for your muscles. Pretend you're wiping water up your body because, in reality, you are wiping the fluid in the lymphatic vessels under your skin.

# Four Tests for Toxins

In my practice, every child with chronic disease gets tested for toxins and heavy metals.

The tests I use include:

1. Urine heavy metal challenge
2. Porphyrin presence in the urine
3. Heavy metal presence in the stool
4. Heavy metal presence in the hair

The best test for heavy metals is a urine challenge. We collect a urine sample and analyze it for heavy metals. Then we give the child the appropriate chelator—an amino acid, herb, or mineral that binds with the heavy metal that's present and facilitates its elimination from the body, usually through urination. Different chelators work with different metals. Besides lead, other metals often found in the urine are mercury, cadmium, aluminum, arsenic, and excess iron and copper.

The second test I always run is called a porphyrin test. This screens for damage caused by toxins. When we test for heavy metals, we are just testing for three or four specific items, such as lead, mercury, cadmium, and arsenic. There are tens of thousands of toxins, and a heavy metal screen looks for just a few. A porphyrin test looks for problems in the formation of hemoglobin and can be used as a marker to measure the complete toxic load. These are the tests I used to diagnose Joanie.

Testing for heavy metals in the stool and hair doesn't give results that are as accurate as the urine and porphyrin tests. They reflect only recent exposure to heavy metals, although they do provide an indication of the amount of toxic buildup in the body. The unfortunate fact about all types of toxin tests is that they are not 100 percent accurate. We always want the best tests that technology can offer us, but everything has its limits. Sometimes the toxin testing does not reveal substances that are present in the body, and other times the test results exaggerate the amount of toxins. Either way, everyone who breathes air, drinks water, or eats food encounters toxic substances, and lessening your family's exposure to them by reducing the number in your home will have benefits.

Toxins will remain in and damage the body until they are removed. In Joanie's case, we needed to chelate the lead and other toxins in order to allow her kidneys and liver to excrete them. Succimer, the prescription medicine approved by the FDA for treating lead poisoning, is commonly used for this. But with Joanie I decided to start with herbs, minerals, and supplements: milk thistle, trimethylglycine (TMG), methylsulfonylmethane (MSM), calcium-D-glucarate, methionine, glutathione, and selenium. Given orally, they are the mildest, most natural approach. Be sure to consult your naturopathic physician before starting any supplement regimen. Just because products are natural doesn't mean they are safe for young children.

But detoxification was only one component of Joanie's treatment. She had not only been exposed to toxins, but also overmedicated with antibiotics for chronic sinus infections. She was also eating a diet high in wheat products, and there was evidence that she might have gluten intolerance.

Once Joanie completed the herbal detox and began to follow a gluten-free diet, her most troublesome physical symptoms disappeared.

# What a Parent Can Do

## Avoid Toxic Products

Open the cupboard under your kitchen or bathroom sink and look at the number of products your children come in contact with daily. I'm talking not just about household cleaners, but also personal care products like soap, moisturizer, and shampoo. These products contain a laundry list of chemicals, such as phthalates and parabens, that may be harmful to your family.

Especially worrisome is the effect that scientists have found these products have on adolescent girls. According to researchers at the nonprofit public health and environmental advocacy organization the Environmental Working Group, teenagers might be especially sensitive to chemicals that disrupt hormones.

**Take Action** Buy or make safe, biobased cleaning products instead of using those with harsh chemicals. (Biobased products are made with primarily renewable plant, animal, or marine materials.) Use natural soaps—olive oil or castile—for washing and bathing.

Avoid products containing fragrance. Whether it's in air fresheners or personal care products, "fragrance" usually means phthalates, which are the potentially toxic synthetic plasticizers added to fragrance to help the scent last longer.

Do not use vinyl shower curtains. The strong smell a new shower curtain has means that it contains phthalates. Use cotton, hemp, or PEVA (polyethylene vinyl acetate) liners instead.

When shopping for cosmetics and personal care products with your adolescent girl, take extra care to read the labels and choose natural brands. Look for products certified as environmentally safe by Green Seal or EcoLogo, and don't use products that list these as ingredients:

Any paraben, any phthalate (DEHP, BBP, DBP, DMP, DEP), DMDM hydantoin, fragrance, triclosan, sodium lauryl sulfate, sodium laureth sulfate, DEA (diethanolamine), TEA (triethanolamine), formaldehyde, any PEG (polyethylene glycol), anything with "glycol"

Before you head to the store, get the details on the safety of thousands of personal care products and cosmetics at the Environmental Working Group's Skin Deep database, www.cosmeticsdatabase.com.

## Stop Using Pesticides

Mice, roaches, bedbugs, and mosquitoes are among the most reviled of nature's pests. However, the poisons used to eradicate them are so highly toxic that they have health implications for our own species, especially our children.

Pesticides have been associated with asthma, cancer, and over- and underactive hormones. In my office, I see 9-year-old girls starting their menstrual periods and 3-month-old babies with thyroid problems. Studies have also shown a link between in utero exposure to organochlorine pesticides and impaired neurodevelopment.

Children, especially boys, who were exposed to high levels of organophosphate metabolites in utero have an increased risk of attention problems, a study published in the journal *Environmental Health Perspectives* reported. For additional information on this topic, visit Physicians for Social Responsibility at www.psr.org.

**Take Action** Forgo insect killers and lawn fertilizers for natural alternatives. Composted kitchen scraps (fruit and vegetable peelings) make a good fertilizer, as do chopped autumn leaves. Spray mild soap on bug-infested leaves and use oil of eucalyptus as an insect repellent on yourself and your kids over the age of 10.

Take all the toxic pesticides and chemicals you have in your home to a household hazardous waste collection facility.

When you enter the house, take off your shoes; the soles of shoes often carry traces of pesticides and other harmful chemicals that remain on rugs and floors, where children and pets play.

Don't buy bug spray that contains DEET, which can be especially dangerous for small children. If you must use it on your children, use only repellents with low concentrations of DEET for short periods of time. Make sure your window screens and windows block the entry of insects.

## Eat for Health

From plastics to additives to colorants, the foods we feed our children often contain potentially harmful substances. Our aluminum cans are lined with bisphenol A, a chemical used in making epoxy resins and plastics (and found in plastic bottles) that's thought to cause a wide variety of health problems. Our meats and milk are laced with antibiotics and growth hormones; our drinking water contains traces of antidepressants and other drugs.

**Take Action** Buy a water filtration system—it can be as simple as a pitcher with a carbon filter—that can remove lead, chlorine, and bacteria from tap water.

Avoid eggs, meats, and dairy products produced with the aid of hormones or antibiotics.

Buy organic fruits and vegetables, especially soft-skinned foods, which harbor the highest levels of herbicides: apples, peaches, strawberries, blueberries, spinach, cherries, imported grapes, potatoes, and lettuce.

Avoid nonstick cookware and use cast iron or stainless steel pans instead.

Avoid storing or reheating foods in plastic containers. The bisphenol A in the container can cause fertility problems, early-onset puberty, and neurological problems.

Cook your own food instead of buying prepared or takeout foods. When you cook it yourself, you avoid many of the synthetic toxins found in processed foods.

Look at labels and avoid as many of these additives as you can:

- **Aspartame:** An artificial sweetener found in gums and candies; implicated as a neurotoxin

- **Artificial Colors:** Can cause rashes, asthma, hyperactivity

- **Butylated Hydroxyanisole (BHA) and Butylated Hydroxytoluene (BHT):** Preservatives added to foods to prevent rancidity; the International Agency for Research on Cancer, part of the World Health Organization, suspects that both BHA and BHT are carcinogenic to humans

- **Monsodium Glutamate (MSG):** A flavor enhancer; thought to damage neurons

- **Potassium Bromate:** Used as a leavening agent in breads; has been linked to cancer

- **Nitrites:** Meat preservatives commonly found in processed meats such as hot dogs, salami, and bacon; have carcinogenic properties

- **Olestra:** A fat substitute added to snacks to make them fat free; causes loose stools and prohibits the absorption of certain nutrients

- **Sulfites:** Preservatives no longer applied to fresh fruits and vegetables to prevent browning, but still used in dried fruits and wines; implicated in asthma

For more information on the levels and sources of pollution in your local area, county, and state, check out www.scorecard.org.

# The Benefits of a Toxin-Free Childhood

My patient Joanie responded remarkably well to the mild chelation therapy, the nutritional supplements, and a glucose-free diet. She became adept at knowing what she could and couldn't eat and needed no enforcer but herself.

The last time I saw her, she had gained a few pounds and was less withdrawn. Her father couldn't hide his delight at her improvement.

A couple of months ago—probably 4 years since our first encounter—I caught sight of a face at a local basketball game and did a double take. Who was this familiar-looking dark-haired girl laughing in the bleachers?

And then I realized that it was Joanie. I barely recognized her: She was healthy, outgoing, her body filled out and her face alive.

I nearly went over to ask how she was doing, but I didn't want to interrupt her evening. In any case, I could see for myself that she was doing fine. I missed much of the ball game that night as I kept looking over at her shining face. Such are the profound and unusual joys of being a doctor. You never know where the fruits of your labors are going to turn up and remind you all over again that nature is the true healer, if we only elicit its power.

# MORE TOXINS YOUR CHILD (AND YOU) SHOULD AVOID

**Cigarette Smoke:** Smoking cigarettes is lethal, but secondhand smoke is also toxic and can damage your child's delicate lungs. It has been implicated in asthma, sudden infant death syndrome, pneumonia, and bronchitis. Besides that, children who regularly breathe secondhand smoke are at increased risk for ear infections.

**Open-Fire Grilled Food:** Charbroiled and blackened food may taste great, but cooking food directly over an open flame to the point where it becomes charred creates cancer-causing chemicals. Don't allow your grilled or broiled food to become blackened.

**Cough Syrups:** Most commercially available cough syrups are brews of artificial sweeteners, colors, alcohol, preservatives, and additives, and they do little to prevent a child's cough. Avoid them and instead choose a natural remedy.

**Radon:** The EPA suggests that all homes be tested for radon, a leading cause of lung cancer. This radioactive gas, which is impossible to smell or see, is caused by the breakdown of uranium in soil, rocks, and water.

**Chemical Laundry Detergents and Dryer Sheets:** The fragrances in these products may be described in poetic terms such as "rainforest fresh," but in fact they're permeated with synthetic chemicals. These additives are harmful not only for the environment, but also for growing children. Use natural detergents and softeners instead.

**Antibacterial Soaps:** These soaps are widely used by parents in order to defend children against germs. In fact, regular vegetable oil–based soaps are far superior to these products, which contain toxic chemicals that are particularly harmful to the nervous systems of developing children.

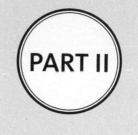

PART II

# TOP 100 PEDIATRIC HEALTH CONDITIONS AND SAFE, NATURAL SOLUTIONS

# TOP 100 CONDITIONS

*Cardiovascular*

**AMERICA'S LEADING CAUSE OF DEATH IS HEART DISEASE;** approximately every minute, it claims a life. But even more shocking is the fact that our children are being diagnosed as having or being at risk for developing this disease at younger and younger ages.

A study published in 2004 in the *Journal of the American Medical Association* (*JAMA*) reported that the top killers of inhabitants of the US in 2000 were tobacco, poor diet and physical inactivity, and alcohol. Fortunately, the damage from these risks can be substantially reduced or, even better, avoided entirely.

One of my patients, 12-year-old Tom, once weighed 200 pounds. He loved to eat and he idolized football linebackers, who often weigh 300 pounds or more. Tom was a lot like his father—they shared not only the same genes, but also, just as importantly, the same habits. Tom's father helped him develop a taste for greasy take-out foods like burgers and pizza, and since Dad never was active or worked out, Tom mimicked his behavior, spending most of his time inside, on the couch.

But when his father, who was only in his thirties, had a heart attack, Tom nearly lost him. The heart attack was a wake-up call for the whole family. After he was released from the hospital, Tom's father changed his diet, began to walk every day, and lost 50 pounds within a few months. Seeing his dad's new lifestyle inspired my patient to make similar changes, and he lost 60 pounds himself. Father and son forged new, healthy habits together.

My patient still loves football, but now he wants to become a running back or a wide receiver. His new habits have decreased his chances of heart disease in the future, and his father's example has been more powerful than anything I ever could have told him.

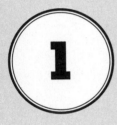

# HYPERTENSION (HIGH BLOOD PRESSURE)

## COMMON SYMPTOMS

Mild hypertension usually has no symptoms, but symptoms in children can include:

Fatigue

Headache

Nosebleeds

High blood pressure, typically an adult condition, is now appearing in more children due to the increasing prevalence of childhood obesity. Your blood pressure depends on the strength of your heartbeat and the diameter of your arteries. The narrower and less expandable your arteries are and the more blood your heart has to pump, the higher your blood pressure.

Previously, hypertension in children was rare and caused by conditions other than obesity, but now, because more children are obese, more have high blood pressure. Children who are obese—many because they have been eating too many sugary, high-fat foods and drinking too much soda—have three times the risk of hypertension as normal-weight children. Even more dangerous, the hearts of more than 40 percent of hypertensive children are enlarged on the left side, which can lead to further cardiac problems down the line.

The blood pressure level is the result of how much blood the heart is pumping and the amount of resistance in the blood vessels. It's similar to how a garden hose works: If you open the spigot to get more water or cover the hose's opening with your finger, the water comes out at a higher pressure. Blood pressure is affected by the volume of a fluid that circulates with the blood, the levels of particular hormones and minerals, and changes in the activity of the sympathetic nervous system in response to stressors. A high blood level of insulin in children who are obese can also elevate blood pressure.

According to the Mayo Clinic, pediatric high blood pressure is defined as "blood pressure that's the same as or higher than 95 percent of children who are the same sex, age and height." Because normal blood pressure levels change for children as they grow, no one measurement can be used for diagnosis.

Even though only an estimated 3 percent of children have high blood pressure, my patient Larry was one of them. Quiet, overweight, and studious, he lived with his grandmother in an inner-city high-rise. His grandmother worked at a senior health clinic and was deeply involved in her grandson's health care. So she was nonplussed when I told her that Larry's blood pressure was sky-high.

"High? Let me see?" She moved closer and watched the numbers as I took it again.

"That's higher than most adults." She turned to Larry. "What've you been eating when I'm not home?" "Nothing," Larry insisted. "Nothing, huh? Well, how could this blood pressure get so high?"

When I took further information about his past health, it turned out that there was a history of hypertension and heart disease on Larry's paternal side. So even though he was living with his health-conscious maternal grandmother, he had a strong genetic basis for heart and vascular problems from the other side of his family—people he barely knew. That is one reason why knowing the total health history of your child is so important.

# 5 Irreversible Conditions Caused by Hypertension

Heart failure

Kidney disease

Blindness

Stroke

Heart attack

# 3 Benefits of Controlling Hypertension

Stroke incidence decreases by 35 to 40 percent

Heart attack incidence decreases by 20 to 25 percent

Heart failure risk decreases by 50 percent

## Natural Prescriptions*

| Diet |
| --- |
| Focus on eating healthy foods, including vegetables, fruits, and whole grains. |
| Remove excess sugar, fat, and salt from the diet. |
| Appropriate fat intake of 25 to 40 percent of the diet, depending on age<br>    1 year of age: 30 to 40 percent<br>    2 to 3 years of age: 30 to 35 percent<br>    4 to 8 years of age: 25 to 35 percent of diet |
| **Vitamins/Supplements** |
| Fish oil EPA + DHA 1 to 2 grams (g) daily |
| Magnesium 200 to 400 mg daily |
| **Naturopathic Remedies** |
| Arginine 1 to 2 g daily |

* Refer to the appendix at the back of the book for a comprehensive list of interactions and condition-based doses.

Many studies have been performed on the effects of fish oil on cardiovascular health in people who have high cholesterol. The major active ingredients in fish oil are EPA (eicosapentaenoic acid) and DHA (docosahexaenoic acid). When you buy a fish oil supplement, check to see if it contains more EPA or DHA. DHA has been found to be more effective than EPA in helping to lower high blood pressure caused by high cholesterol.

Arginine is an amino acid that is converted to nitric oxide in the body. In children with high blood pressure caused by narrow vessels, supplemental arginine can open and relax them, thereby lowering the pressure. Do not give your child arginine if he or she is currently taking a blood pressure medication called an ACE inhibitor.

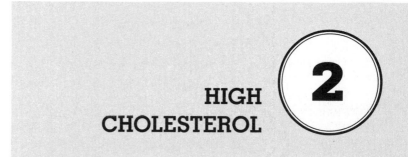

# HIGH CHOLESTEROL 2

## COMMON SYMPTOMS

**Yellow deposits called xanthomas on the skin.**

High cholesterol is usually detected during routine screening and has few symptoms initially. Overweight children should have their cholesterol tested.

When children eat unhealthy foods that are high in sugars and saturated or trans fats over a long period of time, the interiors of their large arteries may become clogged and narrowed by cholesterol deposits by the time they are adults. This condition is called atherosclerosis.

The American Academy of Pediatrics issued cholesterol-testing recommendations in 2008. Children whose parents have premature heart disease (at age 55 or younger in men and age 65 or younger in women) or high cholesterol and children who are overweight (at the 85th percentile or higher on growth charts) should have their cholesterol tested. Testing should begin between the ages of 2 and 10. If your child is overweight or your family has a history of early heart disease, have his or her cholesterol level tested.

*Science Daily* recently reported that a group of researchers had proposed that fast-food chains provide cholesterol-lowering statin drugs to customers free of charge to neutralize the heart disease dangers that come with eating the fatty foods they serve. So, one day you may not even need a prescription to treat your child's high cholesterol. He or she may get a statin along with a Big Mac or Whopper and wash it all down with a sugary soft drink. No more guilt or disease, right?

Ever since conventional medicine created statins, drugs that stop our livers from making too much cholesterol, we've given up on personal responsibility. We take a pill and then eat fast food and desserts and sit in front of the television. But we need to ask ourselves: Does using this approach give us true health? Or does it only temporarily deal with one component of an unhealthy lifestyle? More importantly, is it the kind of example we want to provide for our children?

A permanent cure isn't a drug or coronary artery bypass surgery that reroutes the blood around plugged-up arteries. When we start at the source and change to a healthy diet and daily exercise, the body heals itself. This happens in two ways: When dietary fat intake is lowered, less new cholesterol is deposited in the artery walls, preventing additional plaque and narrowing. Then, over a long time, the walls of the sections of artery that are already narrowed may relax and stretch, allowing more blood to pass and blood pressure to normalize. The risks of heart attack and stroke are dramatically reduced when this occurs. No drugs need to be taken when you've truly resolved the problem. (However, children who have diabetes may need to continue taking the medications to decrease their risks of heart attack and stroke.)

Healthy cholesterol numbers in children vary based on sex and age. Here is a thumbnail guide for adolescents:

| Cholesterol Levels in Adolescents | | |
|---|---|---|
| | Total | LDL |
| Acceptable | Below 170 milligrams per deciliter (mg/dl) | Below 110 mg/dl |
| Borderline | 170–199 mg/dl | 110–129 mg/dl |
| Elevated | 200 mg/dl and higher | 130 mg/dl and higher |

Source: American Heart Association

Niacin, also known as vitamin $B_3$, is an effective vitamin for people with high cholesterol. It increases HDL, the good cholesterol, which transports LDL, the bad cholesterol, from the blood vessels back to the liver to be excreted in the stools. Less cholesterol in blood vessels equals less risk for heart attacks and strokes. Niacin also lowers triglycerides, another kind of fat in the blood.

A research study on plant sterols—substances that occur naturally in plants—gave 41 children with genetically caused high cholesterol 2.3 grams of sterols or placebo for 4 weeks. The plant sterol group of children had their total cholesterol levels lowered by 11 percent and their LDL cholesterol lowered by 14 percent. What a huge drop in cholesterol in 1 month! This, for example, would lower a total cholesterol level of 220 mg/dl to 196, a safer level.

Psyllium is a soluble fiber that binds with cholesterol in the intestines and removes it from the body. Researchers have shown that psyllium lowers cholesterol. Oat bran, which is what Cheerios and similar cereals are made of, is another kind of soluble fiber that does the same thing.

Fish oil is so effective at treating high triglycerides that the FDA has approved a prescription drug made with it. How odd that we think differently about a bottle

## Natural Prescriptions*

| Diet | |
| --- | --- |
| Focus on vegetables, fruits, and whole grains. | |
| Reduce saturated and trans fats in the diet. | |
| Reduce fat content to 25 to 40 percent of diet, depending on age:<br>　1 year of age: 30 to 40 percent<br>　2 to 3 years of age: 30 to 35 percent<br>　4 to 8 years of age: 25 to 35 percent of diet | |
| **Vitamins/Supplements** | |
| Fish oil EPA + DHA 1 to 2 g daily | Vitamin $B_3$ (niacin) 5 to 20 mg daily |
| Pycnogenol 50 to 100 mg daily | |
| **Naturopathic Remedies** | |
| Green tea (decaffeinated) 4 to 6 cups daily | Psyllium 6 g daily |
| Plant sterols 2 to 2.5 g daily | |

* Refer to the appendix at the back of the book for a comprehensive list of interactions and condition-based doses.

of fish oil we find on the shelf at many stores and a bottle of fish oil capsules with a fancy name on it that we pick up from our pharmacists. The fish oil and the "drug" are exactly the same, but your doctor may believe that one works better than the other. This is the future: Natural supplements that have 20 years of research supporting their effectiveness will be co-opted by the pharmaceutical companies as drugs.

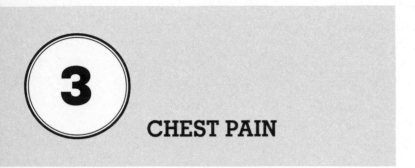

# 3
# CHEST PAIN

## COMMON SYMPTOMS

Pain that radiates to the back, throat, or belly

Superficial or deep pain

Sharp or dull pain

Acute chest pain, which is pain that arises suddenly, is frightening for anyone, especially a child. While a heart attack immediately comes to mind, there are also other possibilities to consider when chest pain is severe.

Skin lesions on the chest can cause pain. Check the skin for abrasions, cuts, signs of trauma, or wounds. If the pain started after a sports injury, get a chest x-ray taken, because ribs can be broken at the breastbone during an impact. If the area is tender to the touch and there was no injury, the pain may be muscular. If an imaging study is needed for some reason, a CT scan can be performed to look for costochondritis, inflammation of the cartilage that attaches the ribs to the breastbone.

The esophagus runs behind the breastbone on its way from the mouth to the stomach. When you have severe heartburn, acid reflux, or gastroesophageal reflux disease, stomach acid has entered the esophagus. In children, this can cause chest pain and a dry, nonproductive cough. An esophageal spasm or stricture—a narrow spot in the esophagus caused by, for example, inflammation or scar tissue—can also cause chest pain.

If a child has had a severe cough, chest pain is to be expected. Lung infections that cause chronic coughing can make the entire rib cage hurt.

Last, but not least, heart problems can cause chest pain. One type is hypertrophic cardiomyopathy, which is enlargement of the heart. In most people with the condition, the wall that separates the ventricles (the two bottom chambers of the heart) enlarges and blocks the blood flow. It is the leading cause of sudden cardiac death during exercise in adolescents. Some children have no symptoms, but the condition may cause trouble breathing, fainting, chest pain (especially during exercise or exertion), or dizziness. Hypertrophic cardiomyopathy has a genetic basis, and if your family includes someone who has the condition, consult your pediatrician about screening for it.

Other types of heart or blood problems can cause chest pain, too. A child may report feeling his heart pounding in his chest or develop tingling in his lips or fingers. If a child begins to lose consciousness, a trip to the emergency room or a call for an ambulance is essential.

Always be cautious and bring a child to the pediatrician if the pain continues for more than a day or seems severe.

## Natural Prescriptions*

| Homeopathic Remedies |
| --- |
| Homeopathic Arnica 30C 5 pellets 3 times daily as needed |

*Refer to the appendix at the back of the book for a comprehensive list of interactions and condition-based doses.*

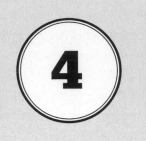

# KAWASAKI SYNDROME

**4**

## COMMON SYMPTOMS

Chest pain

Fever

Horizontal nail lines

Irritability

Red eyes

Skin peeling

Skin rash

Strawberry tongue

Swollen lymph nodes

Kawasaki syndrome causes inflammation of the small- and medium-sized arteries. It is a rare condition most common in young children of Asian descent under the age of 5. When a child has this condition, he or she runs a high fever for 1 or 2 weeks and has a rash on the body or diaper area; red, swollen tongue, hands, and feet; and very red eyes. If you suspect that your child has Kawasaki syndrome, go to the pediatrician right away.

Heart problems are a serious complication of Kawasaki syndrome, and they occur in about 20 percent of those affected. Early treatment in the hospital can prevent the heart and coronary arteries from being damaged. Because of the risk of a heart attack from the syndrome's effects on the heart, be sure to monitor your child closely for signs of heart palpitations or chest pain. Your pediatrician will listen to your child's heart, and an echocardiogram can be performed to assess whether the heart has been damaged.

A deficiency of *Lactobacillus*, the healthy bacteria in our intestines, may occur when a child is actively ill with Kawasaki syndrome. A study performed in 60 children, 20 with Kawasaki syndrome, 20 with fevers for other reasons, and 20 totally healthy, measured the intestinal populations of these bacterial strains and found that 70 percent of the healthy children had normal levels of them, 80 percent of the kids with fever had normal levels, and only 10 percent of the Kawasaki children had normal levels.

After a child has had Kawasaki syndrome, his or her arteries don't adequately dilate. A study performed on 39 children 1 to 10 years after the acute illness showed that intravenous administration of vitamin C temporarily doubled the diameter of the brachial artery, a large artery in the arm.

## Natural Prescriptions*

| Vitamins/Supplements | |
|---|---|
| Probiotics 10 to 20 billion colony forming units (CFU) daily | Vitamin E 200 to 400 IU daily |
| Vitamin C 400 to 2,000 mg daily | |

*\* Refer to the appendix at the back of the book for a comprehensive list of interactions and condition-based doses.*

# ANEMIC JAUNDICE (G6PD DEFICIENCY)

**5**

## COMMON SYMPTOMS

Dark urine

Pallor

Rapid heart rate

Shortness of breath

Yellow skin, mucous membranes, and eyes

G6PD deficiency is a genetic disease in which the body doesn't have enough of the enzyme glucose-6-phosphate dehydrogenase, or G6PD, which helps red blood cells function normally. It is the most common enzyme deficiency in the world and is most prevalent among males of African, Asian, Middle-Eastern, and Mediterranean descent.

Those with G6PD deficiency usually do not show any symptoms of the disorder until their red blood cells are exposed to certain triggers, which include:

- Illness, such as bacterial and viral infections
- Certain pain relievers and fever-reducing drugs, such as nonsteroidal anti-inflammatory drugs (NSAIDs)
- Certain antibiotics (especially those that have "sulf" in their names)
- Certain antimalarial drugs (especially those that have "quine" in their names)
- Certain foods (such as fava beans)

The jaundice that may occur after exposure to these triggers results from the deaths of red blood cells in too great numbers for the liver to process the bilirubin that remains after the cells die.

While we cannot change a genetic condition, we can provide support for the child's sensitive red blood cells. Supplementing with preventive antioxidants on a daily basis and giving extra during a jaundice attack will help limit the oxidative damage these triggers induce in the blood cells.

N-acetylcysteine (NAC) is an antioxidant derived from an amino acid, cysteine, that helps create another antioxidant called glutathione. Researchers at Harvard proved NAC's ability to reduce oxidative damage in the red blood cells of acutely ill G6PD patients. Similarly, vitamin E is an antioxidant that lessens oxidative damage to red blood cells, and in studies it has been shown to extend the lives of red blood cells in those with G6PD deficiency.

## Natural Prescriptions*

| Diet |  |
| --- | --- |
| Avoid fava beans and other legumes (including soy); tonic water; and foods containing sulfites, menthol, or ascorbic acid. | |
| Avoid certain drugs and supplements, notably sulfa antibiotics, aspirin and other NSAIDs, and some remedies used in Chinese herbal medicine, such as *Rhizoma coptidis* (golden thread), *Flos chimonanthi praecocis* (wintersweet flower), *Flos lonicerae* (honeysuckle flower), *Calculus bovis* (dried cow gallstone), and margarita (pearl from oysters and other bivalves). | |
| **Vitamins/Supplements** | |
| NAC 200 to 400 mg by mouth daily | Vitamin E 200 to 400 IU daily |
| Pycnogenol 50 to 100 mg daily | |

*\* Refer to the appendix at the back of the book for a comprehensive list of interactions and condition-based doses.*

# CONGENITAL HEART DEFECTS

**6**

## COMMON SYMPTOMS

Heart palpitations

Fatigue

Lack of endurance

Clubbing of fingers

Trouble breathing

Congenital heart defects—malformations that arise during fetal development—are relatively common in children, occurring in 0.5 percent of full-term babies and 1.3 percent of preterm babies, according to a review of the health records of more than 500,000 infants in northern England.

Any infant who is blue at birth, has trouble feeding, breathes fast, has a heart murmur, or sweats while feeding should be evaluated for a heart defect. While many defects are diagnosed at birth, others may not cause symptoms until a child is old enough to exercise. A child with fatigue while exercising, a heart murmur, or cyanosis—a bluish discoloration of the skin and mucous membranes when crying or exercising—should be referred to a pediatrician for evaluation. A thorough history and physical exam, and perhaps an echocardiogram, is the best noninvasive approach to diagnosing such problems.

## Common Heart Defects

1. Ventricular septal defect. The most common congenital heart defect, this is a hole in the wall separating the lower chambers of the heart, called the ventricles. The heart has to pump harder than normal with this defect, so it may enlarge over time.

2. Coarctation of the aorta. With this condition, the aorta, the largest artery, has a narrow spot that restricts the delivery of oxygenated blood to the lower body. As a result, the heart has to work harder to get blood through the narrow part and the blood pressure above that point increases.

3. Tetralogy of fallot. This condition is made up of four separate defects.
   » A ventricular septal defect (see above)

- » A narrow spot that prevents the free flow of blood from the heart to the lungs for oxygenation
- » The aorta exits the heart directly over the ventricular septal defect
- » The muscle surrounding the right ventricle (the bottom right chamber) is overly thickened

4. Atrial septal defect. This condition, commonly found later in life because it may not cause symptoms until adulthood, is a hole in the wall between the atria, the two upper chambers of the heart. Together with ventricular septal defects, these are commonly called holes in the heart.

5. Patent ductus arteriosus. In this condition, a blood vessel that normally closes within hours after birth remains open, diverting oxygenated blood from the aorta to the pulmonary artery. As many as 20 percent of infants with respiratory distress syndrome have this condition, and premature babies and low-birth-weight babies are more likely to have it. It is sometimes corrected surgically or, in premature babies, treated with intravenous ibuprofen or indomethacin; it may also close on its own, without treatment.

The best way to treat heart defects is to prevent them. Adequate folate is required for the fetal heart to form properly. Women of childbearing age should take folic acid (the supplemental form of folate) or a multivitamin daily. If you wait until you discover you're pregnant to supplement, your child's heart will have already formed, potentially with a heart defect.

While surgery is the best option to correct heart defects, fish oil has been studied to see if it improves heart function in patients whose heart muscles have been damaged by their heart defects, a condition called cardiomyopathy. One study looked at whether fish oil improved the performance of the left ventricle (the lower left heart chamber) in 41 children, 12 of whom were healthy and were given fish oil, 18 of whom had dilated cardiomyopathy (enlarged ventricles that couldn't pump enough blood, causing heart failure) and received fish oil, and 11 of whom had cardiomyopathy but did not take fish oil. After 6 months, left ventricular function had improved by 8.4 percent in the children with heart problems who took fish oil, compared with 2.5 percent in the children with cardiomyopathy who did not take fish oil. The inside diameter of the left ventricle had decreased by 4.4 millimeters (mm) in the children with heart problems who got fish oil and by only 1.9 mm in children with cardiomyopathy who didn't take it.

Other supplements are beneficial after a child has corrective surgery. Since a substantial amount of blood can be lost during surgery, your child may become anemic. Supplemental iron has been shown to boost red blood cell production and correct this anemia.

## Natural Prescriptions*

| Vitamins/Supplements |
| --- |
| For the mother before the birth (used to prevent heart defects): Prenatal multivitamin daily |
| For the child after surgery: Fish oil EPA + DHA 1 to 2 g daily Selenium 45 to 200 mcg daily for 7 days before surgery Vitamin C 250 to 2,000 mg daily Iron 7 to 10 mg daily *Salvia miltiorrhizae composita*, 200 mg/kg (2 g for every 22 pounds) daily |
| **Homeopathic Remedies** |
| Homeopathic Arnica 30C 5 pellets daily |
| **Alternative Treatments** |
| Acupuncture (used to improve surgical outcomes) |

*\* Refer to the appendix at the back of the book for a comprehensive list of interactions and condition-based doses.*

# MEGALOBLASTIC ANEMIA (GIANT RED BLOOD CELLS)

## COMMON SYMPTOMS

Difficulty walking

Fatigue

Lack of endurance

Numbness in hands and feet

Tingling in hands and feet

Megaloblastic anemia is characterized by extra-large red blood cells that result from a deficiency of vitamin $B_{12}$ or folate. This disorder is relatively rare and most often seen by US health care providers in patients of northern European descent. In addition, the children of vegetarian mothers who exclusively breast-feed may develop it.

Iron, vitamin $B_{12}$, and folate are the most important nutrients for building red blood cells. Blood tests for these nutrients and the size and shape of red blood cells can show whether a child has sufficient levels for making strong, healthy red blood cells.

One study looked at 33 children ages 9 to 36 months who had megaloblastic anemia and refused to eat anything but breast, cow's, or goat's milk. They also had low appetite, exhibited developmental delay, and were very pale. Testing revealed that 32 had vitamin $B_{12}$ deficiency, 1 had folate deficiency, and 10 had combined deficiency. Megaloblastic anemia is rare, but if your child refuses to eat anything other than milk for months, severe problems, such as neurological damage, can occur. Have your naturopathic physician monitor your child's treatment to ensure that any deficiencies are properly remedied.

A case report of a 16-month-old girl with megaloblastic anemia described degeneration of her previous neurological development, increased skin pigmentation, and tremor. After testing, it was discovered that she was vitamin $B_{12}$ deficient and that her mother (who was exclusively breast-feeding) had a low but normal level. After appropriate supplementation, the child's anemia, tremor, and skin darkening were cured, although other neurological problems remained.

## 4 Best Tests for Megaloblastic Anemia

Complete blood count
Methylmalonic acid test (for $B_{12}$ deficiency)
Red blood cell folate test (for folate deficiency in red blood cells)
Schilling test (for $B_{12}$ deficiency, to analyze absorption)

## Natural Prescriptions*

| Vitamins/Supplements |
| --- |
| Folic acid (or 5-MTHF) 200 to 400 mcg daily for 2 to 3 months |
| Vitamin $B_{12}$ 5 to 10 mcg daily for 2 to 3 months |

* Refer to the appendix at the back of the book for a comprehensive list of interactions and condition-based doses.

# SUBCONJUNCTIVAL HEMORRHAGE (BROKEN BLOOD VESSEL IN THE EYE)

## COMMON SYMPTOMS

Red spot on the white of the eye (not on the iris or pupil) (but no change in vision)

Vomiting, sneezing, coughing, or constipation

The first case I ever encountered of this scary-looking condition was when a wailing mother carried her 2-year-old into the office.

"Sammy's been hurt—his eye's hemorrhaging. Can you give him something for the pain?"

But once I examined Sammy, I learned that he was in no pain at all and could see perfectly well. What was going on?

He had a benign but frightening-looking condition—a subconjunctival hemorrhage, a broken blood vessel in the eye.

It looked so horrifying because a tiny droplet of blood had spread out underneath the transparent membrane that covers the eye. With the crimson blood displayed against the white of the eye, the minuscule amount of blood looks much worse than it is.

How had it happened?

Sometimes a vessel breaks from something as minor as rubbing the eye or a strong cough or sneeze. Sometimes it occurs spontaneously for unknown reasons.

Most pediatricians will tell you that this condition will go away in a couple of weeks without any treatment, but we can naturally shorten that time using a method called alternating hydrotherapy.

## Natural Prescriptions*

| Alternative Treatments |
| --- |
| ALTERNATING HYDROTHERAPY:<br><br>Sit with your child for 10 minutes with two bowls of water, one hot and one cold. Get two facecloths, one for each bowl of water. Alternate pressing the hot- and cold-water cloths on the closed eyelid. Make sure that the hot water isn't so hot that it burns the child. The hot and cold water will push the blood out of the eye and help the body reabsorb it.<br><br>1. Apply the hot-water facecloth for 2 minutes.<br>2. Apply the cold-water facecloth for 30 seconds.<br>3. Repeat three times.<br><br>This process can be repeated hourly. The more it is done, the faster the child will heal. |

*\* Refer to the appendix at the back of the book for a comprehensive list of interactions and condition-based doses.*

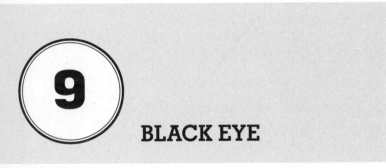

## 9

# BLACK EYE

## COMMON SYMPTOMS

Pain in the eye

Purple skin around the eye

Usually a history of trauma

Usually no change in vision

A black eye is evidence of blood that's collected under the skin around the eye, causing discoloration and swelling. It results from injury to the face or head from a fall, fight, or accident. Black eyes are relatively common and typically are painful only initially.

A black eye can resemble a far more dangerous condition known as orbital cellulitis, in which there is a bacterial infection around the eye. It looks like a black eye, but in reality it's a dangerous infection that can quickly spread through the bloodstream to other organs.

You can tell one from the other because children with cellulitis will seem sick, have a fever, and have severe eye pain, sometimes with eye movement, whereas a child with a black eye has no fever and the pain is mild. If you think your child has orbital cellulitis, call your pediatrician. This condition requires antibiotic treatment. (Remember, always give your child probiotics when he or she is on a course of antibiotics. Make sure your child does not take probiotics and antibiotics at the same time; probiotics should be taken several hours before or after the antibiotic dose is given so that the effectiveness of the medicine is not affected.)

Black eyes will go away over time, but alternating hydrotherapy can expedite healing.

## Natural Prescriptions*

| Vitamins/Supplements |
| --- |
| Bromelain 100 to 200 mg daily |
| Quercetin 200 to 400 mg divided into 2 or 3 doses daily |
| **Alternative Treatments** |
| ALTERNATING HYDROTHERAPY: <br> Sit down with your child for 10 minutes with two bowls of water, one hot, and one cold. Get two facecloths, one for each bowl of water. Alternate pressing the hot- and cold-water facecloths on the closed eyelid. Make sure that the hot water isn't so hot it that it burns the child. The hot and cold water will push the blood out of the eye and help the body reabsorb it. <br> 1. Apply the hot-water facecloth for 2 minutes. <br> 2. Apply the cold-water facecloth for 30 seconds. <br> 3. Repeat 3 times. |

* Refer to the appendix at the back of the book for a comprehensive list of interactions and condition-based doses.

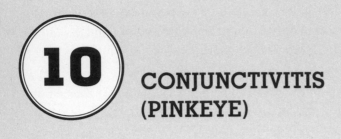

# 10

# CONJUNCTIVITIS (PINKEYE)

## COMMON SYMPTOMS

Discharge from the eye

Itchy eye (in some cases)

No contact lens use, eye trauma, or foreign body in the eye

No pain with eye movement

Reddened white of the eye

Usually no change in vision*

Watery eye

Pinkeye—conjunctivitis—can be caused by bacteria, viruses, substances, or allergies. The viral form is extremely infectious and spreads easily from one person to another. It can affect one or both eyes.

When Judy, the mother of a family I have known for many years, came into my office, I didn't need to ask what was wrong. The skin around one of her eyes was puffy and her eyeball was pink. Right behind her was her daughter, then her son, with the same swollen and pink eyes. The kids' eyes were so itchy that they couldn't help but rub them. Standing there in misery, they looked like members of some odd and miserable clan.

"Let me guess: A kid came to school with pinkeye and spread it."

Judy said, "Yes. We're itching like crazy. The pediatrician says it's viral, so can you help us out since we can't have antibiotics?"

If pinkeye is caused by a virus, not a bacterium, antibiotic medications are of no help. Viral conjunctivitis usually runs its course and clears up on its own, but natural methods such as herbal eyedrops can help with the symptoms.

*Euphrasia* is an herb that is so well known for its benefits in eye conditions that its common name is Eyebright. A research study was performed in which 65 patients with conjunctivitis were given *Euphrasia* eyedrops. Complete recovery after 2 weeks was seen in 82 percent of them and moderate improvement in 17 percent, a tremendous outcome.

*\* If your child has eye pain or a change in vision, consult an ophthalmologist immediately.*

*Ginkgo biloba* eyedrops should be used for seasonal allergic conjunctivitis, such as that caused by hayfever. A study of 60 patients showed that ginkgo and hyaluronic acid solution eyedrops significantly decreased eye swelling, redness, and discharge. Treat the allergy with the natural prescriptions on page 195.

## Natural Prescriptions*

| Naturopathic Remedies |
| --- |
| *Euphrasia* (Eyebright) 3X eyedrops 1 to 5 times a day |
| *Ginkgo biloba* 3X eyedrops, 5 drops, 1 to 5 times a day |
| **Alternative Treatments** |
| WARM PACK:<br>Apply a warm facecloth to the eyelid for 10 minutes 3 times a day. |

*\* Refer to the appendix at the back of the book for a comprehensive list of interactions and condition-based doses.*

# DACRYOSTENOSIS AND DACRYOCYSTITIS (BLOCKED TEAR DUCT)

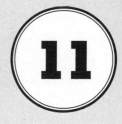

**11**

## COMMON SYMPTOMS

Swelling and redness between the eye and nose

Tearing of one or sometimes both eyes

Excessive tearing of the eye is caused by the eye creating more tears than can drain into the nose through the nasolacrimal duct (also called the tear duct) at the inside corner of the eye. Tears are always being produced to lubricate the eyes, with extra being made when emotion or irritation calls for them. Neither dacryostenosis nor dacryocystitis results from a greater volume of tears being made.

Abby, a beautiful baby girl only 1 week old, was happy and healthy and cooed when she was in her mother's arms. But soon her parents noticed that she was crying all the time. It wasn't regular crying, but simply tears dripping down one side of her cheek all day long. She didn't seem sad. She didn't even seem to notice. This is a symptom of dacryostenosis, a blocked nasolacrimal duct.

When the tear duct is obstructed, tears can't drain from the eyes. This condition—dacryostenosis—occurs mainly in newborn babies and indicates that the nasolacrimal duct didn't finish forming at its far end after birth. Tears can't pass through to the nose and end up falling down the cheek instead.

A related condition is dacryocystitis, which can also occur in newborns whose tear ducts didn't fully form. When fluid collects in a blocked tear duct and is infected by the bacteria that line the mucous membranes of the eyes and nose, it causes inflammation and a red, swollen bump, almost like a pimple, between the eye and nose.

## Natural Prescriptions

### Alternative Treatments

Both of these conditions usually can be remedied by gently rubbing from the inner corner of the eye down the side of the nose three times a day. It may take days or weeks, but eventually the tube should open up and the tearing will stop. However, with dacryocystitis, if the infection seems serious, be sure to visit your pediatrician. Your child may need surgery if the condition doesn't resolve.

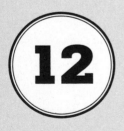

# 12 PINGUECULA AND PTERYGIUM (YELLOW SPOT ON THE WHITE OF THE EYE)

## COMMON SYMPTOMS

Yellow spot on the white of the eye closest to the nose

If the spot extends to the iris, consult an ophthalmologist.

A raised yellow spot on the white of the eye to the left or right of the iris is called a pinguecula. Although the cause is not certain, it's associated with irritation from dust or other airborne particles and chronic exposure to sunlight. It is common in people who live in the desert, spend a lot of time outdoors, or are exposed to air pollution.

A pinguecula is a cosmetic condition and doesn't affect vision or cause any harm. A pterygium, however, is a similar growth, also thought to be caused by sunlight or irritation, that extends onto the iris and may affect the vision, in which case it can be surgically removed.

However, prevention is the best cure for both conditions, so have your children wear sunglasses whenever they are outside and give them antioxidants if you live in the desert or are frequently exposed to airborne particles.

Yellow spots on the eye often occur after microtrauma to the eye. For example, a study of 990 policemen showed that 37.7 percent of those who patrolled on motorcycles had pingueculae whereas only 30.6 percent of their colleagues who worked indoors had them. In another study, surgical analysis of the yellow spot showed that there was decreased antioxidant activity in the tissue. Daily supplementation with common antioxidants may help to prevent these from growing.

## Natural Prescriptions*

| Vitamins/Supplements | |
| --- | --- |
| Alpha-lipoic acid (ALA) 100 mg daily | Vitamin C 1,000 mg daily |
| Selenium 40 to 200 mcg daily | Vitamin E 200 IU daily |
| Vitamin A 1,000 IU daily | |

* Refer to the appendix at the back of the book for a comprehensive list of interactions and condition-based doses.

# 13 OTITIS EXTERNA (SWIMMER'S EAR)

## COMMON SYMPTOMS

Discharge from the ear canal

Painful outer ear and ear canal

Reddened outer ear canal

Swollen outer ear canal

Swimmer's ear is an infection of the outer ear canal. This bacterial—or occasionally fungal or viral—infection is common and often contracted from the surface of bodies of water such as lakes.

An infection of the outer ear canal is quite different from a standard ear infection, called otitis media, which occurs behind the eardrum in the middle ear. In otitis externa, the infecting agent enters the ear canal and causes the symptoms listed above. Temporary hearing problems may occur if the ear canal is completely obstructed. The hearing returns to normal once the infection is gone.

The effects of the powerful oils of tea tree and chamomile on some of the microorganisms that cause swimmer's ear—*Staphylococcus, Pseudomonas, Candida,* and others—have been studied. In one study, tea tree oil was found to kill 71 percent of the bacterial and yeast cultures grown from infecting ear microorganisms. Another study of garlic extract on the most common fungus causing otitis externa showed that it was more effective than a pharmaceutical ear infection formulation.

Also, make sure to keep your child's ears dry. If water does get in the ear canal, put a few drops of distilled white vinegar in the canal right away and let it drain out after a few minutes. It is very important that you do not get any fluid in the ear if the eardrum is perforated or your child has ear tubes.

## Natural Prescriptions*

| Naturopathic Remedies |
|---|
| Do not use any of these to treat otitis externa in children under the age of 1: |
| Tea tree salve applied topically 3 times daily |
| Chamomile oil applied topically 3 times daily |
| Garlic extract salve applied topically 3 times daily |

*Refer to the appendix at the back of the book for a comprehensive list of interactions and condition-based doses.*

# OTITIS MEDIA (MIDDLE EAR INFECTION)

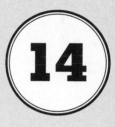

## COMMON SYMPTOMS

Ear pain

Fever

Impaired hearing

Irritability

Loss of appetite

Tugging on ear

Middle ear infections are among the most common health conditions in babies and young children. These infections cause the middle ear space inside the ear to become clogged with fluid and mucus. Inflammation that closes the eustachian tube, which connects the middle ear to the throat, is the main cause.

When I was growing up, the infant son of a family friend seemed to be perpetually fussy. His cries filled the air whenever they came to visit. He always had fevers, and his mother was always carting him off to the doctor. When I was older, I found out that the ailments that dominated his childhood were ear infections.

Certain children seem to be on the ear infection merry-go-round: Every few months, they are back at the doctor, pulling at their ears, fussing and crying, fluid draining from their ears.

The problem is that many of these children have recurrent ear infections that seem to never go away even after endless rounds of antibiotics prescribed by conventional physicians. But even conventional physicians suggest deferring antibiotics for 1 to 3 days if the pain is manageable, because two out of three cases of acute otitis media resolve without antibiotic treatment. Most ear infections are viral. In Europe, it is less common to use antibiotics for ear infections.

The most concerning consequence of untreated ear infections is mastoiditis, which is an infection in the bone behind the ear. While it is rare (fewer than five cases out of every 100,000 people in the US), you should consult your pediatrician if your child develops a tender red bump behind his or her ear. Hearing loss may also occur with untreated ear infections.

The easiest way to prevent the inflammation that can lead to an ear infection is to avoid allergens, such as foods that may cause it in sensitive individuals. In children who are allergic to dairy products, consuming them is the number one cause of ear infection from allergic inflammation. Limit the exposure of children who have environmental allergies to their allergens, and treat the eye and nose symptoms that allergic rhinitis causes with the natural allergy treatments on page 97.

Ear infections are also common in bottle-fed children because the vacuum—negative air pressure—created in the child's mouth by sucking on the bottle travels up the eustachian tube and into the middle ear.

Some children with recurrent ear infections are deficient in a multitude of vitamins. A study of children having ear ventilation tubes inserted showed that 31 percent of them had vitamin D levels insufficient for adults, and 50 percent were deficient.

The blood levels of antioxidants in children who had ear infections in which fluid was trapped in the middle ear were found to be low in another study. Antioxidants include vitamin C, vitamin E, selenium, and zinc.

You may have seen herbal eardrops containing garlic and mullein in the stores. One study of a similar preparation also containing calendula and St. John's wort looked at 103 children with ear infections who were given either the herbal preparation or a pharmaceutical anesthetic eardrop solution to improve ear pain. The herbal drops worked just as well as the pharmaceutical drops!

## Natural Prescriptions*

| Diet | |
|---|---|
| Elimination diet: In dairy-sensitive children, the cornerstone of treatment is to eliminate cow's milk products from the diet. They can have milk substitutes, such as goat's milk, soy milk, coconut milk, goat cheese, soy yogurt, and sorbet (but not sherbet). Many children who are allergic to dairy are also sensitive to eggs, so they should be avoided, as well. Children may also react to wheat or nuts; avoid all foods that your child is allergic to. | |
| **Vitamins/Supplements** | |
| Fish oil EPA + DHA 1 to 4 g daily | Vitamin C 500 to 2,000 mg daily |
| Selenium 40 to 200 mcg daily | Vitamin D 1,000 to 4,000 IU daily for 1 week |
| Vitamin A 100,000 IU in 1 dose | |
| **Naturopathic Remedies** | |
| Garlic and mullein in olive oil eardrops 3 times daily | |

*\* Refer to the appendix at the back of the book for a comprehensive list of interactions and condition-based doses.*

# EARDRUM PERFORATION  15

## COMMON SYMPTOMS

Discharge from the ear canal

Hearing loss

Sudden relief of ear pain

Tinnitus (ringing in the ear)

During an ear infection, the eardrum—a thin membrane at the middle ear's outer limit—may rupture, creating a hole known as a perforation. The pain of an ear infection is caused by pressure from the buildup of fluid in the middle ear, and when the eardrum ruptures, relieving the pressure, the pain disappears immediately. You may notice the fluid from the middle ear dripping out of the ear canal. The child may describe hearing unusual noises.

The eardrum typically heals itself in a few weeks, but you must be careful not to get any water or any other fluid in the ear until it does. Chronic ear infections and eardrum perforations that don't close up may damage the tiny bones in the middle ear and cause partial (or, rarely, complete) deafness. Children who have perforated eardrums cannot submerge in water, get water in their ears while bathing, or use solution-based eardrops (suspension eardrops are still sometimes used).

Ear ventilation tubes that an ENT physician surgically implants are inserted into the eardrum through a perforation; ear fluid can then drain, preventing infection. If your child has ear tubes, the same precautions must be taken to avoid getting water in the ears. After the tubes are removed, natural therapies to heal the eardrum should be started.

## Natural Prescriptions*

| Vitamins/Supplements |
| --- |
| Glutamine 500 mg 1 to 3 times daily for children over 10 years of age |
| **Homeopathic Remedies** |
| Homeopathic Symphytum 30C 5 pellets daily before bedtime |

* Refer to the appendix at the back of the book for a comprehensive list of interactions and condition-based doses.

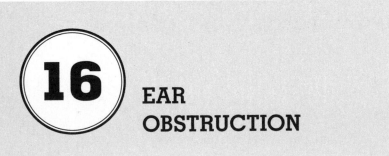

# 16 EAR OBSTRUCTION

## COMMON SYMPTOMS

Loss of hearing          Tugging on the ear

Kids often think ear canals are great places to put beads, pebbles, peas, corn kernels, and even bugs. This can be uncomfortable and impair hearing. Most children won't tell you their hearing is compromised, but you may notice that they're turning up the volume on the TV.

Your pediatrician can examine the ear canal for an obstruction and remove the offender. Commonly, earwax obstructs the ear canal and is difficult to remove. An easy way to naturally remove earwax is to pour warm olive oil into the ear.

## Natural Prescriptions*

| Naturopathic Remedies |
| --- |
| Olive oil, warmed and poured into the ear for earwax removal. Leave it in the ear for 5 minutes, then drain and flush out the ear with hydrogen peroxide or an over-the-counter ear cleaner. Or, have your naturopathic physician flush out the earwax and examine the ear canal to make sure no infection or damage has occurred. |
| Have your pediatrician check for eardrum perforation before putting anything in the ear canal. |

*Refer to the appendix at the back of the book for a comprehensive list of interactions and condition-based doses.*

# BENIGN PAROXYSMAL POSITIONAL VERTIGO

**17**

## COMMON SYMPTOMS

Nausea

Symptoms occur when the head is moved in specific ways

Vertigo

Vomiting

Benign paroxysmal positional vertigo (BPPV) is created by tiny crystals of calcium carbonate that have been displaced in the inner ear. Normally, the inner ear allows you to sense movement and your position in space, but if crystals migrate within the inner ear, they affect balance and cause vertigo—the sense that everything is spinning.

BPPV is a cause of vomiting and dizziness in children. When the child moves his head, such as when rolling over in bed, sitting up, or leaning forward, he becomes dizzy and vomits. Epley's maneuver can resolve the symptoms of BPPV if that's in fact the problem, but before trying it, have your child evaluated by your pediatrician if he or she has vertigo.

Epley's maneuver has been tested many times and its effectiveness has been proven. One study of 81 people showed improvement in 1 month in 89 percent of patients treated once with Epley's and in only 10 percent of a control group that got no treatment. A meta-analysis, a type of study that looks at the combined results of many studies, revealed that most people experienced relief within 1 week after initiating treatment with Epley's maneuver.

## Natural Prescriptions*

| Alternative Treatments |
| --- |
| EPLEY'S MANEUVER:<br>This condition can be cured by returning the little crystals to the part of the ear they came from with a treatment called Epley's maneuver.<br>1. Start with your child sitting on the bed. Rotate his head 45 degrees toward the affected ear.<br>2. Lay him on his back on the bed with his head off the side and still turned toward the affected ear. Hold for 30 seconds.<br>3. Turn his head toward the other side until that ear is parallel to the floor. Hold for 30 seconds.<br>4. Roll his body in the same direction so he is lying on his side with the unaffected ear toward the floor. Hold for 30 seconds.<br>5. Help him sit up on the edge of the bed, still facing the same direction.<br>6. Repeat this a few times a day until the vertigo stops. |

* Refer to the appendix at the back of the book for a comprehensive list of interactions and condition-based doses.

# LABYRINTHITIS (OTITIS INTERNA)

## COMMON SYMPTOMS

Nausea

Trouble balancing

Trouble walking

Vertigo

Vomiting

Labyrinthitis is inflammation of the inner ear, usually due to an infection. Its symptoms can mimic those of benign paroxysmal positional vertigo.

Sixteen-year-old Barbara came into my office with her mom one day. She hadn't been to school for a month, and she was in danger of having to skip the entire school year. She had been nauseated and vomiting every day for the past month.

Barbara had been to her pediatrician, then to an ENT, then to two different neurologists. She had had numerous blood tests and two MRIs. No one could tell her what was wrong with her. In my office, she sat right next to the sink in case she became ill and had to vomit. When I asked her to stand and close her eyes, she fell.

I diagnosed Barbara with labyrinthitis, an infection of the inner ear, which controls balance. Two weeks before her nausea and vomiting began, she had had a cold. It went away pretty quickly, and then she developed these new symptoms.

The inner ear rarely becomes infected, but when it does, the symptoms are severe. Most children have severe vertigo (the sense that everything is spinning) and vomiting. This infection usually appears several weeks after a chest cold or middle ear infection. An affected child will probably lie in bed all day, unable to go to school because the vertigo is so extreme.

We had a strict deadline. If Barbara missed 2 more weeks of school, she would have to repeat the grade. Barbara and her mother were nervous and looking for answers, and her conventional doctors hadn't given them any.

The natural prescriptions for labyrinthitis are extremely effective: vitamins A and D, echinacea, and two other herbs.

We started immediately, and I called Barbara the following week to see how she was. Her mother picked up because Barbara wasn't there. Her mother explained that she had gone back to school 2 days before. She was so busy catching up with homework, friends, and her boyfriend that she hadn't had the opportunity to call me. But Barbara was completely cured.

## Natural Prescriptions*

| Vitamins/Supplements | |
|---|---|
| Vitamin A 100,000 IU in 1 dose | Vitamin D 1,000 to 4,000 IU daily |
| **Naturopathic Remedies** | |
| *Echinacea purpurea* tincture, 1:2.5 ratio, 1 teaspoon 3 times daily | Lemon balm tincture, 1:5 ratio, 1 teaspoon 3 times daily |
| Garlic in food, 1 to 3 cloves daily | |

*\* Refer to the appendix at the back of the book for a comprehensive list of interactions and condition-based doses.*

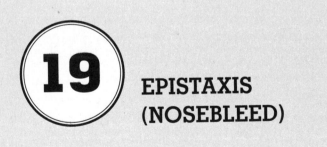

# 19 EPISTAXIS (NOSEBLEED)

## COMMON SYMPTOMS

Blood draining from the
   nose (blood going forward)

Funny taste in the back
   of the mouth (blood
   draining backward)

Nausea

Stomachache

Bloody noses are common childhood occurrences and usually originate from the septum, the wall that divides the nose into two passages. Most nosebleeds are from the front part of the nose, but posterior nosebleeds, which start deep within the nose, cause blood to drain down the throat. Posterior nosebleeds may need to be packed to stop the bleeding, so consult your pediatrician. When nosebleeds are recurrent; associated with bruising, bleeding gums, or black stools; or not a result of trauma, they may be a sign of a clotting disorder.

During a nosebleed, have the child pinch his nose and lean forward so he swallows less blood. It's easy to do, and the bleeding should stop in a minute. But what if it doesn't stop? And how many bloody noses are too many?

One day, I had a meeting scheduled with one of my colleagues. I went to her office and was told she was seeing a patient. Fifteen minutes passed, which turned into 30. I knew something was wrong and finally walked into her office. As I opened the door, I saw bloody tissues nearly covering the floor. Her patient, a 12-year-old girl, was looking so sad as she tried to stop her nosebleed. I walked out and went to a nearby pharmacy for the number one remedy for bloody noses: homeopathic phosphorus.

I came back and gave her five pellets, and within 30 seconds, the bleeding stopped and she hugged me in relief! Homeopathic phosphorus should be kept in every family's first aid kit.

Still, a parent may wonder, how many bloody noses are too many? If a child bangs his face, a nosebleed is common and expected, but what if the bleeding occurs without any trauma? If the capillaries in the nose are weak, they can rupture without a bump or fall. Vitamin C and flavonoids strengthen capillaries so they'll break less often and cause fewer chronic nosebleeds. Flavonoids are compounds made by plants that have positive health effects in humans.

A study of 100 people showed that 4 to 6 weeks of flavonoid supplementation significantly reduced nosebleeds, bruises, and other symptoms of weak capillaries. Flavonoids are found in plant foods, including the white part of citrus fruits that's known as the pith. When we peel an orange or grapefruit, we normally throw away the healthiest part. Cut the white part away from the rind (don't eat the peel) and mix it in with other foods. It's a little sour on its own, but packed with nutrients.

## Natural Prescriptions*

| Vitamins/Supplements |
| --- |
| Vitamin C 500 to 2,000 mg daily |
| Flavonoid supplement (such as rutin or quercetin) 250 to 500 mg divided into 2 or 3 doses daily |
| **Homeopathic Remedies** |
| Homeopathic Phosphorus 200C 5 pellets in 1 dose |

*\* Refer to the appendix at the back of the book for a comprehensive list of interactions and condition-based doses.*

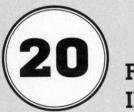

# 20 RHINITIS (NASAL INFLAMMATION)

## COMMON SYMPTOMS

Congestion            Headaches

Cough                 Nasal discharge

Fever                 Sneezing

Rhinitis is inflammation and swelling of the nasal passages that causes a runny, stuffy nose. There are two types: allergic rhinitis and nonallergic rhinitis. The latter is commonly associated with upper respiratory infections in children. Allergic rhinitis occurs with exposure to allergens, such as pollen or foods, and follows the release of histamine.

A multitude of natural remedies help runny noses and other symptoms of rhinitis. Probiotics improve the symptoms of allergic rhinitis. They cannot prevent an attack, but they should be taken at the first sign of symptoms, such as a runny nose or itchy eyes. Low blood levels of antioxidants predispose kids to either allergic or nonallergic rhinitis, so you should supplement with them.

A large study analyzing the effect of probiotics on rhinitis had 1,223 mothers take probiotics or placebo during the last month of pregnancy and their infants take probiotics or placebo for the first 6 months of life. The children were then evaluated at 5 years old. While probiotics did not reduce the occurrence of allergies compared with placebo in the study as a whole, they did reduce them somewhat in children delivered by Caesarean section.

Most young children, whose immature anatomy allows them to breathe through the nose while swallowing as they nurse, have trouble breathing when they are congested. Your pediatrician or pediatric pulmonologist can perform breathing tests, such as peak flow measurement, to analyze your child's lung capacity and function. One study gave 16 patients 2 grams of vitamin C along with histamine (to provoke an allergic reaction), and 1 hour later, it took a lot more histamine to reduce their lung capacity.

Your child may be taking antihistamines, such as Benadryl, for rhinitis, but did you know that a plant called stinging nettle does the same? Research studies have shown that it is an antihistamine that prevents inflammation.

## Natural Prescriptions*

| Vitamins/Supplements | |
|---|---|
| Bromelain 80 to 320 mg daily | Probiotics 2 to 10 billion CFU daily |
| Mixed carotenoids 1,000 to 5,000 IU daily | Quercetin 200 to 400 mg divided into 2 or 3 doses daily |
| Mixed tocopherols (one of which is vitamin E) 100 to 400 IU daily | Vitamin C 500 to 1,000 mg daily |
| **Naturopathic Remedies** | |
| Stinging nettle leaf (*Urtica*) 100 to 500 mg daily | |
| **Homeopathic Remedies** | |
| 5 pellets daily of Sulphur 30C, Pulsatilla Nigricans 30C, Medorrhinum 30C, Tuberculinum 30C, Natrum Muriaticum 30C, Phosphorus 30C, Sepia 30C, Arundo Mauritanica 30C, Calcarea Carbonica 30C, Phosphoricum Acidum 30C, or Thuja Occidentalis 30C | |

* Refer to the appendix at the back of the book for a comprehensive list of interactions and condition-based doses.

# 21

## SINUSITIS

**COMMON SYMPTOMS**

Congestion          Runny nose

Fever               Tooth pain

Headache

Sinusitis is a common condition in which inflammation causes congestion in the sinuses and nasal passages. The mucus trapped by the congestion then provides a breeding ground for bacteria, viruses, or fungi. Sinusitis is most often caused by common cold viruses, but it may also be caused by bacterial infections, fungi, allergies, anatomical abnormalities, and noncancerous growths in the nose called polyps. In children between the ages of 5 and 10, sinusitis often occurs with upper respiratory tract infections.

Our sinuses contain healthy bacterial flora, just like the good bacteria in our intestines (such as *Acidophilus*). Only 3 to 5 percent of sinusitis cases are caused by bacteria, yet antibiotics are commonly prescribed to treat them. And, if your child is taking antibiotics for another reason, that may affect the healthy flora in his or her sinuses, increasing the likelihood of later infection. Instead, treat sinusitis with natural remedies, which are very effective in treating the majority of cases.

My patient Mary's headaches wouldn't stop. It hurt behind and between her eyes. She couldn't do her homework, and she didn't want to go to school. Her headaches grew progressively worse, and they didn't stop for months. The migraine medicine her pediatrician prescribed didn't work, and she was developing a stomach ulcer from all the ibuprofen she was taking.

When most people think of sinusitis, they think of congestion and a runny nose, but many people get headaches with chronic sinusitis. Sinus headaches are also common in children who live in damp areas, because mold can cause an allergic reaction that leads to sinus problems.

The best natural therapy for any form of sinusitis is to wash the nasal passages to help the connecting sinuses drain the mucus that is causing the headache. Also called nasal lavage, nasal washing is commonly performed in many cultures as a daily habit, like brushing the teeth. Neti pots are small pitchers that many people use to wash the nasal passages, but I prefer using a water bottle with a sports top. Pouring the water through the nostrils will clear the nose of mucus and allow the sinuses to drain better, speeding healing.

The sinus wash should be saline water (mix warm tap water with sea, pickling, or canning salt, not table salt, and baking soda), and you can also add probiotics, N-acetylcysteine (NAC), or *Hydrastis*. NAC is a modified form of cysteine, an amino acid that is an extremely powerful mucus fighter. It will dissolve the mucus and make it drain out of the nose more easily. *Hydrastis* (goldenseal) may also be included; it is an antimicrobial herb that may kill organisms living in your sinuses.

It surprises me sometimes to see what scientists study. One study compared the effectiveness of two different concentrations of salt in a nasal lavage solution used by children who had chronic sinusitis. A study of 30 children divided into two groups tested a high-salt (hypertonic) saline wash and a normal saline solution used three times a day for 4 weeks. Both groups' nasal discharge improved, but the hypertonic salt group had less coughing and better sinus x-ray findings compared to the group using normal saline. Another study showed that nasal lavage reduced nasal discharge and edema (swelling caused by fluid in the tissues) after sinus surgery.

## Natural Prescriptions*

| Vitamins/Supplements | |
| --- | --- |
| Bromelain 80 to 320 mg daily | Multivitamin, 1 daily |
| Fish oil EPA + DHA 1 g daily | NAC 100 to 600 mg by mouth daily |
| **Naturopathic Remedies** | |

NASAL LAVAGE:

Nasal lavage, or nasal irrigation, is an effective therapy that may reduce antibiotic and decongestant use. Water is instilled into the nostril, usually with a small pitcher called a neti pot, though a baster or water bottle with a sports top can also be used. Water flows through the nasal passages, washing away mucus and microorganisms and allowing the sinuses to drain more freely. Salt (make sure it is noniodized salt) is added to the water to make it more like the cells in the nose; baking soda may also be added as a buffering agent if the salt alone bothers your nose.

Other therapeutic substances that can be added to the salt solution for extra benefit when treating sinusitis:

Goldenseal (*Hydrastis canadensis*) 5 drops          NAC 5 drops

*\* Refer to the appendix at the back of the book for a comprehensive list of interactions and condition-based doses.*

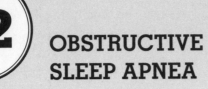

# OBSTRUCTIVE SLEEP APNEA

## COMMON SYMPTOMS

Daytime sleepiness

Loud snoring

Mouth breathing

Pauses in breathing during sleep

Sleep apnea has become common in children and is linked to daytime attention problems. It is characterized by repeated episodes of upper airway obstruction each night, usually causing a reduction in blood oxygen saturation.

My client Harry was brought in by his mother for classic adolescent behavior. He couldn't pay attention; he was moody; and he was so sleepy during the day that he fell asleep at his desk. This constellation of symptoms had elicited the typical diagnosis from his pediatrician—ADHD, what else?—along with a prescription for the typical strong medication.

Harry's mother had no problem with giving Harry this medication, except for one fact: It didn't work, and it also made her son more depressed than before. That's when they came to see me.

Harry was relatively fit physically, on the slender side, with an ashen, pale face. As I examined him, I noticed two things: Harry breathed through his mouth and his tonsils were enlarged.

"Does Harry snore?" I asked his mother.

"He certainly does," she says. "We can hear him all over the house."

We don't normally think of sleep apnea as a problem in children, but it is becoming increasingly common, and it turned out to be Harry's problem.

Sleep apnea can cause temporary cessation of breathing. When this occurs for too long, the amount of oxygen in the blood decreases. During overnight sleep studies conducted at a sleep laboratory, a child's blood oxygen level is measured to evaluate sleep apnea. A tiny airway transports air from the nose through the throat and down into the lungs. If anything along that pathway makes the airway narrow or close, it's difficult for the air to pass through. Because of this, the airflow gets stronger and causes the tissues at the back of the throat to vibrate, making the sound of snoring. Each time the blood oxygen level gets too low—potentially hundreds of time each night—the child wakes up so briefly that he or she usually doesn't even realize it. These repeated awakenings throughout the night make a child wake up very tired and with an early morning headache.

In some children with enlarged tonsils and adenoids, pediatricians recommend removing them so they no longer obstruct the airflow. In children whose airways are obstructed by other tissues in the throat, a continuous positive airway pressure (CPAP) machine may be used. Every night, the child must wear over the mouth and nose a mask that forces air into the throat, preventing the tissues from obstructing the airway. If your child has allergies, treating them may improve sleep apnea; see page 102 for natural remedies.

The natural cure is much simpler: Decrease inflammation (which causes swelling) in the nose and throat, and the air will move through the airway more easily. I have prevented hundreds of tonsillectomies and cured cases of sleep apnea by reducing this inflammation.

Enlarged tonsils or adenoids are the most common cause of sleep apnea in children. Have your naturopathic physician evaluate your child for food allergies and sensitivities as well as environmental allergies, because they are a common cause of tonsil enlargement.

If you are allergic to dairy products, think about the last time you had ice cream or yogurt. Were you clearing your throat? Did you feel congested? In my dairy-allergic patients, milk, cheese, yogurt, and ice cream are the leading food causes of snoring. Stop feeding a dairy-allergic child dairy for 2 weeks and snoring will magically disappear.

Natural anti-inflammatory herbs can also be beneficial. Try the spice turmeric, right out of your kitchen cabinet. Put $1/4$ teaspoon of it in some dinner foods, and its potent anti-inflammatory effect should work that night. Have pineapple for dessert; the anti-inflammatory enzyme bromelain that it contains will also reduce snoring.

## Natural Prescriptions*

| Diet |
|---|
| Avoid dairy if your child is allergic to it or has an intolerance to it. |
| **Vitamins/Supplements** |
| Bromelain 80 to 320 mg daily |
| **Naturopathic Remedies** |
| Turmeric standardized extract 400 to 600 mg daily |

*Refer to the appendix at the back of the book for a comprehensive list of interactions and condition-based doses.*

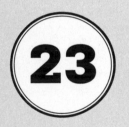

# 23 PHARYNGITIS (SORE THROAT)

## COMMON SYMPTOMS

Fatigue

Fever

Sore throat

Swollen lymph nodes in the neck

White patches on swollen, red tonsils

A sore throat, the primary symptom of pharyngitis, causes pain and irritation and hurts more when swallowing or talking. Most cases are from a viral infection, but bacterial infections, postnasal drip, and even gastroesophageal reflux disease (GERD) can also cause it. Naturally, removing the offending source and boosting the immune system are key in stopping sore throat pain.

In the initial phase (the first week) of a sore throat, start giving the herb elderberry, also known as sambucus. It's available as a sweet syrup that kids love. It helps strengthen the immune system and often stops a cold in its tracks. Once your child no longer has a fever, you can stop giving him or her the elderberry.

If the sore throat persists, then bring out the rest of the arsenal by adding other herbs such as echinacea and astragalus. Echinacea boosts the number of white blood cells, the soldiers of the immune system, and astragalus also strengthens immunity.

If a sore throat is linked to a cold or cough, resist using over-the-counter cold medications whenever possible. These medications have potential side effects, including rapid heart rate and convulsions. The FDA recommends that parents avoid using cough and cold medicines to treat children younger than age 2.

Early in every episode of sore throat, have your naturopathic physician test your child for strep throat. If he or she does have it, antibiotics are needed to prevent kidney problems and rheumatic fever.

## MYTHS ABOUT ECHINACEA*

**MYTH:** Echinacea kills germs.
**FACT:** Echinacea's primary effect is strengthening the immune system so it kills the germs.
**MYTH:** You should give echinacea throughout the cold and flu season.
**FACT:** Echinacea should be used only when a child has a fever or cold. It can be given for up to 4 weeks if the child has a lingering fever. When health returns, stop giving echinacea and allow the immune system to react on its own.

*Echinacea purpurea root, aerial parts, and seed

If your child will eat garlic, have him eat as much as he wants. Because it is one of nature's strongest antimicrobials, eating enough garlic makes colds and flus disappear overnight.

Another wonderful herb for treating sore throats is *Salvia officinalis,* also called sage. A throat spray preparation of this herb was studied in almost 300 patients with sore throat, and it dramatically reduced the pain.

A research study on *Salvia officinalis* in 286 patients with viral pharyngitis compared the spray to placebo. The herbal spray significantly improved their pain compared to placebo.

## Natural Prescriptions*

| Vitamins/Supplements | |
| --- | --- |
| Vitamin A 100,000 IU in 1 dose | Vitamin E 100 to 400 IU daily |
| Vitamin C 500 to 2,000 mg daily | Zinc 10 to 20 mg daily |
| Vitamin D 1,000 to 4,000 IU daily | |
| **Naturopathic Remedies** | |
| Astragalus root tincture, 1:2 ratio, 30 drops 2 times daily | |
| *Echinacea purpurea* root, aerial parts, and seed in glycerite or tincture, 30 drops 3 times daily | |
| Elderberry glycerite, 1:4 ratio, 30 drops 3 times daily | |
| Garlic 1 to 3 cloves, minced, daily | |
| *Salvia officinalis* 15 percent spray every 2 hours | |

*\* Refer to the appendix at the back of the book for a comprehensive list of interactions and condition-based doses.*

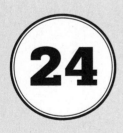

# 24

# STREP THROAT

## COMMON SYMPTOMS

Discharge from red, swollen tonsils

Fatigue

Fever

Painful throat

Possibly a full-body rash

Swollen lymph nodes in the neck

Strep throat is a throat infection caused by streptococcal bacteria that makes your throat feel very sore and scratchy. Compared to a viral throat infection, strep throat symptoms are generally more severe. It can occasionally cause dangerous complications, including kidney problems and rheumatic fever. We want to make sure we treat this condition quickly so dangerous aftereffects don't occur.

## The Myth About Recurring Strep Throat

Does your child regularly get strep throat? When he's tested, does the result always come back positive? He may be a carrier of the strep bacterium, *Streptococcus*.

We all know that bacteria reside in our intestines—strains of *Lactobacillus, Bifidus,* and other microbes that are beneficial. But these bacteria also live in our throats, noses, and sinuses. They help our immune systems defend against invasion.

A small percentage of children have strep bacteria all the time. If your child gets strep throat repeatedly, have him tested when he's at peak health. If the test returns positive, this means that strep bacteria live naturally in him and another virus or bacterium caused his sore throat or infection.

While antibiotics are recommended for strep throat, I suggest using natural remedies in conjunction with them. A special herbal formula of *Hydrastis,* echinacea, myrrh, and *Phytolacca* works wonderfully to kill bacteria and decrease the pain of strep throat. Probiotics should also be given to anyone taking antibiotics. Research also shows that garlic mouthwash kills *Streptococcus*.

## Natural Prescriptions*

| Naturopathic Remedies |
| --- |
| Berberine, echinacea, myrrh, and *Phytolacca* tincture 30 drops 3 times daily—This can be purchased as a combination product. If it is not available, mix equal parts of each herb. |
| Garlic 1 to 3 cloves, minced, daily |

* Refer to the appendix at the back of the book for a comprehensive list of interactions and condition-based doses.

# 25
# POSTNASAL DRIP

## COMMON SYMPTOMS

Coughing that is worse at night

Coughing to try to clear the mucus

Mucus in the throat

Nasal congestion

Sore throat

Like a faucet that never turns off, postnasal drip results when the nose and sinuses produce too much mucus, often in response to allergens. A sore throat results.

Many people experience this sore throat in the morning, and it then gets better after a little coughing, only to return the next morning. Allergy and sensitivity testing can be performed to discover whether a food or environmental allergen is at fault, or you can try a hypoallergenic diet to see if that helps.

Andy was a freshman in college who had never gotten sore throats—until he went to college. He came in to see me a month after he started school, complaining of morning sore throats.

I ran a complete allergy and sensitivity test protocol on him and discovered that he was allergic to dust mites. I deduced that they might be in his dorm-room mattress, which are notorious for their prolonged use. Andy was repelled by the thought that he was breathing in these microscopic mites all night and that they were causing his postnasal drip. But the fact is, these mites are everywhere and live in our pillows and mattresses by the millions, eating the dead skin cells that flake off us. Upon learning this, Andy bought mattress and pillow covers, and his sore throat was cured by the next week.

Much of the research on clearing mucus has been done in children with cystic fibrosis, a genetic condition that makes mucus thick and sticky. N-acetylcysteine (NAC), a form of the amino acid cysteine, shows the most clinical effectiveness. You don't need to have cystic fibrosis to experience the benefits of NAC. It is the best natural way to break down and dissolve the mucus that is causing postnasal drip. Taking a couple of capsules of NAC in the morning should help get rid of the mucus and resolve a sore throat within a half hour. Drinking plenty of fluids will also thin the mucus that drains as postnasal drip.

## OPTIONAL TESTS TO ORDER FOR POSTNASAL DRIP

Environmental allergy panel (IgE)
Food allergy panel (IgE)
Food sensitivity panel (IgG)

## Natural Prescriptions*

| Naturopathic Remedies |
| --- |
| NAC 100 to 600 mg by mouth in the morning |

*\* Refer to the appendix at the back of the book for a comprehensive list of interactions and condition-based doses.*

# TONSILLITIS

## COMMON SYMPTOMS

Cough
Fever
Red, swollen tonsils
Sore throat

Trouble swallowing
White or yellow discharge
from the tonsils

Tonsillectomy (surgically removing the tonsils) once was common in children.

Up until the 1960s, the tonsils were considered expendable organs that had no physiological reason for existence. If they became inflamed, the common practice was to take them out. But our bodies were designed the way they are for a reason, and tonsils have their own important role: They are made up of lymphatic tissue, which is a part of the immune system that is designed to store antibodies that are activated and released at the start of an infection.

The tonsils also store white blood cells and act as our first line of defense against germs entering through the mouth or nose by trapping them. Often when we get a sore throat, the tonsils become infected as well. Usually this infection, called tonsillitis, is not a concern, but occasionally, the tonsils can swell to a size large enough to block a child's airway. This can be extremely dangerous, and they will need to be reduced in size or taken out altogether. Any tonsillar discharge should be cultured, and sensitivity testing conducted to determine the appropriate antibiotic to use. In my office, we try to avoid sending a child for surgery unless it's medically necessary, so we've put together the best natural remedies to cure tonsillitis.

Blood levels of trace minerals such as zinc, copper, and magnesium may be altered in children with chronic or recurrent tonsillitis compared to those in healthy children. One study showed that the mean blood level of zinc was significantly lower in tonsillitis patients, but the mean levels of copper and magnesium were significantly higher. The researchers couldn't say whether the differences were caused by or predisposed patients to tonsillitis, but having your child's nutritional status evaluated and treating for any deficiencies found may be an easy way to prevent and treat tonsillitis.

Antioxidants such as vitamins A, C, and E as well as glutathione are important for the functioning of the immune system. They are also important for healing after surgery. If your child currently has tonsillitis or has just gone through a tonsillectomy, give him or her plenty of antioxidants to improve healing.

Astragalus is an herb commonly given to children to boost immunity. A study of 27 children showed that it may also improve the immune response in children with recurrent tonsillitis.

In children who do have tonsillectomies, the oxidative stress that tonsillitis and surgery cause can be limited with antioxidants like vitamin C. A study of children having their tonsils surgically removed showed that their antioxidant levels were significantly lower than healthy children's before surgery and had not rebounded to normal levels by 1 month after surgery.

## Natural Prescriptions*

| Alternative Treatments |
|---|

ALTERNATING HYDROTHERAPY:

Sit down with your child for 15 minutes with two bowls of water, one hot, and one cold. Get two facecloths, one for each bowl of water. Alternate pressing the hot- and cold-water facecloths to the areas where the child has pain. Make sure the hot water isn't so hot that it burns the child.

    1. Apply the hot-water facecloth for 3 minutes.
    2. Apply the cold-water facecloth for 30 seconds.
    3. Repeat 3 times.

| Vitamins/Supplements | |
|---|---|
| Copper 200 to 2,000 mcg daily | Vitamin B$_2$ (riboflavin) 10 to 20 mg daily |
| Magnesium 50 to 350 mg daily | Vitamin C 500 to 2,000 mg daily |
| Vitamin A 100,000 IU in 1 dose | Vitamin E 100 to 400 IU daily |
| Vitamin B$_1$ (thiamine) 5 to 10 mg daily | Zinc 5 to 20 mg daily |

| Naturopathic Remedies |
|---|
| Astragalus root tincture, 1:2 ratio, 30 drops 2 times daily |

* Refer to the appendix at the back of the book for a comprehensive list of interactions and condition-based doses.

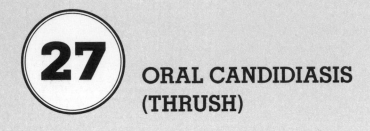

# 27 ORAL CANDIDIASIS (THRUSH)

## COMMON SYMPTOMS

Low fever

Not eating

Painful swallowing

White coating on the tongue

White dots in the mouth

A frantic mother called me in the middle of the night. Her 2-month-old daughter hadn't eaten in 24 hours—no breast milk or formula. The mom was panicked about what to do.

I drove over to the family's house and looked in the child's mouth to see the telltale white dots of thrush. Thrush is caused by a fungus, *Candida,* that grows inside the mouth and may even extend to the throat. It makes swallowing very painful, and babies often stop eating because of the pain.

Dehydration is a major concern in infants, who require frequent breast milk or formula. I gave the baby natural medicines and she was eating the next morning.

The mother remained baffled: Where had the yeast come from? If a child is breast-feeding, the mother often has a yeast infection of her breasts. I saw redness around the mother's nipples and told her that the yeast was actually growing on her breasts, which is how the child had contracted it. We started antifungal therapies for the mother as well so the child would not get thrush again.

While thrush is more common with breast-feeding, if a child contracts thrush from being bottle fed, clean the bottle nipples more often and with hotter water and extra soap.

Natural removal of thrush is quite simple. Probiotics should be started first to introduce healthy bacteria that will fight the *Candida* in a microscopic turf war. Wet your pinky finger and get some probiotic powder on it. Then stick your finger in the child's mouth while he or she is feeding, or place some on your nipple if your child is breast-feeding.

The same technique should be used to give a little baking soda. Thrush thrives in an acidic environment, and creating an alkaline environment with baking soda will inhibit it.

Garlic destroys a large number of microorganisms that cause disease. A study of 56 patients with thrush showed that 14 days of garlic paste applied to the mouth was as effective as a solution of the antifungal drug clotrimazole.

A similar study on the use of gentian violet in AIDS patients proved it to be as effective as the drug ketoconazole (Feoris, Nizoral) and almost five times as effective as nystatin (Mycostatin, Pedi-Dri) in combatting oral thrush (but not esophageal thrush).

## Natural Prescriptions*

| Vitamins/Supplements |
| --- |
| Probiotics 10 to 20 billion CFU 4 times daily |
| Baking soda (sodium bicarbonate) ¼ tsp gargled or swallowed in water or formula 4 times daily |
| **Naturopathic Remedies** |
| These remedies can be used individually or simultaneously to treat oral candidiasis:<br>    Garlic paste applied topically 2 times daily<br>    Lemon juice, 1 tbsp diluted in 8 oz water and applied topically, gargled, or swallowed 2 times daily<br>    Lemongrass infusion applied topically or gargled 2 times daily |

* Refer to the appendix at the back of the book for a comprehensive list of interactions and condition-based doses.

# Gastrointestinal

The gastrointestinal tract starts at the mouth and leads to the esophagus, stomach, small and large intestines, and, finally, the rectum and anus. The gastrointestinal system also includes the liver and pancreas, which make digestive juices, and the gallbladder, which stores what the liver makes until it is needed. This intricate system converts food into fuel so we can survive. If the stomach and intestines aren't working properly, we can't absorb vitamins, minerals, and other nutrients. Children who have gastrointestinal problems can also have other health problems that are caused by a lack of nutrients.

The gastrointestinal system is associated with two other body systems: the immune system and the nervous system. Some of the tissues that make up the immune system are located within or near the intestines. These tissues are collectively known as gut-associated lymphoid tissue, and they are the first line of defense against any bacteria and viruses that we swallow—an immune system headquarters, in a way. When it's working correctly, it is a wonderful defense system, but when you have acute or chronic intestinal inflammation, it causes the immune system to go into overdrive and worsen inflammatory conditions throughout the body. It can also increase the risk of autoimmune diseases, in which the immune system attacks the body itself.

The gastrointestinal system's actions are orchestrated mainly by the separate nervous system in the intestines—the enteric nervous system or the "second brain." You've heard of the brain-gut connection. Why do we have "gut feelings," and why do we register emotional sensations in our stomachs? It's because the enormous number of nerves that line the entire gastrointestinal system respond to and influence emotion.

Another factor that influences the workings of the gastrointestinal system is our population of intestinal flora. You've seen commercials for brands of yogurt that have healthy probiotics such as *Lactobacillus* strains. They explain that adding healthy bacteria can help your stomach and intestines. There are trillions of healthy bacteria that live along our intestinal linings; in fact, 90 to 95 percent of the bacteria in our bodies are beneficial intestinal flora.

These bacteria are keeping us alive. They produce vitamins, regulate our bowels, and, most importantly, make up part of our defense systems, keeping us from getting infections so easily. Quite simply, without enough of these organisms, we would be sick all the time. In fact, my patients who don't have sufficient levels of these healthy bacteria are chronically ill and frequently have diarrhea. Excessive use of antibiotics affects the kinds of intestinal bacteria we have. These drugs don't care what bacteria they kill, good or bad. When they have killed off too many beneficial flora, patients get antibiotic diarrhea.

## top 3 Unknown Facts about the Gastrointestinal System

It is the center of the immune system.

It has a large number of nerves and produces chemicals that help messages move from nerve cell to nerve cell

It contains trillions of healthy bacteria that keep us alive.

## Digestion 101

In our fast-paced world, our lifestyles prevent many of us from having proper digestion. This can lead to stomach pain, changes in bowel habits, and heartburn. Teaching our children proper eating habits is essential for them to lead a healthy lifestyle later on.

Proper digestion begins with a proper mental state. Our nervous systems need to be in a relaxed state in order to digest properly. When we are rushing to soccer practice, watching television, or eating on the run, we are in a fight-or-flight mode of action. Many cultures start the meal with grace. In addition to recognizing our thankfulness for the food, this pause relaxes the digestive system. Digestive juices begin to flow when we sit and concentrate on the task at hand, which is eating—not driving or watching TV.

The second part of proper digestion is chewing. While most of us think we chew our food, if you take a minute to notice, you'll see that you swallow large unchewed pieces of food. If you don't chew your food well, you won't obtain the nutrients from the large pieces. Chewing food breaks it into smaller pieces so the digestive enzymes in your saliva can penetrate it better and start breaking it down on a molecular level. Try chewing each bite 21 times. That may seem like a lot, but your food should be mush when you swallow it, not big pieces that your stomach can't handle. (This is also great for people who are trying to lose weight, because chewing longer gives your brain time to realize that you've eaten enough, so you take in fewer calories.)

The rest of digestion occurs in the stomach and intestines with help from the liver and pancreas, which add bile and enzymes to digest our food. The bacteria in our intestines also help digest our food by producing enzymes as well as vitamins for us to absorb. Intestinal inflammation can prevent us from completely digesting our food and may lead to nutritional deficiencies.

Last, but not least, the remains pass through the colon, or large intestine, on their way to the rectum so we can empty our bowels through the anus. Our stools are composed of waste products that the body wants to get rid of, along with dead bacteria from our flora and undigested food. The gastrointestinal tract is a large tube passing through us from mouth to colon. Along the way, the body has to actively absorb nutrients through the intestinal wall to get good things into the body, or else they will be dumped right out. So if undigested food passes out in our stools, we're not receiving any benefit from it.

The consistency of stools is based on hydration status, mineral levels, and the amount of muscle movement in the colon's walls. When we have diarrhea or constipation, we need to look at the amount of fluids we're drinking, the minerals we're taking, any infections we may have, and how well the muscles in the walls of our colons are working. Stools also provide important information that we can examine through lab testing. We can see if your gastrointestinal system is digesting and absorbing the three major nutrients in foods: proteins, fats, and carbohydrates.

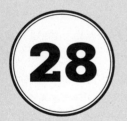

# 28

## ABDOMINAL PAIN

### COMMON SYMPTOMS

| | |
|---|---|
| Bloating | Flatulence |
| Burping | Foul-smelling stools |
| Constipation | Stomach cramping or pain |
| Diarrhea | |

Severe abdominal pain is often associated with emergency conditions that can be identified with lab testing and imaging studies. If your child is in severe abdominal pain, go to the emergency room. If no acute conditions are detected, body levels of toxic substances and food sensitivities should be checked.

The major symptom of gastrointestinal problems is pain. If your child has stomach pain, there are a myriad of mild or serious conditions that might be causing it. The correct condition needs to be diagnosed before we can start treating it. Sometimes, infection with a bacterium, virus, parasite, or fungus can cause the pain, or sometimes it's even an ulcer. If pain is severe and sudden, consult your pediatrician.

Let's take a look at common reasons for abdominal pain by age:

## Infant

**Common:** Infectious gastroenteritis caused by parasites, viruses, bacteria, or fungi; food allergy or sensitivity; colic; abuse; urinary tract infection (UTI)

**Rare:** Intestinal obstruction, intussusception, incarcerated hernia, pancreatitis, sepsis, testicular torsion, volvulus

## Toddler

**Common:** Infectious gastroenteritis, food allergy or sensitivity, otitis media, constipation, trauma, abuse, pneumonia, UTI

**Rare:** Appendicitis, pancreatitis

## Adolescent

**Common:** Gastroenteritis, food allergy or sensitivity, dysmenorrhea, constipation, trauma, irritable bowel syndrome, sickle cell anemia, pelvic inflammatory disease, UTI, appendicitis

**Rare:** Inflammatory bowel disease, ovarian cyst, ulcer

## Natural Prescriptions*†

| Vitamins/Supplements |
| --- |
| To treat and prevent abdominal pain caused by parasites, viruses, ulcers, bacteria, and fungi:<br>    Probiotics 10 to 20 billion CFU daily |
| If antibiotics are being used, probiotics must be given at times alternating with them.<br>    Digestive enzymes 1 or 2 capsules with each meal |
| To treat abdominal pain caused by an ulcer:<br>    Glutamine 500 mg twice daily |
| **Naturopathic Remedies** |
|     Garlic 1 to 3 cloves daily |

\* *Refer to the appendix at the back of the book for a comprehensive list of interactions and condition-based doses.*

† *Treatment is based on the diagnosis. Consult your naturopathic physician before using these remedies.*

# 29 FOOD ALLERGIES AND SENSITIVITIES

## COMMON SYMPTOMS

| | |
| --- | --- |
| Anxiety | Rash |
| Constipation | Stomach pain |
| Diarrhea | Tantrums |
| Flatulence | Trouble breathing |
| Foul-smelling stools | |

We are all familiar with food allergies, the most common of which are to peanuts, eggs, dairy products, and shellfish. Symptoms can range from slight eczema, stomachache, and runny nose all the way to an extreme anaphylactic reaction, in which the child's airway may close.

I remember a mother telling me a story about her son who was extremely allergic to dairy. His doctor had eaten some yogurt for lunch and forgotten to wash his hands afterward, and when he touched the child, the anaphylactic reaction occurred. The child began to wheeze and had to be taken to the hospital. While a reaction this extreme rarely happens, it is possible; however, most dairy reactions result from food intolerances (such as lactose intolerance).

An allergy is a reaction of a specific type of antibody called immunoglobulin E (IgE). IgE attacks foods that your child is allergic to, creating the allergic symptoms we're all familiar with. If your allergist orders blood work that tests for allergies to both foods and environmental substances (pets, dust mites, trees, grasses, molds, etc.), he or she is testing for IgE antibodies to these substances. When the IgE antibody level is elevated, it means that your child is either already allergic or likely to become allergic to that specific food or environmental substance.

Food sensitivity is a reaction of a different type of antibody called immunoglobulin G (IgG). These are the same antibodies that become active when your child has a bacterial or viral infection. In fact, when we test for strep infections, hepatitis viruses, or mono, we test for the IgG antibodies to those organisms. Food-sensitivity testing analyzes the IgG antibodies to certain foods. If the level generated by a particular food is high, it means your child's immune system sees that food as the enemy and mounts an attack whenever he or she eats it.

What does this mean for your child? When the immune system attacks a food with IgG antibodies, certain symptoms can result, including abdominal pain, colic, hyperactivity, joint pain, irritable bowel syndrome (IBS), and ADHD. In my office, we test every child's immune system for IgG to determine food sensitivities and for IgE to identify food allergies.

When we receive our results, we have parents stop feeding their children all foods that the kids' immune systems attack with either IgE or IgG antibodies. The results are often nothing less than miraculous. I have seen IBS, eczema, ADHD, and arthritis completely disappear when children eat foods that their immune systems like and avoid foods that their immune systems can't tolerate. It's simple and powerful.

Many children also have a genetic intolerance to certain foods, which means that they cannot appropriately digest those foods. This is most common with dairy, because many people do not produce enough of an enzyme (lactase) that is required to digest milk sugar (lactose). Children who have food intolerances can experience gastrointestinal symptoms such as changes in bowel habits, gas, and bloating. You can tell your child has lactose intolerance if you start giving him or her lactose-free milk products, such as the Lactaid brand, and the gastrointestinal symptoms go away.

## Natural Prescriptions

| Diet |
|---|
| Once testing has determined what foods a child is allergic to, sensitive to, or can't tolerate, a variety of diets may be established, including: |
| Elimination diet (see page 5) |
| Lactose-reduced diet |
| Low-carbohydrate diet |

# 30
# CELIAC DISEASE

## COMMON SYMPTOMS

Abdominal pain

Diarrhea

Failure to thrive or delayed growth

Celiac disease is an autoimmune disorder that causes an inflammatory response to gluten in the small intestine. Gluten is a protein in many grains, such as wheat, barley, and rye. I like to think of it as the "glue" that develops to make dough sticky during kneading. Children whose immune systems attack them when they eat gluten will experience not only diarrhea, but also intestinal inflammation that prevents nutrient absorption, leading to failure to thrive, iron-deficiency anemia, muscle wasting, and short stature from not being able to grow as well. They may also experience gastrointestinal bleeding and joint difficulties.

Children must avoid eating gluten if they have celiac disease. Supplementing with certain digestive enzymes that help break down gluten can alleviate symptoms somewhat, but they are not a substitute for complete avoidance.

We are currently experiencing an epidemic of undiagnosed celiac disease. Any child with frequent diarrhea should be tested for it. Your pediatrician will test for antiendomysial antibodies, antitissue transglutaminase antibodies, and antigliadan antibodies. The pediatrician may even order an endoscopy to confirm a diagnosis of celiac disease, as well as a colonoscopy to make sure there are no other bowel problems.

Probiotics and enzymes can help digest gluten. A study of probiotics added to wheat flour during cereal processing and a separate study on enzymes extracted from germinating wheat showed that both helped break down the toxic substance in gluten and lessened the effects of the substance on laboratory cultures of small intestinal tissue.

## Natural Prescriptions*

| Diet |
| --- |
| Gluten-free diet: Gluten-free grains include rice, quinoa, and amaranth. All are very tasty, although they are unfamiliar to many people, and they should be dressed with a little olive oil and some spices. |
| **Vitamins/Supplements** |
| Digestive enzymes 1 or 2 capsules with each meal |
| Probiotics 10 to 20 billion CFU daily |

* Refer to the appendix at the back of the book for a comprehensive list of interactions and condition-based doses.

# 31

## CONSTIPATION

### COMMON SYMPTOMS

Delay in bowel movements       Stomach pain

Difficulty in passing stools

Constipation—delayed or difficult defecation—is common in children and often caused by dehydration, diet (frequently dairy products), supplements, medications, or health problems such as hypothyroidism.

When I was in medical school, I attended rounds at the children's hospital. An 8-year-old boy hadn't gone to the bathroom in 2 weeks. His mother had tried enemas, laxatives, and everything else. We had also given him medications to help him go, with no success. Finally, one morning, his bowels moved. Everyone was excited and relieved. When we suggested that the mother talk to our nutritionist on staff about how to prevent the problem from happening again, she said, "No thanks, we're going to McDonald's to celebrate!"

I wanted to tell her that fast food was probably where the problem had started, but she wasn't ready. We need to understand that our health today is a result of our choices yesterday. Especially with the digestive system and changes in bowel habits, we need to look first at everything our children put in their mouths, including foods, beverages, and medicines.

"Transit time" is the term used to describe the number of hours it takes for food to go from your mouth to the other end. Children who are constipated commonly have long transit times of days or weeks. A study of 48 children with chronic constipation gave them toilet training and a fiber supplement made of cocoa husk or a placebo for 4 weeks to test the ability of that type of fiber to decrease transit time (make the bowels move faster). When all the children's results were considered, the trend toward faster times seen in the supplement group was statistically insignificant. However, when only the children with the slowest transit times were assessed, the placebo group went an average of 9 hours sooner and the fiber group was able to move food more than 45 hours faster.

A study of the effects of a mixture of probiotics on improving constipation in children revealed that they doubled the number of bowel movements per week from two to four.

## Foods

Dairy products can cause constipation, especially in children younger than 2 years old. Stop giving your child cow's milk, cheese, yogurt, and ice cream for a week to help relieve constipation.

## Beverages

In addition to withholding dairy, make sure your child is drinking enough water. Divide your child's weight by 2 to determine the number of ounces of water he or she should be drinking every day. For example, a 32-pound child should drink 16 ounces (2 cups) of water daily.

Constipation often occurs when a breast-fed child is switched to formula made of cow's milk. This is less likely to happen when it is a soy or hypoallergenic formula.

## Supplements

Certain minerals are constipating, including calcium and iron. Have your child stop taking these supplements for a week if he or she is constipated.

## Castor Oil

Castor oil is an old-fashioned remedy for constipation, but a teaspoon of it can cause you to double over in pain and run for the bathroom. While I suggest oral castor oil only for extreme circumstances, when rubbed topically in a clockwise fashion on the belly, it works wonderfully for constipation. This is especially effective for infants; take a little castor oil and rub it on their bellies clockwise before they go to bed. It soaks through the skin and makes the intestines move the stool out. It's easy and painless. (But watch out, castor oil can stain clothes!)

## Natural Prescriptions*

| Diet | |
|---|---|
| Elimination diet: Rid the diet of cow's milk and bananas for 2 weeks (see page 5 ) | |
| Add fiber in the form of vegetables, fruits, whole grains, and legumes. See the table in Chapter 1 for some guidelines. | |
| Ensure that your child drinks plenty of water. Divide his or her weight by two to find the number of ounces of water that should be drunk. For example, a 64-pound child should drink 32 ounces of water daily. | |
| **Vitamins/Supplements** | |
| Magnesium 100 to 250 mg daily | Probiotics 4 to 20 billion CFU daily |
| **Naturopathic Remedies** | |
| Castor oil rubbed clockwise on the abdomen | |

*\* Refer to the appendix at the back of the book for a comprehensive list of interactions and condition-based doses.*

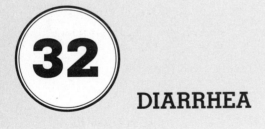

# 32 DIARRHEA

## COMMON SYMPTOMS

Abdominal pain

Increase in frequency
of bowel movements

Loose or watery stools

An increase in the fluid content or "looseness" of the stools, generally in conjunction with an increase in bowel movement frequency (usually more than three times in a 24-hour period), compared to the normal bowel pattern can be considered diarrhea.

Diarrhea is most commonly caused by infectious organisms, but diet and medications also are frequently at fault. It may also be due to celiac disease, irritable bowel syndrome, or anatomical abnormalities. Whenever there's a change in the stools, we need to look first at possible intestinal infections along with everything a child eats, drinks, and takes as a medicine or supplement.

Diarrhea may be a common condition of childhood, but if it goes on for more than 3 days, a child can become dangerously dehydrated and develop an electrolyte imbalance, in which the blood levels of essential minerals such as sodium, magnesium, and potassium aren't in the proper proportions. If your child has changes in his or her mental status (confusion, impaired memory, change in alertness), it may indicate dehydration. Bring your child to the emergency room to be rehydrated with electrolytes.

Antibiotics may be necessary to treat severe infections, but the mineral zinc is so effective in treating diarrhea that the World Health Organization suggests it as one of the major diarrhea treatments. A Harvard study on supplementing with zinc found that it reduced the number of episodes of diarrhea experienced by children infected with one of two gastrointestinal parasites.

In a study of 82 children with chronic diarrhea, IgG antibodies to one or more foods were found in 96 percent of them. The most common sensitivities were to milk (68 percent) and eggs (62 percent). Removal of these foods from the diet improved the diarrhea in 79 percent of those children.

Probiotics are readily available. Most research studies recommend giving 5 to 40 billion CFU daily to encourage normal stools in smaller doses. If less is given, the probiotics may not be effective.

## Foods

Dairy products are common causes of diarrhea in lactose-intolerant children (in fact, they can cause both constipation and diarrhea). Children who have celiac disease can have diarrhea after eating gluten-containing grains such as wheat.

Foods infected with bacteria (the classic mayonnaise at the picnic) or viruses (the buffet line that's been sneezed or coughed on) can cause infectious diarrhea, which should be treated the way gastroenteritis is.

## Beverages

Make sure your child is drinking enough water during an episode of diarrhea. Dehydration is a distinct danger with diarrhea. Have your child avoid drinking caffeine, which can cause diarrhea in those who are sensitive to it.

## Supplements

Supplementing with certain minerals, including magnesium and potassium, can cause diarrhea. Stop giving your child these supplements for a week if he or she has diarrhea.

Infectious diarrhea can be treated with hyperimmune bovine colostrum, which contains antibodies that attack the agent that is causing the gastroenteritis. The antibodies in the colostrum do not attack the flora that is currently established in the intestines. However, it will attack the bacteria in probiotic supplements that are given concurrently. I learned this from a colleague who took probiotics and colostrum on his honeymoon to Mexico. He used them at the same time and found that the colostrum attacked the probiotics, and then his body wanted to get rid of it all as quickly as possible. You can imagine the results. Children who are allergic to dairy products should not take colostrum.

## Natural Prescriptions*

| Diet | |
| --- | --- |
| Rehydrate with water and electrolyte-enhanced drinks such as sports drinks if there is severe vomiting or diarrhea. | |
| Avoid milk and eggs if IgE or IgG testing indicates allergy, sensitivity, or intolerance. | |
| **Vitamins/Supplements** | |
| Berberine 400 mg daily | Glutamine 0.3 g/kg (3 g for every 22 pounds) daily |
| Calcium 200 to 500 mg daily | Probiotics 20 to 40 billion CFU daily |
| Fiber 5 to 15 g 3 times daily with plenty of water | Zinc 10 to 20 mg daily |

*Refer to the appendix at the back of the book for a comprehensive list of interactions and condition-based doses.*

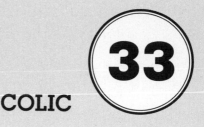

# COLIC

## COMMON SYMPTOMS

Abdominal pain after eating

Crying in the late afternoon and evening after eating

Improvement after passing flatus

Tensed abdomen after eating

Colic is diagnosed in an infant who cries excessively and is irritable for longer than 3 hours a day on 3 days a week for at least 3 consecutive weeks. Colic affects many children between the ages of 2 weeks and 4 months—up to 25 percent, by some reports. Children usually curl their legs to their bellies, clench their fists, and tense their abdominal muscles during an episode of colic. No one knows what causes the excessive crying and irritability of colic.

Janarleen was so upset because her daughter wouldn't stop crying all day every day and screaming throughout the night. Why wouldn't she stop? The only thing that made it better was rocking her, burping her, and letting her release some gas. But then it would just start again.

Colic can be so tough on children, and also on the families who don't get any sleep night after night. What surprises me most is that the answer for some of these infants is so easy and so obvious that we don't see it.

The answer is food allergies and food sensitivities in children who have these conditions. When a child can't digest a food or his or her immune system attacks the food, it creates tremendous pain in a sensitive stomach. Take a good look at everything your child is eating, and if you're breast-feeding, take a good look at everything you're eating, too.

If your child is lactose intolerant or has a dairy allergy or sensitivity (see Condition 29, Food Allergies and Sensitivities), you must switch to another kind of milk (such as soy, goat, or hypoallergenic cow's milk). If your child is sensitive to wheat or has celiac disease, you must stop feeding him or her wheat cereals and switch to a rice cereal.

If the child is breast-feeding, you as the mother need to be tested for your own IgE and IgG antibodies to foods and stop eating anything that your immune system doesn't like. When your immune system attacks food, the IgE and IgG antibodies enter your breast milk and can cause colic in your child. Alcohol and caffeine also get into the breast milk and cause colic as well. If you're breast-feeding, keep the foods you eat simple. Spicy foods can also cause colic. Some pediatricians believe acid reflux can also cause colic.

Probiotics are beneficial for most digestive complaints, even in infants. A study compared probiotics to simethicone, the active ingredient in Alka-Seltzer and similar antigas products, in 90 colicky breast-fed infants over 4 weeks. The number of minutes per day the kids taking probiotics cried was reduced from 159 minutes to 51 minutes (more than $1\frac{1}{2}$ hours less crying!) by the end of the 4 weeks. The infants in the drug group reduced their crying only from 177 minutes to 145 minutes daily.

Similar studies were performed giving herbal oils to colicky infants for 1 week. A combination of chamomile, fennel, and lemon balm oils shortened crying from 201 minutes daily to 77 minutes (that's more than 2 hours less).

## Natural Prescriptions*

| Diet | |
| --- | --- |
| Elimination diet (especially milk and soy in infants sensitive to them; see page 5). Consult your naturopathic physician to assist with nutritional guidelines. | |
| **Vitamins/Supplements** | |
| Probiotics 5 to 10 billion CFU daily | |
| **Naturopathic Remedies** | |
| Fennel tea $\frac{1}{4}$ cup 3 times daily | Chamomile tea $\frac{1}{4}$ cup 3 times daily |

* Refer to the appendix at the back of the book for a comprehensive list of interactions and condition-based doses.

# GERD/REFLUX/ HEARTBURN

## COMMON SYMPTOMS

Burning pain in the chest

Burping

Crying at night

Children of all ages suffer from upset stomachs, but currently there's a tendency to diagnose as gastroesophageal reflux what in the past would have been considered colic.

A class of drugs called proton-pump inhibitors are commonly prescribed for reflux in children. But there are issues with these medications because they stop the stomach from producing any gastric acid at all. Furthermore, the side effects of these drugs when taken for longer than 8 to 12 weeks include iron-deficiency anemia. They're approved for use in children for a maximum of 8 to 12 weeks, and one recent review study indicated that they are ineffective in children ages 1 month to 1 year.

Acid reflux, heartburn, and GERD (gastroesophageal reflux disease) are all very similar conditions in which acid leaves the stomach and enters the esophagus. For GERD, the most serious of the conditions, in which there is damage to the esophagus, proton-pump inhibitors are the most effective treatment.

The problem is that we need stomach acid to begin digesting food so the intestines can absorb vitamins and minerals such as iron and B vitamins. If you give these drugs to your child for more than 3 months, you're putting your child at risk for iron-deficiency anemia, pernicious anemia, and protein deficiency.

Let's locate the real cause of the problem. There's a little muscle between the stomach and the esophagus known as the esophageal sphincter. It acts like a valve to prevent the stomach contents from backing up into the esophagus. If this muscle relaxes, acid and food go into the esophagus and cause heartburn. If we can keep that muscle closed, no reflux—or symptoms—occurs!

Certain foods, such as mint, coffee, and alcohol, may make this sphincter not close as tightly, which makes reflux more likely, or they may make reflux worse. If you are breast-feeding, your child can also get reflux from these foods through your breast milk. Stop eating and drinking these triggers and see if the reflux goes away. Also be sure to avoid medicines that contain alcohol, such as herbal tinctures.

Jane was a 4-year-old girl with constant reflux. She came into my office pale and exhausted, with the complaints of a person far older than her years. She couldn't sleep at night because her stomach's burning was just too severe. She had been on esomeprazole (Nexium), a proton-pump inhibitor, for 2 years, but it barely managed her pain.

Jane had iron-deficiency anemia. Her mother was astounded. "But she eats meat and hamburgers all the time!"

I explained to her that the medicine Jane was taking was keeping her body from digesting some foods and absorbing some nutrients. It was making her so anemic and exhausted that she couldn't play outside with her friends. The drug was causing her anemia and we needed to stop it, but we also had to stop the reflux pain.

Another way in which Jane was like an older person was that she had started drinking coffee at an early age because she was so tired and loved the taste. We switched her to green tea and gave her iron supplements to cure her anemia. Within a week, she was a different person—a child again—energetic and outside playing with her friends. Her mother reported that her daughter had finally returned to her happy childhood.

## Natural Prescriptions*

| Diet | |
|---|---|
| Mothers who are breast-feeding should stop drinking caffeine immediately. | |
| Breast-feeding mothers and young children with reflux should be tested for IgG food sensitivities. | |
| **Vitamins/Supplements** | |
| Apple cider vinegar ¼ tsp before meals | Deglycyrrhizinated licorice (DGL) 300 mg 3 times daily |

*Refer to the appendix at the back of the book for a comprehensive list of interactions and condition-based doses.*

# IRRITABLE BOWEL SYNDROME

## 35

### COMMON SYMPTOMS

Abdominal pain

Bloating

Constipation, diarrhea, or alternating constipation and diarrhea

Gas

Mucus in the stools

No other diagnosis to explain symptoms

Irritable bowel syndrome (IBS) is made up of a constellation of symptoms, and it affects millions of people. Among children, it is most common in those of junior high and high school age. Approximately 14 percent of high school students and 6 percent of junior high students have the symptoms of IBS. The syndrome is considered a diagnosis of exclusion, which means that when the pediatricians can't figure out what's wrong with your child, they say, "IBS." On one hand, this diagnosis is a good thing, because it means that your child doesn't have celiac disease or a more severe condition such as ulcerative colitis or Crohn's disease. On the other hand, your doctor hasn't determined what is causing your child's pain.

Luckily, when we understand how digestion works, we know where to look and can discover the actual cause of pain. There are four major causes of IBS:

1. Poor digestion
2. Imbalanced intestinal flora
3. Food allergies and sensitivities
4. Emotion and stress

Jack, 13, had horrible abdominal pain. He had seen his pediatrician and gastroenterologist, both of whom had shoved tubes and cameras in places where no child should be invaded. The doctors had told him he had IBS and that he'd have to live with it. They tried several drugs to stop the pain, but they didn't work. Then Jack came to see me.

Our complete testing included looking at how Jack digested food. Did he have enough probiotics and enzymes? Did his immune system react to certain foods and cause his inflammation and pain? Or was there some emotional trauma that he was holding on to?

For Jack's immune system, wheat was the enemy. Even though he didn't have celiac disease, wheat was still problematic for him, and it was causing his IBS. Jack also had low levels of digestive enzymes. I told him to stop eating wheat for 2 months and to take supplemental digestive enzymes or to eat foods with high levels of these enzymes, such as pineapples and papayas.

He came back in 3 weeks with a big smile on his face. All of his pain had disappeared. He had found it embarrassing at first to eat different foods at school, but he soon learned that he'd rather be different than doubled over in pain.

Adjusting a child's diet is extremely important in treating IBS. A study looking at the effect of a very-low-carbohydrate diet on IBS patients who mainly got diarrhea showed that 77 percent of them improved. Another study showed that removing from the diet those foods that IgG antibodies were present for improved symptoms.

Melatonin is a supplement that has been shown to have benefits in some adults with IBS. Although no studies on melatonin's effects in children with IBS have been performed, it is a safe, natural remedy you can try. Mostly known for being beneficial for insomnia, melatonin supplementation was shown in a research study to also cause a 44 percent improvement in IBS patients' quality of life after they'd taken it for 8 weeks.

Many research studies report the benefits of probiotics in treating IBS. A review looking at some of these papers concluded that probiotics decreased inflammation, improved the environment within the colon, and positively affected intestinal transit time.

And don't forget exercise! One study of 25 adolescents with IBS showed that 4 weeks of practicing yoga at home daily by following a video significantly improved gastrointestinal symptoms as well as lowered anxiety.

## Natural Prescriptions*

| Diet | |
|---|---|
| Depending on the cause, one of the following diets may be helpful:<br>    Elimination diet (for all forms of IBS; see page 5)<br>    High-fiber diet (for IBS with constipation or alternating diarrhea and constipation)<br>    Lactose-restricted diet (for IBS with diarrhea or alternating diarrhea and constipation) | |

| Vitamins/Supplements | |
|---|---|
| Digestive enzymes 1 or 2 capsules with each meal | Probiotics 10 to 20 billion CFU daily |
| Fiber, insoluble | Tryptophan 1 to 5 g daily |
| Melatonin 3 mg daily | |

| Naturopathic Remedies |
|---|
| Peppermint oil 1 enteric-coated capsule 3 times daily |
| Artichoke leaf extract with 13 to 18 percent caffeoylquinic acids, 200 to 500 mg daily |

| Alternative Treatments |
|---|
| Exercise |

* Refer to the appendix at the back of the book for a comprehensive list of interactions and condition-based doses.

# GASTROENTERITIS (STOMACH BUG)  36

## COMMON SYMPTOMS

Abdominal pain

Diarrhea

Fever

Increase in frequency of bowel movements

Loose or watery stools

Vomiting

Gastroenteritis is inflammation of the intestines usually due to a virus that gets passed around schools or day care centers, though it can also be caused by a bacterium contracted from foods at buffets or left out in the sun. Neither kind of gastroenteritis is fun for anyone because each produces lots of stomach pain and diarrhea. Food poisoning sometimes has similar symptoms, perhaps with vomiting. Consult your pediatrician to determine what's causing the trouble.

One form of bacterial gastroenteritis caused by infection with an organism called *Clostridium difficile* is associated with long-term use of antibiotics. Remember our intestinal flora, the good bacteria that help protect us and reinforce our immune systems? When we take antibiotics, the drugs kill both good and bad bacteria. This lowers the population of the good flora and allows other—bad—organisms to invade and take hold in our intestines. There are as many as 3 million cases of *C. difficile* infection in hospitalized patients in the United States every year, along with 20,000 in the general population, and it is very difficult to treat.

Many studies have investigated the effects of probiotics on gastroenteritis. One study showed that a mixture of three strains of probiotics stopped diarrhea in children with rotavirus infection in 76 hours compared to 115 hours for placebo. Another study of children infected with nonrotavirus agents showed that diarrhea resolved within 6 days in 76 percent of the children treated with one probiotic strain compared to 49 percent of the placebo group. A third study of children with rotavirus infection revealed that improvement began as quickly as the second day of therapy with a probiotic mixture consisting of nine different strains.

## Natural Prescriptions*

| Vitamins/Supplements | |
| --- | --- |
| Probiotics 10 to 20 billion CFU daily (in some research studies, patients were given 180 to 360 billion CFU daily) | |
| Vitamin A 200,000 IU in 1 dose | |
| Zinc 10 to 20 mg daily | |
| **Naturopathic Remedies** | |
| Berberine 2 capsules 1 to 3 times daily | Olive leaf 250 to 1,000 mg daily |
| Garlic (raw, as much as can be tolerated) | |

* Refer to the appendix at the back of the book for a comprehensive list of interactions and condition-based doses.

# GASTROINTESTINAL CANDIDIASIS

**37**

## COMMON SYMPTOMS

Abdominal pain                    Gas

Foul-smelling stool               Red skin around the anus

One form of candidiasis is a unique gastroenteritis in which too much of the fungus *Candida,* or yeast, grows in the intestines. Although *Candida* normally lives in the gastrointestinal tracts of most people, when there's too much of it, it can cause colic symptoms as well as increase the risk of eczema. Gastrointestinal candidiasis is more common in children with immunoglobulin A (IgA) deficiency, which is also present in many autistic children.

*Candida* overgrowth can affect us in multiple parts of the body. In the mouth, we call it thrush; it can grow on the skin as a diaper rash; adolescent girls can have it as vaginal yeast infections; and we can also have too much *Candida* in our intestines. This is common in children with poor immune systems caused by IgA deficiency as well as in children with autism. IgA is the antibody that's specific to the gastrointestinal tract and mucous membranes. When the body's production of it is low, intestinal immunity is poor and gastroenteritis infections can begin overnight.

Many children with intestinal candidiasis have symptoms that include reddened skin around the anus, thrush, diarrhea, and hyperactivity. The treatment can initially cause a worsening of symptoms known as a Herxheimer reaction, which may also cause a wide range of flulike symptoms, emotional disturbances, and skin breakouts. However, this shouldn't last longer than a few days, and the child should get better with continued treatment.

In vitro studies (which are performed in a container in a laboratory rather than in a person or animal) have shown that many botanical compounds inhibit the growth of yeasts, especially *Candida*. Olive leaf is prescribed most in my office because children like its taste and don't mind taking it, and because it delivers results. Currently, at the University of Bridgeport, I am conducting an in vitro study that is showing that olive leaf kills *Candida* just as effectively as the antifungal medication nystatin.

## Natural Prescriptions*

| Vitamins/Supplements |
| --- |
| Probiotics 10 to 20 billion CFU daily |

| Naturopathic Remedies |
| --- |
| Black walnut hull tincture, 1:1 ratio, 1 drop for each 10 pounds of weight, in a glass of water 3 times daily |
| Caprylic acid 250 to 500 mg daily |
| Garlic 1 to 3 cloves daily |
| Olive leaf 250 to 1,000 mg daily |

\* Refer to the appendix at the back of the book for a comprehensive list of interactions and condition-based doses.

# 38 ACUTE PANCREATITIS

## COMMON SYMPTOMS

Fever

Jaundice (yellow skin and whites of the eyes)

Severe abdominal pain that comes on quickly

If the skin at the center of your child's abdomen darkens in color, go to the emergency room immediately. It is a sign of internal bleeding.

Pancreatitis is inflammation of the pancreas that most often occurs in children after an abdominal trauma such as being hit when playing sports, being struck by the handlebars of a bicycle in an accident, or being punched during a fight. It may also result from certain viral infections.

Patients with pancreatitis are often hospitalized for intravenous (IV) feeding so the pancreas doesn't have to produce digestive enzymes. Conventional medical therapies are necessary to treat this condition, but natural therapies can be added to speed healing during the recovery period.

Fish oil is beneficial as an anti-inflammatory therapy in pancreatitis. In a study in which 60 patients were receiving the usual treatment for acute pancreatitis, half were also given IV fish oil. After the fourth day of supplementation, all signs of the systemic inflammatory response syndrome that sometimes develops in pancreatitis patients were gone, in contrast to the other patients. The patients who were given fish oil recovered faster than those who weren't.

Glutamine, the primary amino acid used for food by the cells of the intestines, can be given to pancreatitis patients. A research study in 50 patients with severe pancreatitis who were being fed intravenously showed that adding glutamine to the nutrition solution shortened hospital stays compared to the usual IV feeding formulation.

## Natural Prescriptions*

| Vitamins/Supplements |
| --- |
| Chlorophyll 5 to 20 mg daily |
| Fish oil EPA + DHA 4 g daily |
| Glutamine 0.3 g/kg (3 g for every 22 pounds) daily |
| Probiotics 10 to 20 billion CFU daily |

* Refer to the appendix at the back of the book for a comprehensive list of interactions and condition-based doses.

# PEPTIC ULCER

## COMMON SYMPTOMS

Black or tarry stools          Upper abdominal pain

Nausea          Vomiting

Janet was 14 years old and hated eating because it hurt her stomach so much. Her parents and friends urged her to eat, but she just couldn't bear the pain. She was losing weight and she could hardly pay attention in class anymore.

Her parents had taken her to the pediatrician and to the gastroenterologist. The camera that was put down her throat showed that she had a peptic ulcer, a bad one. No wonder she was in so much pain. But it wouldn't go away. The antibiotics, the over-the-counter stomach medicines—nothing seemed to work, and that's why Janet and her parents came to see me.

As soon as I heard the word "ulcer," I knew how much pain Janet was in. Anyone who's had an ulcer knows the terrible pain it causes in the belly. But with a smile on my face, I told Janet to get ready to feel better. I told her that I can treat ulcers better than anyone else, and I promised her that by the weekend, she could eat as much as she wanted without any pain.

Understandably, Janet and her parents thought I was crazy. Luckily, I have the power of naturopathic prescriptions at my disposal. Glutamine, and lots of it, is the best natural cure for any ulcer. I've seen it cure ulcers in just a few days, and Janet's was no exception. She called me over the weekend in tears of joy. I could barely understand what she was saying. Then I understood that she was eating her second or third breakfast. She was so hungry, and so grateful to be eating without pain.

Ulcers are open sores that form in the mucous lining of the stomach, upper small intestine (the duodenum), or esophagus.

Ulcers are not common in children, but they can occur with infection by the bacterium *Helicobacter pylori* or with regular use of NSAIDs. Ulcers usually temporarily feel better with food. Knowing how long after meals the pain recurs helps the doctor determine where in the gastrointestinal tract the ulcer is located. A bleeding ulcer can be life threatening and must be treated in the hospital. If your child is in severe abdominal pain, bring him or her to the emergency room.

The natural cure for ulcers is one of the most miraculous I have ever seen. Normally, children may be on antibiotics and other medications that may not work for weeks, but 3 days of the natural cure therapy should be enough to make any ulcer a thing of the past.

Glutamine is an amino acid used as fuel for cells that divide rapidly, like the intestinal cells. Since we grow new stomach and intestinal mucous cells every 3 or so days, with the correct nutrients it shouldn't take long to seal up a hole in the stomach. Usually an ulcer takes 3 days. You can take glutamine as a powdered supplement mixed into water (it has no taste) or juice a raw cabbage, which has the greatest amount of glutamine of any food.

## Natural Prescriptions*

| Diet |
| --- |
| Juiced cabbage head daily (The glutamine in cabbage may interact with cancer therapies. Consult your oncologist before use.) |
| **Vitamins/Supplements** |
| Glutamine 500 mg 2 times daily |

*Refer to the appendix at the back of the book for a comprehensive list of interactions and condition-based doses.*

## Inflammatory Bowel Disease

Inflammatory bowel disease (IBD) is a group of severe intestinal conditions that tremendously worsen children's quality of life. The two major conditions of IBD are Crohn's disease and ulcerative colitis. They usually require a lifetime of medications, but adding the correct natural remedies to your child's conventional therapies will alleviate his or her pain.

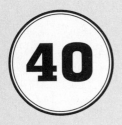

# 40

# CROHN'S DISEASE

**COMMON SYMPTOMS**

| | |
|---|---|
| Abdominal pain | Fever |
| Diarrhea | Rectal bleeding |
| Fatigue | Weight loss |

Crohn's disease is chronic inflammation of any part of the gastrointestinal tract, usually the small intestine. Its cause is unknown. If your child has Crohn's disease, he or she must regularly see a gastroenterologist (and be taken to the emergency room when symptoms are serious), but a naturopathic physician can help with additional therapies.

Because Crohn's disease involves inflammation, we treat it naturally by decreasing inflammation in the gastrointestinal tract. As you've learned, a major source of inflammation is food. Following certain dietary suggestions, as well as discovering what your child's food allergies and sensitivities are, are the first steps in decreasing symptoms. Supplements that have anti-inflammatory properties are also beneficial.

Researchers at Duke University who used laboratory cultures to study the effects of bromelain on the inflammatory substances released by mucus taken from the colons of Crohn's patients found that it reduced their production.

The University of Chicago Children's Hospital performed a study on four children with active Crohn's disease by giving them a *Lactobacillus* probiotic. Within 1 week of starting the probiotic, improvements were seen, and after 4 weeks, ratings of the children's symptoms had improved by 73 percent.

## Natural Prescriptions*

| Diet | |
|---|---|
| Avoid meats, fatty foods, and desserts, which seem to worsen Crohn's. | |
| Eat ample fiber, vegetables, fruits, olive oil, whole grains, and nuts to improve it. | |
| Get food allergy and sensitivity testing. | |
| **Vitamins/Supplements** | |
| Bromelain 250 to 1,000 mg daily | Butyrate 4 g daily |
| Fiber (both soluble and insoluble) 5 to 15 g daily—Consult the table in Chapter 1 to see how many vegetables, fruits, whole grains, and legumes your child should have. | |
| Fish oil EPA + DHA 3 g daily | N-acetyl glucosamine (NAC) 3 to 6 g daily |
| Glutamine 5,000 mg daily | Probiotics 10 to 20 billion CFU daily |
| L-carnitine 500 to 2,000 mg daily | Vitamin D 1,000 to 5,000 IU daily |
| **Naturopathic Remedies** | |
| Turmeric standardized extract 400 to 600 mg daily | |

* Refer to the appendix at the back of the book for a comprehensive list of interactions and condition-based doses.

# 41 ULCERATIVE COLITIS

## COMMON SYMPTOMS

Abdominal pain

Anorexia

Bloody diarrhea

Fatigue

Twenty percent of cases of ulcerative colitis—inflammation of and sores in the lining of the large intestine—appear before the age of 20.

Matt was entering his junior year of high school when he began having blood in his stool, first a little, then more. His pediatrician said it was just hemorrhoids, but it got increasingly worse. The sight of blood in his stool made Matt anxious. *How could this only be hemorrhoids?* he wondered.

Eventually, he went to a pediatric gastroenterologist who gave him a colonoscopy and diagnosed ulcerative colitis (UC). The drugs the doctor gave Matt helped somewhat, but they had side effects that made him feel horrible. He wondered if this was how his life would be forever. He was only 16 and felt like an invalid because of a humiliating disease he couldn't even talk about.

Matt came to see me, and we added a full natural protocol to help his UC. Since it is a condition of inflammation, natural remedies that decrease it are the most effective in improving symptoms. Matt changed his diet based on his food allergy and sensitivity testing. Natural anti-inflammatory medicines improved his symptoms so that he could reduce his medication dosages to amounts that caused no side effects. He felt comfortable in school again and played sports without fear of having to run to the bathroom.

While glutamine is the fuel for the stomach and intestinal cells, butyrate, also called butyric acid, helps to fuel the large intestine's cells. In a study of 51 patients with ulcerative colitis of the rectum, adding topical butyrate to the standard topical anti-inflammatory medication put six patients in remission compared with only one in the placebo group.

Curcumin also helps keep inactive UC from becoming active again. A study of 89 patients with inactive UC gave them curcumin or a placebo in conjunction with their regular antiinflammatory medications. During the 6 months of therapy, only 4.7 percent of the people taking curcumin relapsed, while 20.5 percent taking the placebo relapsed.

Probiotics added to steroid and anti-inflammatory medications can also put ulcerative colitis patients into remission. In a study of 29 children with UC, 14 were given 450 billion to 1,800 billion bacteria and 15 were given a placebo daily in conjunction with the standard medications. The probiotic group had a 93 percent remission rate compared to only 36 percent of the placebo group.

Please note that if your child has UC, he or she must be seen regularly by a gastroenterologist; however, a naturopathic physician can help with additional natural therapies.

## Natural Prescriptions*

| Diet | |
|---|---|
| Elimination diet (based on allergy and sensitivity testing; see page 5) | |
| Peanut-free diet | |
| **Vitamins/Supplements** | |
| Bromelain 250 to 1,000 mg daily | Probiotics 10 to 20 billion CFU daily |
| Butyrate 500 to 1,000 mg daily | Vitamin C 500 to 2,000 mg daily |
| Fish oil EPA + DHA 3 g daily | Vitamin D 1,000 to 4,000 IU daily |
| **Naturopathic Remedies** | |
| Curcumin 500 to 1,000 mg daily | |

* Refer to the appendix at the back of the book for a comprehensive list of interactions and condition-based doses.

# HERNIA

## COMMON SYMPTOMS

Protrusion around
the belly button

Protrusion around
the groin

If the protrusion becomes discolored,
go to the emergency room
immediately

A hernia is a weakness in the abdominal wall through which a portion of an abdominal organ, usually the small intestine, pushes and causes a protrusion.

Hernias are very common in either the belly button area (where they are called umbilical hernias) or in the groin (inguinal hernias). Some children are born with hernias. Umbilical hernias usually resolve within 5 years and don't require surgery unless they're larger than 1 inch, growing in size, or persist after 5 years. As long as they don't change color, they're perfectly safe. If they darken in color over a day or two, bring your child to the pediatrician immediately. Inguinal hernias always require surgery.

While there's not much to do about an umbilical hernia except wait for it to heal on its own or, if necessary, get surgery to avoid the possibility of a strangulated bowel, we can prevent them before the child is born. The B vitamin folate is essential to the growing fetus not only to prevent spina bifida but also to prevent hernias. Folate acts as a zipper in the front and back of the developing child in the womb. Without folate, the child doesn't form in the back (spina bifida) or the front (hernia, cleft lip, heart malformations). If a woman is of childbearing age, she should always be taking a multivitamin or a prenatal multivitamin, which contains double the level of folic acid, the synthetic form of folate found in supplements.

The Centers for Disease Control and Prevention analyzed more than 3,100 children and found that mothers who took multivitamins beginning 3 months before and continuing through the first trimester had a 60 percent reduction in the incidence of having children with the birth defect omphalocele, a hole in the abdominal wall at the belly button that allows the organs to herniate.

## Natural Prescriptions*

| Vitamins/Supplements |
| --- |
| For the mother before conception and throughout pregnancy:<br>Folic acid 400 to 1,000 mcg daily<br>Multivitamin 1 daily |

* Refer to the appendix at the back of the book for a comprehensive list of interactions and condition-based doses.

# Neurological

What accounts for the explosive increase in autism and ADHD? What's happening to our children's brains? Skeptics say we're now simply handing out diagnoses to kids who would have been categorized as "mentally challenged" in the past, but ask teachers and look in schools: These disorders are spreading like wildfire; they're everywhere.

There are two important issues to consider when we look at chronic disorders of the nervous system: nutrition and inflammation. A growing brain needs the proper nutrients to function and create adequate levels of the different brain chemicals to work properly. Any inflammation of the brain is like a sprained ankle. When your ankle is sprained and swollen, you can't use it; the same thing happens with the brain. You can't use an inflamed brain. It doesn't learn.

The common brain nutrients that are effective in a majority of these neurological conditions are fish oil, B vitamins, and amino acids, and they work in conjunction with specific diets.

- **Fish Oil:** The omega-3 fatty acids EPA and DHA that are found in fish oil have two benefits in neurological conditions. First, they have anti-inflammatory properties, so they reduce inflammation in the brain and throughout the body. They also provide healthy fat that wraps around each neuron. Nerves are insulated with a blanket of fat called the myelin sheath. Look at the electrical cord on your computer, lamp, or any electronic device. Can you see the metal wire inside? No; it's insulated for safety, but also to keep the electronic signal in the wire. Fish oil wraps nerves in fat to insulate and ensure proper conduction, improving learning and brain function.

- **B Vitamins:** B vitamins are crucial for brain function, most importantly for creating neurotransmitters, such as serotonin, dopamine, and epinephrine. There are a myriad of other chemicals that the brain secretes and that affect how often our nerves fire and what parts of our brains are active. Without B vitamins, we cannot create many of these neurotransmitters, and our brains will not function optimally.

- **Amino Acids:** Proteins are created from tiny substances known as amino acids. Certain amino acids are the building blocks of neurotransmitters. If you were to try to make a peanut butter sandwich and you didn't have any bread, you wouldn't get very far. This happens in children with neurological conditions.

If they eat only carbohydrates and don't eat any protein, they won't have the amino acids necessary to make neurotransmitters such as serotonin and melatonin. While this does not fix all neurological conditions, a lack of protein will make most neurological conditions worse.

- **Specific Diets:** Certain foods should be avoided and others encouraged in children with neurological conditions. Children with ADHD and autism often have food allergies and sensitivities, meaning that their immune systems create inflammation when they eat those foods. The foods are different for each child, so testing must be performed, but commonly they are wheat, dairy, food colorings, monosodium glutamate (MSG), and food preservatives and flavorings. A high-fat diet is often suggested for people with epilepsy.

# ATTENTION DEFICIT HYPERACTIVITY DISORDER

## COMMON SYMPTOMS

Behavioral problems at home and at school

Daydreaming

Difficulty focusing

Excessive talking

Fidgetiness

Hyperactivity

Inability to concentrate on or finish homework

Insomnia

Peer problems

Attention deficit hyperactivity disorder (ADHD) can be caused by genetics, exposure to environmental toxins and heavy metals, alcohol or tobacco use during pregnancy, poor nutrition, or food sensitivities. Children with the disorder often show symptoms primarily related to one or more of the three key behaviors that define it—inattention, hyperactivity, and impulsivity.

Brian, one of my patients, was an 8-year-old who had trouble sitting still. His mother had taken him to another doctor who'd put him on methylphenidate (Ritalin), but it seemed to make him more hyperactive. Brian was smart, but he got bad grades because he couldn't concentrate on his homework, and his teachers were always reprimanding him.

I tested Brian for a variety of issues, including the vitamins, proteins, and toxins present in his body. I determined that he would benefit from nutritional supplementation and changes to his diet that would support proper brain function and nervous system health.

Fish oil is one of the most common naturopathic prescriptions for ADHD. A study of 75 children taking omega-3 and omega-6 oils revealed that the symptoms of the 26 percent of the children who had primarily symptoms of inattention were reduced by 25 percent after 3 months of treatment. After 6 months of treatment, 47 percent of all the children taking the supplement showed improvement.

A group of scientists in France has been studying how supplementing with vitamin $B_6$ and magnesium affects children's neurological conditions. In one study, a specific ratio of the two—which you can purchase as Metabolic Maintenance's InGear—was administered to children with ADHD and found to significantly improve hyperactivity and aggressiveness after at least 2 months of treatment.

Herbal formulas have also been proven to be beneficial in children with ADHD. One study tested a combination of 200 mg of North American ginseng and 50 mg of *Ginkgo biloba* in children between the ages of 3 and 17. After 4 weeks, 44 percent of the participants had significant improvement in symptoms involving social problems and 74 percent had improved symptoms of hyperactivity and impulsivity.

## Natural Prescriptions*

| Diet |
|---|
| Elimination diet (see page 5) |
| Oligoantigenic diet |

| Vitamins/Supplements |
|---|
| Acetyl L-carnitine 500 to 1,500 mg 3 times daily |
| Fish oil EPA + DHA 2 to 4 g daily |
| Magnesium[†] 6 mg/kg daily (60 mg for every 22 pounds of body weight) |
| Phenylalanine 100 mg daily for every 10 pounds of body weight |
| Tyrosine 500 to 1,000 mg daily |
| Vitamin $B_6$[†] (pyridoxine) 0.6 mg/kg daily (6 mg for every 22 pounds of body weight) |
| Zinc[†] 10 to 20 mg daily |

| Naturopathic Remedies |
|---|
| Chamomile tea 2 cups daily |
| *Ginkgo biloba* leaf extract, 50:1 ratio, 24 percent ginkgo heterosides, 6 percent terpene lactones, 50 to 200 mg daily |
| *Panax* (Asian) *ginseng* root extract, 13 percent ginsenosides, 200 mg daily |

* Refer to the appendix at the back of the book for a comprehensive list of interactions and condition-based doses.

† Refer to the table on pages 28–31 to determine the correct dosage for different ages.

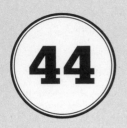

# 44

## AUTISM

## COMMON SYMPTOMS

Compulsive behaviors

Delayed development of motor skills

Delayed development of speech

Disinterest in physical contact

Disinterest in socializing

Echoing the speech of others

Tics

Toe walking

Trouble sleeping

Autism refers to a group of developmental disorders with a wide spectrum of symptoms that make it difficult for a child to communicate with others. The causes of autism are multiple and not agreed upon, but they include: genetics, inflammation of the nervous system, the cellular composition of each child, and immune system imbalances. Toxicity from heavy metals, dioxins, or other substances is usually present.

Josh changed one day at 18 months of age, after he had his vaccinations. Just after being immunized, he spiked a fever and began having diarrhea. The next day, he stopped talking. He quit saying "Mama," and he ceased laughing and looking into his parents' eyes. Josh's mother cried in my office as she told me the story of her son's change, which had taken place before her very eyes.

Regardless of the conclusions of scientific studies, court cases, and specialists, hundreds of mothers have told me this exact story. They've lost their children to autism, and they don't know what to do to bring them back. Pediatricians shrug off those parents, and millions of families are left with no answer, just an upheaval that leaves a questionable future for the child, couples divorced, and siblings ignored in the daily grind of caring for a child with autism.

It's time to step up and change things. In 20 years, these hundreds of thousands of children with autism will be adults with autism. Who will care for them then? Their families? Will they be institutionalized? Or will we have found a cause and a cure?

In my office, we are doing everything we can to reverse autism. While we don't use the word "cure," what we do lets children speak again, mainstream in school, play sports, and, most importantly, look in their mothers' eyes and say, "I love you, Mommy."

Our therapies revolve around nutritionally supporting the brain, avoiding foods to which the child has allergies and sensitivities, and removing toxins such as mercury and arsenic. A supplement I created called Spectrum Awakening, which contains vitamins, minerals, and amino acids, is the most popular one in my office. Parents were looking for an all-in-one supplement they could give instead of having to dole out 5 or 10 different ones. It naturally nourishes the brain to help calm the nervous system. Most cases of ADHD and autism respond immediately. If you give only one supplement, give this one.

Magnesium and vitamin $B_6$ have been used to treat autism for decades. A group of scientists in France found in a 2-year clinical trial of 33 children that using these two nutrients improved social interactions in 70 percent and communication in 73 percent.

A carnosine study in 31 children with autistic spectrum disorders revealed that 400 mg twice daily for 8 weeks significantly improved symptoms on the Gilliam Autism Rating Scale, including improvements in behavior, socialization, and communication, as well as significant improvement in the Receptive One-Word Picture Vocabulary Test.

## Natural Prescriptions*

| Diet | |
| --- | --- |
| Gluten-free or casein-free diet (for children who have gluten or milk allergy or sensitivity) | |
| **Vitamins/Supplements** | |
| Digestive enzymes 1 or 2 capsules with each meal | Tryptophan 1,000 mg daily |
| Essential amino acid combination 500 to 2,000 mg daily | Vitamin A 2,000 IU daily |
| Fish oil EPA + DHA 2 to 4 g daily | Vitamin $B_6$ 0.6 mg/kg (6 mg for every 22 pounds) daily |
| Gamma-aminobutyric acid (GABA) 750 to 1,500 mg daily | Vitamin $B_{12}$ 1,000 mcg daily |
| Magnesium 6 mg/kg (60 mg for every 22 pounds) daily | Vitamin E 200 to 400 IU daily |
| Probiotics 20 to 40 billion CFU daily | Zinc 10 to 20 mg daily |
| Spectrum Awakening ¼ tsp 3 times daily | |
| **Alternative Treatments (Detoxification based on testing)** | |

* Refer to the appendix at the back of the book for a comprehensive list of interactions and condition-based doses.

# DEPRESSION

## COMMON SYMPTOMS

| | |
|---|---|
| Crying | Irritability |
| Desire to be alone | Sadness |
| Indifference | Suicidal thoughts or actions |

A serious condition marked by low mood and difficulty with everyday life, depression is commonly caused by stressful or traumatic events; hormonal changes, including those caused by endocrine-disrupting chemicals; nutritional deficiency; or neurotransmitter imbalance.

Tom was 12 years old and depressed. Really depressed. He wasn't just down in the dumps about a bully at school or his sister stealing his toys. Instead, he talked seriously to his parents about sadness and suicide. These are words you never want to hear from your child, but Tom's parents had to listen and try not to cry.

The emotions of depression are serious, and a psychologist or psychiatrist should always be involved when a child talks about suicide or sadness. Usually, it is a stressful or traumatic event that causes childhood depression. Problems cited by California teens who were polled about factors contributing to depression included worries about appearance, popularity, family problems, and friendships and romances.

Proper counseling is essential for emotional healing. Most kids are put on antidepressants by psychiatrists, but these can lead to weight gain and suicide in some children, and Tom's parents didn't want them.

Puberty is the most common time for significant mood changes like depression to occur because of the changes in hormone levels. Add to those natural changes the extra hormones that are encountered in the environment—estrogens in foods like dairy products and the endocrine-disrupting chemicals found in shampoos, toothpastes, and plastics—and the result may be depression.

It turned out that Tom was filled with endocrine-disrupting chemicals that were affecting his testosterone level and making him depressed. We started him on a natural detoxification protocol, and after a month, he started to brighten up. He began to play baseball and spend time with his sister again. As our treatment continued, he turned back into the Tom that his mother remembered.

A study in Japan involving 3,067 boys and 3,450 girls ages 12 to 15 determined that 22.5 percent of the boys and 31.2 percent of the girls had depressive symptoms. When the researchers looked at the students' fish intake, they saw that boys who consumed less fish, EPA, and DHA were more likely than those who ate more to have depressive symptoms, but this association was not seen in girls.

The same researchers also looked at the children's B vitamin intake. The lower the amounts of folate and vitamin $B_6$ ingested, the greater the likelihood of depressive symptoms in both boys and girls.

Make sure to have a crisis hotline number on hand for emergencies.

## Natural Prescriptions*

| Vitamins/Supplements | |
|---|---|
| 5-HTP 50 to 100 mg daily | Magnesium 200 mg daily |
| B complex vitamin daily | Phenylalanine 100 mg daily (for every 10 pounds of body weight) |
| Fish oil EPA + DHA 2 to 4 g daily | |
| **Homeopathic Remedies** | |
| Homeopathic Ignatia Amara 30C, 5 pellets twice daily | |
| Homeopathic Natrum Muriaticum 30C, 5 pellets twice daily | |

* Refer to the appendix at the back of the book for a comprehensive list of interactions and condition-based doses.

# HEADACHE

## COMMON SYMPTOMS

Head pain

Nausea and vomiting

Sensitivity to light

There are three common types of headaches:

**Food-sensitivity headaches** can start immediately after the food is eaten or up to 2 days later.

**Tension headaches** have a distinct pattern of starting or worsening in the afternoon and with stress, but not occurring on weekends, when school is out. Children with poor posture may also have chronic contraction of the shoulder, neck, and jaw muscles.

**Migraines** are unique and often begin with a visual aura that may include floaters crossing the field of vision or flashing lights. Only classic migraines, not all kinds of migraines, have this visual aura "prodrome." Patients may also have nausea and vomiting and be bothered by light.

Andrea was home from school again. Another headache, the sixth this month. Andrea's mother didn't know what to do. There was no pattern, no specific day or time. There were just headaches. The neurologist had given her medicine. Sometimes it helped, sometimes it didn't. What Andrea really wanted was an answer. Why did she have so many headaches? Her doctors never ventured an answer.

On the day of Andrea's first appointment with me, she had a headache and wanted to cancel. She arrived but with a tortured look on her face.

The number one cause of chronic headaches is food allergies and sensitivities. I tested Andrea and discovered eggs were giving her headaches.

Andrea stopped eating eggs for breakfast, although she thought it was silly. But the next morning, there was no headache, nor did she have one in the following days or weeks. Andrea was astounded. Why hadn't her doctors told her this? A simple change in diet, and her headaches vanished completely. No medications had been able to accomplish as much as this small dietary adjustment.

When I saw Andrea a few months later, she had a smile on her face. She'd had several hard-boiled eggs on Easter and gotten another headache. But she knew what the cause was, and she knew she could stop eating eggs and the headaches would disappear again. She had the answer, and she was in control.

A study was performed to see if supplementing with coenzyme Q10 (CoQ10) could prevent migraine headaches. Of 1,500 patients ranging from 3 to 22 years old, 33 percent were found to have low levels of CoQ10. They were advised to take a CoQ10 supplement of 1 to 3 mg/kg daily (roughly 50 mg for a 50-pound child), and in those who later returned for reassessment, the number of headaches each month had decreased from 19 to 13. The severity of the headaches as measured on a headache disability scale decreased from 47 to 23, showing a distinct improvement.

Melatonin was given daily to 21 children between the ages of 6 and 16 who had recurrent headaches. After 3 months, 67 percent of them reported that they had had 50 percent fewer headaches and 19 percent had had no headaches at all.

## Natural Prescriptions*

| FOR FOOD-SENSITIVITY HEADACHE | |
|---|---|
| **Diet** | |
| Elimination diet (see page 5): Foods commonly associated with these headaches are chocolate, nuts, cheeses, dairy, eggs, wheat, and wines. | |
| FOR TENSION HEADACHE | |
| **Vitamins/Supplements** | |
| Magnesium 200 to 400 mg daily | Melatonin 3 mg daily |
| **Alternative Treatments** | |
| Massage | Topical heat or cold |
| FOR MIGRAINES | |
| **Vitamins/Supplements** | |
| CoQ10 100 to 300 mg daily | Magnesium 200 to 400 mg daily |
| Fish oil EPA + DHA 2 to 4 g daily | Vitamin B$_2$ (riboflavin) 40 mg daily |
| **Naturopathic Remedies** | |
| Butterbur extract, 15 percent petasins, 50 to 150 mg daily | Feverfew 20 to 100 mg daily |

* Refer to the appendix at the back of the book for a comprehensive list of interactions and condition-based doses.

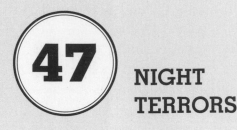

# NIGHT TERRORS

## COMMON SYMPTOMS

Dilated pupils

Screaming during sleep

Disorientation upon awakening

Night terrors are recurrent periods of intense fear and crying while sleeping, sometimes accompanied by sleepwalking. They are not normal nightmares, and during a night terror, the child is hard to wake up.

Night terrors affect many children and families by keeping them up at night. Some children have night terrors frequently and consistently; others have them only occasionally, perhaps monthly. For children who have daily night terrors, even sleep provides no respite.

The screams of Jody's son, Tyler, would awaken her in the middle of the night. Tyler had a blood-curdling scream that always started her heart racing in seconds. Jody would turn on the lights and shake him. He'd bolt straight up in bed, staring at something she couldn't see. His pupils would be dilated, the nightmare still unfolding.

I gave Tyler a homeopathic remedy and the night terrors began to abate.

When I saw him a couple of weeks later, I said, "How are your dreams?" and he replied, "I don't have to hide under the covers anymore!"

## Natural Prescriptions*

| Homeopathic Remedies |
| --- |
| Homeopathic Aconite 30C, 5 pellets daily before bedtime |
| Homeopathic Chamomilla 30C, 5 pellets daily before bedtime |
| Homeopathic Phosphorus 30C, 5 pellets daily before bedtime |

* Refer to the appendix at the back of the book for a comprehensive list of interactions and condition-based doses.

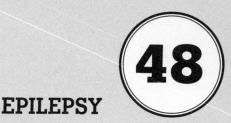

# EPILEPSY

## COMMON SYMPTOMS

Loss of consciousness          Recurrent seizures

Watching a child convulse uncontrollably during a seizure is terrifying for parents. Seizures are electrical storms in the brain. No one understands exactly what causes them. For some kids, it's head trauma, for others it's Lyme disease or toxins.

While all children with epilepsy should be on medications to prevent seizures, there are some natural remedies we can add to their current protocols that may help. Giving nutrients that insulate the nerves and feed the brain is our best option to enhance their lives.

Amino acid levels may be abnormal in children with seizures. These amino acids are essential to the production of brain chemicals. Levels of the amino acids taurine and gamma-aminobutyric acid (GABA) are often low in people with seizures, but there is no scientific evidence that supplementing with them will decrease seizure activity. Have your naturopathic physician check your child's amino acid and neurotransmitter levels. Check with your neurologist before supplementing with amino acids, and don't let your child stop taking his or her seizure medications without the neurologist's approval.

## Natural Prescriptions*

| Vitamins/Supplements | |
| --- | --- |
| Fish oil EPA + DHA 2 to 4 g daily | Taurine 500 mg 3 times daily |
| GABA 750 to 1,500 mg daily | |

*\* Refer to the appendix at the back of the book for a comprehensive list of interactions and condition-based doses.*

# 49 STRESS AND ANXIETY

## COMMON SYMPTOMS

Anorexia or compulsive eating

Clinging to parents

Desire to be alone or to always
be with others

Insomnia

Nervousness

Necessary for adaptation and survival by instigating fight-or-flight reactions, stress has taken on a new dynamic for children in today's world. Issues involving puberty often cause stress reactions in the body, as can the physical stresses of living in a polluted, uncertain environment.

Audrey shouldn't have been familiar with this level of stress. Her parents were both doctors and her older sister was a popular prom queen, but Audrey struggled not just in school, but also in every part of her life. First, she couldn't sleep; then she stopped eating. Worst of all, she started fighting with her family. They had put so much pressure on her to excel that her fuse grew shorter until she finally exploded. Audrey, at her core, felt unloved by her family, as though she wasn't good enough.

I tested her level of the stress hormone cortisol and found that it was low. In children, the cortisol level is abnormally low when anxiety has been present for a long time, and she had been having these feelings for months.

I talked to her parents about loving their daughter for who she was and helping her flourish to reach her potential without putting extra pressure on her. Once that change was combined with following the naturopathic prescriptions I gave her, Audrey bounced back within several months.

A group of 105 children about to undergo surgery were studied to compare the effects of melatonin and the tranquilizing drug midazolam on their anxiety levels before being anesthetized. Anxiety improved equally in both groups, and melatonin lessened postoperative excitement and improved sleep 2 weeks after surgery compared to midazolam.

## Natural Prescriptions*

| Vitamins/Supplements | |
|---|---|
| Melatonin 1 to 3 mg daily | Vitamin B$_5$ (pantothenic acid) 2 mg daily |
| Phosphatidylserine 100 to 250 mg daily | Vitamin C 500 to 2,000 mg daily |
| **Naturopathic Remedies†** | |
| Passionflower tea 1 cup, 2 times daily | Siberian ginseng 500 mg daily |
| *Rhodiola roseu* 100 mg daily | Valerian 500 mg daily |
| **Alternative Treatments** | |
| Aerobic exercise | Tai chi |
| Counseling | Yoga |
| Meditation | |

*Refer to the appendix at the back of the book for a comprehensive list of interactions and condition-based doses.*

† *Use one herb at a time. Don't combine them without consulting your naturopathic physician.*

# INSOMNIA  50

## COMMON SYMPTOMS

Difficulty falling asleep       Difficulty staying asleep

Insomnia causes children to be frequently unable to fall asleep and/or stay asleep, or to not be refreshed by sleep. It is called primary insomnia when no underlying physical or mental condition causing it can be identified. This occurs when, for example, a child drinks too much caffeine or watches a scary movie and then can't calm down. It can also happen when a child is under a lot of stress and too many stress hormones are released.

Secondary insomnia happens as a result of a medical condition, such as depression. In addition, insomnia can be acute or chronic. Acute insomnia goes away when the immediate factor causing it is eliminated; chronic insomnia goes on for a longer time.

When Bobby walked into my office, he was tripping over his feet. He was so exhausted that he kept nodding off during our meeting. The problem was that he couldn't sleep. Insomnia affects many children and their families, because when kids don't sleep, parents don't, either.

I gave Bobby melatonin, a natural supplement that helps people fall asleep. Melatonin is created by the pineal gland in the brain. I call it the Big Ben hormone because it sets our sleep cycles, and when we don't produce enough of it, we may need to supplement. Some melatonin supplements are made from the pineal glands of animals, and that kind shouldn't be taken because they might contain viruses. Most melatonin sold in the US is synthetic, and that's what you should get.

Bobby's mother called me the next day, a Saturday. Bobby hadn't slept for a solid 10 hours straight for months, but he was still asleep when she called me, and it was nearly noon.

Duke University recently reviewed 20 research studies that evaluated the effect of melatonin on chronic sleep-onset insomnia in children with ADHD. They found that it is effective and well tolerated in doses of 3 to 6 mg given before bedtime.

While it is effective for many children, there is concern that melatonin at dosages of more than 0.3 mg per day may cause seizures.

Try each of these remedies for a week at a time to see which one works best for your child.

## Natural Prescriptions*

| Vitamins/Supplements | |
| --- | --- |
| 5-HTP 50 to 100 mg before bedtime | Melatonin 0.3 to 3 mg before bedtime |
| GABA 750 mg before bedtime | Taurine 1,000 mg before bedtime |
| Magnesium 65 to 350 mg before bedtime | |
| **Naturopathic Remedies** | |
| Chamomile tea 1 cup before bedtime | Valerian tea 1 cup before bedtime |

* Refer to the appendix at the back of the book for a comprehensive list of interactions and condition-based doses.

## HEAD BANGING 51

### COMMON SYMPTOMS

Purposefully banging the head on a surface such as the wall, crib, or floor

Head banging is when a child purposefully and repetitively bangs his or her head. This commonly occurs in children with autism, but most children are doing it to relax (to help themselves sleep, for example) or because of pain from an ear infection. Bring your child to the pediatrician to look in his or her ears. When there's ear pressure, there may be pain or discomfort. Your child may be head banging to try to dislodge whatever's causing the plugged sensation.

## Natural Prescriptions*

| Diet |
| --- |
| Avoid dairy products in children who are sensitive to them. |
| **Homeopathic Remedies** |
| Homeopathic Tuberculinum 30C, 5 pellets once a week |

* Refer to the appendix at the back of the book for a comprehensive list of interactions and condition-based doses.

## Endocrine

When we hear the word "hormone," we commonly think of estrogen, progesterone, and testosterone. These are well-known hormones that pertain to sexual development, but there are many others that control metabolism, the amount of sugar in the blood, digestion, growth—almost every action in the body.

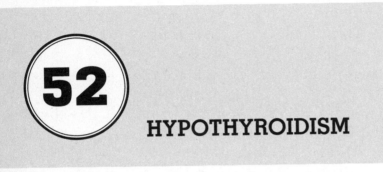

# 52

# HYPOTHYROIDISM

## COMMON SYMPTOMS

Constipation

Dry skin

Fatigue

Intolerance to cold

Menstrual problems

Weight gain

In this condition, the thyroid gland is underactive and doesn't produce enough thyroid hormones. Most cases of hypothyroidism arise after inflammation of the gland damages it. Hashimoto's disease, in which the immune system attacks the thyroid, is the most common form. Congenital hypothyroidism is the most common cause in infants, occurring in 1 out of every 3,500 newborns in the US.

Once your pediatrician determines the cause of your child's hypothyroidism, proper treatment can begin. Thyroid hormones are produced from certain nutrients, and giving more of these will cause the thyroid to be more productive.

While iodine (I call it the thyroid mineral), which is found in seawater, seaweed, soil and groundwater near the ocean, and, in many countries, iodized salt, is necessary to produce thyroid hormones, other minerals, such as bromine, and chlorine can interfere with iodine.

We receive a constant stream of chlorine in our tap water. Towns and cities put it in public water supplies to kill bacteria. When we drink this, we not only kill good bacteria in our intestines, but also interfere with iodine, which in turn affects the thyroid.

Potassium bromate, a chemical compound that includes bromine, is added to some bread products for texture and taste. This substance also interferes with iodine's effect on the thyroid. You can test for your child's levels of iodine, bromine, and chloride (a compound containing chlorine) to determine if iodine therapy is necessary.

An interesting review article highlighted the population of Japan, where there are few cases of hypothyroidism. In that country, people commonly consume 25 times the amount of iodine than people do in the US, where hypothyroidism is extremely prevalent. The Japanese normally eat 1,000 mcg of iodine daily, but the RDA for American children is only 90 mcg through age 8 and 120 mcg for 9 to 13 year olds. In addition, because consumers can now buy noniodized table salt, some are not getting it through that route.

## Natural Prescriptions*

| Vitamins/Supplements | |
|---|---|
| Iodine 50 to 900 mcg daily | Tyrosine 500 mg daily |
| Selenium 20 to 200 mcg daily | Vitamin A 200,000 IU in 1 dose |
| **Naturopathic Remedies** | |
| Seaweed (kelp) 2 Tbsp daily | |

* Refer to the appendix at the back of the book for a comprehensive list of interactions and condition-based doses.

## Diabetes Mellitus

Millions of people have diabetes mellitus, a condition of excess sugar in the blood. In type 1 diabetes, this excess sugar results from the immune system having mistaken the insulin-producing cells in the pancreas for enemies and destroying them. Insulin is the hormone that escorts sugar from the blood into cells so it can be used for energy. In type 2 diabetes, the body's muscle, fat, and liver cells are resistant to insulin and the pancreas can't make enough of it to get the sugar into the cells. Eventually, repeated spikes in blood sugar levels and changes in how the body metabolizes lipids (fats, cholesterol, and other substances) damage the eyes, kidneys, arteries, and other parts of the body. Although it takes decades for these complications—which include cardiovascular disease and kidney disease—to occur, many people who have diabetes of either type develop nerve problems, blindness, and other problems. They can even end up losing parts of their bodies, such as their feet.

The Centers for Disease Control and Prevention suggests that people who have diabetes eat fewer refined carbohydrates, less salt, and more fiber to help avoid those drastic consequences. Make them less likely for your child by feeding your family the appropriate diet and following the correct naturopathic prescriptions.

# 53 TYPE 1 DIABETES MELLITUS

## COMMON SYMPTOMS

Blurred vision

Fatigue

Increased thirst

Increased urination

Weight loss

This form of diabetes is actually an autoimmune disease in which the immune system has attacked and destroyed the specific part of the pancreas that makes insulin. It arises from multiple genetic, microbial, and environmental factors and may be triggered in infants by an immunological reaction to cow's milk.

Insulin is necessary to bring sugar from the bloodstream into our cells. Without insulin, we don't have energy. What if the gasoline in our cars sat in the fuel tanks and never got to the engines? They wouldn't run. Insulin takes our fuel and brings it into our cells, which burn it for energy.

Type 1 diabetes used to be known as juvenile diabetes because the symptoms tend to arrive during adolescence (although it can appear at any age). Most children with it will have to be on pharmaceutical insulin for the rest of their lives. However, naturopathic treatments can decrease the amount of insulin needed and reduce the need for medications for related problems.

In a study performed in Norway, the families of 545 children with type 1 diabetes and 1,668 healthy children were asked about their use of cod liver oil during the child's first year of life. The children who were given it had a significantly lower risk of type 1 diabetes.

A similar study in Finland analyzed the health records of more than 10,000 children and discovered that vitamin D supplementation decreased the risk of type 1 diabetes. Because about a third of Finland is north of the Arctic Circle, the country gets much less sunlight than most of the world does, making low vitamin D levels more common. However, many of our kids spend too much time inside playing video games and don't get outside enough. Have your child's vitamin D level tested to see if a supplement is necessary.

## Natural Prescriptions*

| Diet | |
|---|---|
| Low-glycemic-index diet (low in refined, processed foods and high in fruits, vegetables, and fiber) | |
| **Vitamins/Supplements** | |
| Alpha-lipoic acid 100 mg daily | Vitamin $B_3$ (niacin) 2 to 30 mg daily |
| Chromium 50 to 200 mcg daily | Vitamin C 250 to 1,000 mg daily |
| Fish oil EPA + DHA 500 to 2,000 mg daily | Vitamin D 600 to 4,000 IU daily |
| Magnesium 100 to 400 mg daily | Vitamin E 100 to 400 IU daily |
| **Naturopathic Remedies** | |
| Milk thistle, 80 percent silymarin, 200 mg daily | |

* Refer to the appendix at the back of the book for a comprehensive list of interactions and condition-based doses.

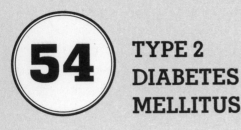

# TYPE 2 DIABETES MELLITUS

## COMMON SYMPTOMS

Fatigue

Frequent urination

Increased urination

Weight loss

The prevalence of this form of diabetes is increasing enormously in children, faster than a rocket to the moon. It's almost always brought on in susceptible kids by obesity caused by poor diet and lack of exercise. It used to be called adult-onset diabetes, but now, with the increased incidence of childhood obesity, the prevalence of corn syrup– and sugar-laden foods, the copious amounts of calories children are eating, and the hours they spend sitting in front of television and computer screens, children are getting type 2 diabetes at increasingly younger ages.

It's time to take a stand against the poor nutrition that is all too common in our society and is slowly killing our children. Some schools are removing soda machines from their campuses. The subject of passing a tax on soda comes up repeatedly. I say, "fantastic!" We tax cigarettes to dissuade people from smoking because we know it has catastrophic health consequences, and we should do the same for sugary foods. The government subsidizes our farmers to grow corn, much of which is made into high-fructose corn syrup. They should instead start subsidizing them to grow vegetables and fruits for our children.

If your child has diabetes, he's on a road to a lifetime of disease and sickness. You need to stop that car immediately, turn it around, and drive in the other direction. Change the whole family's eating habits. If your kids see you do it, odds are that they will do it, too (until they're teenagers). Everyone should eat vegetables and fruits. Dessert should be a special treat once a week. Allow three bites of any sugary snack. Don't just inhale (or let your child inhale) a whole slice of cheesecake. Chew and savor just a few bites instead.

You also have to start exercising with your children. Go on hikes or bike rides or play ball. Time is short with school and jobs and life, but if you don't do it now, when will you?

Cinnamon has been studied in a multitude of research trials. A recent summary of this research stated that 1 to 6 g ($\frac{1}{3}$ to 2 teaspoons) of cassia cinnamon daily for 40 days decreased the blood sugar level by 18 to 29 percent, total cholesterol by 12 to 26 percent, and LDL (bad) cholesterol by 7 to 27 percent. Can you think of a tastier medicine?

Magnesium levels were tested in 24 obese children who didn't have type 2 diabetes and 24 lean children. The obese children had significantly lower magnesium levels than their lean counterparts. They also had higher insulin levels, which may eventually lead to a diagnosis of diabetes.

## Natural Prescriptions*

| Diet | |
|---|---|
| Low-glycemic-index diet (low in refined, processed foods and high in vegetables, fruits, and fiber) | |
| **Vitamins/Supplements** | |
| Alpha-lipoic acid 100 mg daily | Vitamin D 400 to 4,000 IU daily |
| Chromium 50 to 200 mcg daily | Zinc 5 to 20 mg daily |
| Magnesium 100 to 200 mg daily | |
| **Naturopathic Remedies** | |
| Cassia cinnamon 1 to 2 g ($\frac{1}{3}$ to $\frac{2}{3}$ tsp) 3 times daily | |
| *Gymnema,* 75 percent gymnemic acids, 100 mg 2 times daily | |
| Milk thistle, 80 percent silymarin 200 mg daily | |
| *Panax* (Asian) *ginseng* root extract, 15 percent ginsenosides, 200 mg daily | |

* Refer to the appendix at the back of the book for a comprehensive list of interactions and condition-based doses.

# Exanthems (Viral Rashes)

Viral exanthems are rashes that erupt with some viral infections. When the virus starts, it may produce symptoms that look like a regular cold or sore throat with a mild fever. Then, after a few days, a red rash appears on the torso, arms, legs, and face of the child. Since the most common medicines in the pediatrician's cabinet are antibiotics that kill bacteria but not viruses, most doctors will tell you to give your child chicken soup, TLC, and lots of fluids. Where modern medicine succeeds at killing bacteria, it falters at killing viruses.

Measles, mumps, and rubella are specific exanthematous diseases that have almost disappeared since the introduction of vaccines against them. Most young pediatricians graduating from medical school haven't even seen them. But other viruses, such as those that cause the conditions fifth disease and roseola, are still present because modern medicine has not developed vaccines for them.

Due to the public's concern that the MMR (measles, mumps, rubella) vaccine might be associated with some cases of autism (an assumption that has never been medically proven), many parents are opting not to vaccinate their children or choosing to delay the vaccination schedule. Children who aren't vaccinated have a greater risk of catching viral exanthems, but the risk is still low because other schoolchildren have been vaccinated, creating herd immunity.

Research studies have shown conflicting results about vaccines' association with autism and their safety in general, and undoubtedly there will be more research in the future to fuel the controversy. On February 22, 2011, the US Supreme Court ruled that lawsuits cannot be filed against vaccine manufacturers for serious side effects arising from their products. Instead, claimants seeking compensation must continue to go through a special "vaccine court" that Congress set up in 1986 to prevent juries from granting such large awards that vaccine makers might drop out of the market.

Naturopathic medicine has the best antiviral therapies known to humankind. Any viral illness I see in my office is cured within a couple of days. Whether it's roseola, herpes simplex, or mono, I guarantee parents that we can shut down a virus twice as fast as when a child simply rests at home for a week. Our viral influenza prevention program is extremely successful as well, and it utilizes the same antiviral treatments that we use for viral exanthems.

Vitamin A supplementation is a naturopathic treatment I often use. It is such a fantastic antiviral therapy that the World Health Organization recommends two doses of it be given during active measles infection in developing countries, where vitamin A deficiency is common, to reduce the likelihood of eye damage and death. An extraordinarily effective immune-system booster, vitamin A can be helpful in treating most viruses.

There are concerns that, because it is a fat-soluble vitamin, it may be toxic. The vitamin A treatment for viruses is a high dose, and it should be used only for a period of 1 to 3 days. It should be given only under the supervision of a physician, and your child's vitamin A level should be monitored. Giving a high dose of vitamin A for a longer period of time is risky. Pregnant women should get no more than about 10,000 IU of vitamin A per day from all sources, including foods, because more may cause birth defects. They should avoid multivitamins and prenatal multivitamins containing more than 5,000 IU of vitamin A.

# MEASLES

## COMMON SYMPTOMS

Body rash

Fever

White spots on the inside of the cheek (Koplik's spots)

Formerly known as "first disease," because in 1627 it was the first viral exanthem identified by physicians, this systemic viral illness is highly contagious and brings on a characteristic rash that usually appears about 14 days after exposure.

Measles starts as an upper respiratory infection with fever, sore throat, and cough for 2 to 4 days, followed by a full-body rash that sometimes lasts 4 to 7 days. What's unique about measles is that white spots called Koplik's spots form on the insides of the cheeks. Don't confuse these with thrush, which may look similar but usually doesn't cause a fever. Measles can be dangerous if complications such as severe diarrhea and pneumonia develop.

Researchers at Harvard looked at the dietary vitamin A intake of more than 28,000 children in Sudan beginning when they were 6 months old and continuing until they were 6 years old. The children were given either 200,000 IU of vitamin A plus 40 IU of vitamin E or only 40 IU of vitamin E at three separate times over the study period. They found that those with the higher vitamin A intake had less risk of measles, diarrhea, and cough in combination with fever.

Another study showed that the measles vaccine lowered the vitamin A level for at least 6 weeks after vaccination. You should supplement with vitamin A after each vaccination your child gets except DTaP (for diphtheria, tetanus, and pertussis).

## Natural Prescriptions*

| Vitamins/Supplements |
| --- |
| Immediately after diagnosis or when symptoms appear in children ages 6 to 12 months: Vitamin A 100,000 IU in 1 dose followed 4 weeks later by 100,000 IU in 1 dose |
| Immediately after diagnosis or when symptoms appear in children over 1 year old: Vitamin A 200,000 IU in 1 dose followed 4 weeks later by 200,000 IU in 1 dose |

* Refer to the appendix at the back of the book for a comprehensive list of interactions and condition-based doses.

# 56

# RUBELLA

## COMMON SYMPTOMS

Body rash      Malaise

Fever

Rubella, also known as German measles, was the third childhood viral exanthem described by scientists, in 1881. It is sometimes called third disease. *Rubella* is a Latin word meaning "little red." It is a stereotypical example of an exanthem that starts with a cold and leads to a rash. There's no unique symptom that makes it stand out from any other exanthem, and in children symptoms are usually mild. However, if an unvaccinated pregnant woman contracts this virus in the first trimester, the fetus is at high risk for premature delivery, eye problems, heart problems, mental retardation, and even death.

## Natural Prescriptions*

| Vitamins/Supplements |
| --- |
| Beta-glucan 500 to 1,000 mg daily |
| Immediately after diagnosis or when symptoms appear in children ages 6 months to 1 year: Vitamin A 100,000 IU in 1 dose |
| Immediately after diagnosis or when symptoms appear in children over 1 year old: Vitamin A 200,000 IU in 1 dose |
| **Naturopathic Remedies** |
| Honey 1 tablespoon daily (children more than age 1) |
| Lemon balm 100 to 500 mg daily |

*Refer to the appendix at the back of the book for a comprehensive list of interactions and condition-based doses.*

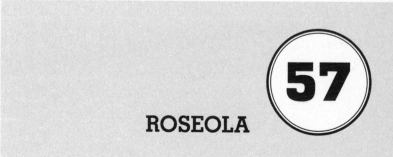

# ROSEOLA 57

## COMMON SYMPTOMS

Body rash          Fever

Cough

Jillian brought her 2-year-old daughter in to see me.

"Dr. Skowron," Jillian asked, "do antibiotics kill viruses?"

"Of course not," I told her. "Antibiotics only kill bacteria."

"Well, my daughter's doctor said she had roseola, which is a virus, and then he gave me antibiotics. Why would he do that?"

I wish I had the answer to that question, I told Jillian, because the overprescription of antibiotics is creating drug-resistant bugs like MRSA (methicillin-resistant *Staphylococcus aureus*) and VRE (vancomycin-resistant *Enterococcus*). There's no point in giving antibiotics for a viral infection, and that's why we use our naturopathic prescriptions to cure them.

Roseola is another common viral exanthem, probably the most common since the introduction of the MMR vaccine. There is no vaccine for roseola, which is caused by human herpes virus 6.

Its symptoms are those of a standard viral exanthem, with fever, cough, and then a rash on the trunk, neck, and arms. Seizures due to the high fever characteristic of roseola occur in 5 to 10 percent of children with this infection.

## Natural Prescriptions*

| Vitamins/Supplements |
| --- |
| Immediately after diagnosis or when symptoms appear in children ages 6 months to 1 year: Vitamin A 100,000 IU in 1 dose |
| Immediately after diagnosis or when symptoms appear in children over 1 year old: Vitamin A 200,000 IU in 1 dose |
| Vitamin C 500 to 1,000 mg daily |
| **Naturopathic Remedies** |
| Lemon balm 100 to 500 mg daily |
| Licorice (*Glycyrrhiza*) 100 to 500 mg daily |

* Refer to the appendix at the back of the book for a comprehensive list of interactions and condition-based doses.

# FIFTH DISEASE (ERYTHEMA INFECTIOSUM)

**58**

## COMMON SYMPTOMS

Bright red rash on
the cheeks

Fever

Headache

Malaise

Sore throat

This virus was the fifth exanthem described, in 1905. Caused by a parvovirus, the disease has the symptoms that most exanthems do, with a fever first and then a full-body rash. What is unique about fifth disease is that the rash starts on the cheeks, which turn bright red before the rash spreads across the body. This is known as a "slapped-cheek rash" because it looks as though the child was slapped hard across the cheeks.

## Natural Prescriptions*

| Vitamins/Supplements |
| --- |
| Immediately after diagnosis or when symptoms appear in children ages 6 months to 1 year:<br>Vitamin A 100,000 IU in 1 dose |
| Immediately after diagnosis or when symptoms appear in children over 1 year old:<br>Vitamin A 200,000 IU in 1 dose |
| Vitamin C 500 to 1,000 mg daily |
| **Naturopathic Remedies** |
| Lemon balm 100 to 500 mg daily |

*\* Refer to the appendix at the back of the book for a comprehensive list of interactions and condition-based doses.*

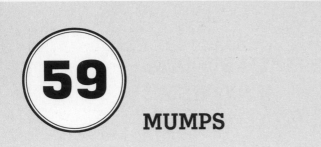

# MUMPS

## COMMON SYMPTOMS

Fever

Swollen salivary glands

Pain and swelling at the jaw,
especially with a sour taste

Mumps is an infection characterized by enlargement of the three pairs of salivary glands, especially the parotid glands, which are below and in front of the ears. It is contagious 6 days before to 9 days after swelling. Mumps is caused by a particular virus, but parotid swelling can also occur when the gland is infected with an influenza virus or bacterium or when an obstruction keeps the saliva from leaving the gland. Vaccination is now commonly performed to prevent mumps.

Before 1967, when the mumps vaccine was made available, it was fairly common to see kids looking like Alfalfa in that episode of the old show *The Little Rascals* in which he had big, swollen cheeks and an ice bandage wrapped around his head. Now, we rarely see this. As noted, however, other organisms, and even something as tiny as a sesame seed, can get stuck in the salivary glands and cause swelling that looks like mumps.

In boys who have gone through puberty, mumps can cause testicular inflammation and swelling, which may then cause one or occasionally both of the testicles to shrink (atrophy). This occurs in approximately 33 percent of cases in postpubescent boys. Fertility usually is not affected. Meningitis is another less common complication.

## Natural Prescriptions*

| Vitamins/Supplements |
| --- |
| Immediately after diagnosis or when symptoms appear in children ages 6 months to 1 year:<br>Vitamin A 100,000 IU in 1 dose |
| Immediately after diagnosis or when symptoms appear in children over 1 year old:<br>Vitamin A 200,000 IU in 1 dose |
| **Naturopathic Remedies** |
| Lemon balm 100 to 500 mg daily |

*Refer to the appendix at the back of the book for a comprehensive list of interactions and condition-based doses.*

# CHICKEN POX

## COMMON SYMPTOM

Itchy rash all over

A common viral infection until a vaccine became widely available in 1995, chicken pox in childhood is characterized by an extremely itchy rash. After the active illness is over, the virus—varicella zoster—stays in the body and may reactivate to cause shingles in adulthood. The FDA has not yet evaluated the effect of the chicken pox vaccine on shingles, so your child may still get shingles even if he or she has had the vaccine.

Bobby's mother brought him into my office. The 4-year-old couldn't stop scratching. They'd just come from a visit with the pediatrician, who had given her cortisone cream for the rash because it looked like poison ivy. It was the dead of winter, and Bobby's mother was certain that Bobby hadn't touched poison ivy.

I asked Bobby to show me where it itched. He took off his shirt and showed me 10 red dots across his chest that he kept scratching.

I asked Bobby's mom, "Has he had chicken pox yet?"

She replied, "Of course not, he's had the chicken pox vaccine."

Bobby was among the 2 percent of children who've been vaccinated against chicken pox but still get a mild and short-lived case of it. Because the vaccine isn't 100 percent effective, we see many children come in with low-grade chicken pox that has been misdiagnosed by their conventional doctors. If you've had chicken pox, as most adults have, you know what it looks like and how much it itches. But don't think that just because your child had the vaccine, he or she is immune. In addition, we have no idea how the vaccine will affect cases of shingles in the future because there has been no long-term testing.

A research study evaluated the relationship between the incidence of shingles in 726 adults and their intake of fruits and vegetables. The more fruit they ate, the lower their risk of the virus reactivating—it's as simple as that. People who ate less than one piece of fruit weekly had more than three times the risk compared to people who ate more than three pieces daily. A similar effect was seen with vegetables.

## Natural Prescriptions*

| Vitamins/Supplements | |
|---|---|
| Alpha-lipoic acid 100 mg daily | Vitamin A 200,000 IU in 1 dose immediately after diagnosis or when symptoms appear |
| CoQ10 10 to 20 mg for every 22 pounds daily | Vitamin C 500 to 1,000 mg daily |
| Digestive enzymes 1 or 2 capsules with each meal | Vitamin E 200 to 400 IU daily |
| Selenium 50 to 200 mcg daily | Zinc 10 to 20 mg daily |
| **Naturopathic Remedies** | |
| *Ganoderma lucidum* (a medicinal mushroom also called reishi mushroom) 4 percent triterpenes, 10 percent polysaccharides, 100 to 500 mg daily | |
| **Homeopathic Remedies** | |
| Homeopathic Hypericum 30C, 5 pellets 3 times daily | |
| **Alternative Treatments** | |
| Tai chi | |

*Refer to the appendix at the back of the book for a comprehensive list of interactions and condition-based doses.*

# SHINGLES

# 61

## COMMON SYMPTOMS

A band of painful blisters in a
discrete area of the body

Occurrence during a
time of high stress

Once your child is infected with the chicken pox virus, it lives within nerve cells, lying dormant forever. Although it's uncertain what reactivates the virus, having an impaired immune system seems to be a risk factor.

Because the virus lives in one of our nerves, it causes skin problems in the places where that particular nerve's connections run. Shingles is a band of blisters that appears on the chest or back. They are very painful, not itchy like chicken pox.

Although shingles is uncommon in children, it can occur. Teenagers may get shingles if they have an immune deficiency or are under extreme stress. We have no idea how the chicken pox vaccine will affect pediatric shingles. Since it is caused by a virus, antibiotics are ineffective and naturopathic remedies reign supreme.

## Natural Prescriptions*

| Vitamins/Supplements |
| --- |
| Immediately after diagnosis or when symptoms appear in children ages 6 months to 1 year: Vitamin A 100,000 IU in 1 dose |
| Immediately after diagnosis or when symptoms appear in children older than 1 year old: Vitamin A 200,000 IU in 1 dose |
| **Naturopathic Remedies** |
| Lemon balm 100 to 500 mg daily |
| **Homeopathic Remedies** |
| Homeopathic Hypericum 30C, 5 pellets daily |

* Refer to the appendix at the back of the book for a comprehensive list of interactions and condition-based doses.

# 62 HERPES SIMPLEX (COLD SORE)

## COMMON SYMPTOMS

Occurrence during a time
of stress

Painful sore, most often
on the lips

Tingling on mucous membrane
where sore later forms

A common infection that can appear at any time of life, including during childhood, herpes simplex virus type 1 normally affects the mouth but can also affect the face and neck. It is common in children who participate in school wrestling programs. The virus is transmitted through direct contact. Once a person contacts herpes, it remains with him or her for life.

There are two strains of the virus, one typically affecting the mucous membranes around the mouth (herpes simplex type 1) and the other most often found on the genitals (herpes simplex type 2), although either virus can infect either area. Contagious and easily spread, they usually are contracted through saliva or sexual contact with someone with an active lesion. A child may also contract herpes during birth, especially if his or her mother is having an active genital outbreak.

The most infectious time is when there is an active sore. If there is no active lesion, passing the virus is less likely, but still possible. In the period just before a sore appears, known as the prodrome, many people feel tingling or pain at the site where the sore will appear, which it usually does within a day or two. Sores occur in the same general area every time.

The herb lemon balm was tested on 66 patients with herpes simplex type 1. They applied a lemon balm cream to active lesions four times a day for 5 days. The patients experienced significant improvements in itching, tingling, burning, swelling, redness, the size of the area involved, and blisters compared to controls.

The effectiveness of another herb, propolis, was compared to that of a common antiviral drug, acyclovir, in patients with genital herpes simplex type 2. After 10 days of treatment, 80 percent of the people using propolis had healed compared to only 47 percent of the acyclovir group.

## Natural Prescriptions*

| Vitamins/Supplements |
| --- |
| Copper 500 to 1,000 mcg daily |
| Lysine 1,000 mg daily to prevent and 1,000 to 3,000 mg daily to treat |
| Vitamin A 100,000 IU in 1 dose |
| Vitamin C 100 to 1,000 mg daily |
| Vitamin E 200 to 400 mg daily |
| Zinc 10 to 20 mg daily plus topical cream daily |
| **Naturopathic Remedies** |
| Lemon balm 100 to 500 mg daily |

*Refer to the appendix at the back of the book for a comprehensive list of interactions and condition-based doses.*

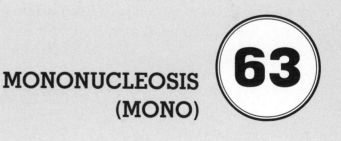

# MONONUCLEOSIS (MONO) 63

## COMMON SYMPTOMS

Extreme fatigue        Sore throat

Fever

Justin and his dad walked up to me in a health food store.

"We heard you're the best naturopathic physician in the area, and my son just got diagnosed with mono," Justin's dad said.

Justin had just started high school and made the football team. Now a virus threatened to sideline him for up to 3 months. Mono is usually caused by infection with the Epstein-Barr virus, and it can be life-changing for some children who need to remain in bed for months because of the extreme fatigue they experience. Many have to take leaves of absence from school or college, which interferes not only with life plans, but also with the important social experience of growing up with a group of friends.

I thanked Justin's dad for the compliment and told him that naturopathic prescriptions are the best antiviral medicines known to humans. I also gave my pep talk on the efficacy of vitamin A as an antiviral.

Justin came to my office to pick up his prescription, took what was listed on it, and called me only 3 days later.

"The mono is gone!" Sure enough, Justin had only had to stay in bed for the weekend. The fatigue disappeared as if by magic, and he was well on the road to complete recovery.

## Natural Prescriptions*

| Vitamins/Supplements |
| --- |
| Immediately after diagnosis or when symptoms appear in children ages 6 months to 1 year: <br> Vitamin A 100,000 IU in 1 dose |
| Immediately after diagnosis or when symptoms appear in children over 1 year old: <br> Vitamin A 200,000 IU in 1 dose |
| Vitamin C 500 to 1,000 mg daily |
| Vitamin D 1,000 to 4,000 IU daily |

* Refer to the appendix at the back of the book for a comprehensive list of interactions and condition-based doses.

# PERTUSSIS (WHOOPING COUGH)

**64**

## COMMON SYMPTOMS

Difficulty breathing

Fatigue

Fever

Long fits of coughing that end with a "whoop" sound during inhalation

Vomiting

A highly contagious bacterial infection of the respiratory system that can last for up to 6 weeks, whooping cough is making a comeback. Despite widespread vaccination, children can still contract it because, even with boosters the vaccine's protection isn't complete or lifelong. Likewise, having it already does not guarantee a person immunity. Since 2000, the annual incidence of whooping cough in the US has hovered at around four or five cases for every 100,000 people, and it reached 6 per 100,000 in 2007. In 2009, there were 17,000 cases reported in the country. Thirty million to 50 million cases are diagnosed each year worldwide.

The symptoms of pertussis are variable, from mild upper respiratory symptoms to severe illness, and usually feature unique coughing spells that may last for a couple of minutes. When the child finally is able to draw a breath, there may be a high-pitched "whoop" sound because the airway is still partially closed. Children can even turn blue during these coughing fits because of the lack of oxygen. Antibiotics are necessary for treatment, but naturopathic remedies can be added to speed healing.

## Natural Prescriptions*

| Vitamins/Supplements |
| --- |
| Iron 10 to 40 mg daily |
| **Naturopathic Remedies** |
| *Withania* (also called ashwagandha) 500 to 1,000 mg daily |

* Refer to the appendix at the back of the book for a comprehensive list of interactions and condition-based doses.

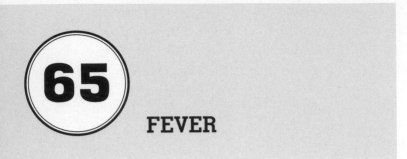

# FEVER

## COMMON SYMPTOMS

Temperature above 100°F, which can be associated with:

Abdominal pain

Cough

Diarrhea, nausea, or vomiting

Ear or other infection

Nasal discharge

Sore throat

Urinary symptoms

Fevers can be scary. Your child feels as if she's burning up. She's listless and just wants to sleep. As parents, you may find yourself falling into our society's symptom-suppressing paradigm. Children's Tylenol! Stop the fever!

Let's stop for a moment and think about the body's immune system. We're designed to overcome colds and other infections. We create antibodies that attack bacteria and viruses and usually provide us with lifelong immunity. But when we haven't encountered these microorganisms before—as is especially the case when we're young, before our immune systems fully develop—we have another defense: heat.

How do you sterilize a needle? Heat. Why do we cook meat to a high temperature? To kill the bacteria. The body has an internal oven that responds when we're sick by turning up the thermostat to kill the bugs. The body is trying to heal itself with this amazing defense system, so why are we purposefully suppressing it?

Many parents have "fever phobia" and are scared that a fever is dangerous. However, in a March 2011 revision of its fever treatment policy, the American Academy of Pediatrics emphasized that a fever is not an illness itself but rather the body's reaction to fight an infection. Fever-reducing medications such as acetaminophen (Children's Tylenol) may help a child feel better, but there is no evidence that a high fever causes brain damage. (However, a child whose body temperature is higher than 105°F due to hyperthermia, which can occur with heat stroke, for example, may experience serious physical effects such as convulsions and coma. Go to the emergency room immediately.) Most infection-related fevers of up to 103°F (oral temperature) are safe in children over the age of 3 months, and fevers of up to 100.5°F are okay in children younger than that. If your child's fever is higher, bring him or her to your pediatrician immediately.

There is no evidence that giving fever reducers to a child lowers the risk of injury or death from the illness causing the fever or of having febrile seizures in subsequent illnesses (except perhaps in children who are critically ill or respond poorly to increased demands on their metabolisms). The healthiest thing for our children is to let them run fevers until the germs are killed. We can use natural remedies to help alleviate discomfort, and this takes diligence and continuous monitoring.

If you choose to give a fever-reducing drug, don't be fooled when the fever comes back in 4 hours, when the drug wears off. The body is still trying to fix itself. The germs are still there, and you may be keeping your child sicker for a longer period of time. When you monitor a fever and let the heat kill the germs, your child returns to health faster and will have a stronger immune system that can prevent chronic diseases from developing in the future.

## Natural Prescriptions*

| Homeopathic Remedies |
| --- |
| Homeopathic Belladonna 30C, 5 pellets 3 times daily |
| **Alternative Treatments** |
| WARMING SOCKS (to stimulate the immune system and reduce fever):<br>1. When your child is ready for bed or a nap, wet a pair of cotton socks with cold water.<br>2. Wring them out and put them on his feet.<br>3. Cover those socks with a pair of dry, wool socks. |
| WARMING BATH (to stimulate the immune system and reduce fever):<br>1. Prepare bathwater at 99° to 100°F.<br>2. Put your child in the bath untils he becomes chilled. Closely monitor the temperature of the water throughout the bath, adding more warm water as necessary. You do not want it to go below 99°F, because it could send her into shock.<br>3. As soon as she starts to shake, take her out. |

* Refer to the appendix at the back of the book for a comprehensive list of interactions and condition-based doses.

# BRUXISM (TEETH GRINDING)

## COMMON SYMPTOMS

Jaw pain          Worn-down teeth

Muscle spasms

An unconscious, regularly occurring clenching or grinding of the teeth that may be intermittent or continual and tends to peak between the ages of 7 and 10, bruxism can wear down and loosen teeth, cause gum recession, and cause morning tension headaches.

Grinding and clenching can be caused by nervous tension, neuromuscular disorders, misaligned teeth, allergies that cause mouth breathing, and nutrient deficiencies. Regardless of the cause, the muscles of the jaw clench and won't relax.

Have your child's amino acid levels checked by your naturopathic physician to see if they need to be adjusted. Amino acids are the building blocks of neurotransmitters (brain chemicals) and directly affect muscular contraction, including spasms of the jaw muscle. When using amino acids as therapy, try GABA (gamma-aminobutyric acid) and theanine first. If that makes it worse, try phenylalanine and tyrosine. Some children do better with one combination or the other.

In a small study, 10 adult patients with bruxism were given the drug levodopa (L-dopa). Although the body makes L-dopa itself, the drug L-dopa has serious side effects, including involuntary movements (called dyskinesia). To make L-dopa naturally, the body coverts the amino acid phenylalanine into tyrosine, which is then converted to L-dopa. In the study, L-dopa decreased the average number of bruxism episodes per hour of sleep.

## Natural Prescriptions*

| Vitamins/Supplements |
| --- |
| Magnesium 200 mg daily |
| Phenylalanine 500 to 1,000 mg + tyrosine 500 to 1,000 mg daily |
| Theanine 100 to 500 mg + GABA 750 mg daily |

*Refer to the appendix at the back of the book for a comprehensive list of interactions and condition-based doses.*

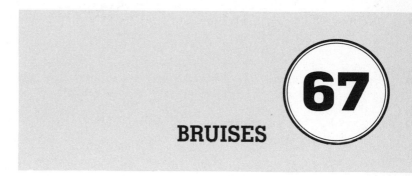

# BRUISES 67

## COMMON SYMPTOM

Discoloration under the skin

When my 2-year-old nephew came over to my house for a visit once, the adults all cringed as we helplessly watched him jump off the couch and hit his head on the floor. Childhood comes with a few bumps and bruises. When a blood vessel is broken, the blood seeps out inside the body, and we see it first as a red discoloration under the skin. Then, a day or so later, it turns bluish. After about a week, it changes to yellow or green, and it's usually gone a couple of weeks later.

Bruises are to be expected in childhood, but we must watch to make sure a child isn't getting too many, because this may indicate the presence of a serious blood disorder such as hemophilia or perhaps something mild, such as weak capillary blood vessels or skin. Some people tend to bruise easier than others. While this is not a serious health condition, it may indicate a deficiency in nutrients that create strong blood vessels or ensure adequate clotting.

I recommend treating bruises with homeopathic arnica in both oral and topical preparations. No research studies have been performed on arnica's effects on pediatric bruises, but many studies have looked at its effects on the bruises from cosmetic surgery, such as laser surgery and face-lift. A study in which 26 facial plastic surgery patients were treated with either homeopathic arnica or placebo before surgery and for 3 days afterward found that the arnica made the area of bruising smaller than that in the other patients, although there were no differences in the degree of coloration or in how long it took to go away.

Treating bruises naturopathically will help children heal much faster so they can get back to jumping off the couch into a pile of fluffy pillows, like my nephew does now.

## Natural Prescriptions*

| Diet |
| --- |
| Eat the pith of an orange or grapefruit every day to prevent and treat easy bruising. |
| **Vitamins/Supplements** |
| Bromelain 100 to 200 mg daily |
| Vitamin C 500 mg daily |
| **Homeopathic Remedies** |
| Homeopathic Arnica 30C, 5 pellets daily |
| **Alternative Treatments** |
| ALTERNATING HYDROTHERAPY:<br><br>Sit down with your child for 10 minutes with two bowls of water, one hot, and one cold. Get two facecloths, one for each bowl of water. Alternate pressing the hot- and cold-water facecloths on the bruise. Make sure that the hot water isn't so hot that it burns the child. The hot and cold water will push the blood out of the skin and help the body reabsorb it. |

* Refer to the appendix at the back of the book for a comprehensive list of interactions and condition-based doses.

# FIBROMYALGIA

**COMMON SYMPTOMS**

Fatigue

Sleep disturbance

Tender points pain at
multiple locations

Fibromyalgia is a condition that causes widespread pain and fatigue. The pain emanates from multiple defined focal "tender points" and spreads to the muscles, particularly those of the shoulders, back, hips, and legs, which seem to ache the most.

Maya came to my office right after school. She was sad because she'd had to quit the soccer team. Her body just hurt too much. It had reached the point where she was in tears from the pain. She thought it was from playing too hard.

When I diagnosed fibromyalgia, she said, "I thought only older people got that." "Not anymore," I told her.

I put her on a program that included specific foods, vitamins, supplements, and herbs. I also suggested that she do some stretching exercises and light aerobic exercise, such as walking, on a daily basis. A month later, she had finished the treatment program and was back on the soccer field, scoring the winning goal.

## Natural Prescriptions*

| Diet | |
| --- | --- |
| Elimination diet (based on IgG and IgE food sensitivities and food allergies; see page 5) | |
| **Vitamins/Supplements** | |
| Bromelain 50 to 100 mg daily | Fish oil EPA + DHA 500 to 1,000 mg |
| Calcium 200 to 1,000 mg daily | Magnesium 200 mg daily |
| CoQ10 100 mg daily | Zinc 10 mg daily |

*\* Refer to the appendix at the back of the book for a comprehensive list of interactions and condition-based doses.*

# 69 JUVENILE RHEUMATOID ARTHRITIS

## COMMON SYMPTOMS

Joint pain          Joint swelling

Joint stiffness

Inflammation, pain, tenderness, and decreased range of motion of at least one joint for at least 6 weeks are the hallmarks of juvenile rheumatoid arthritis (JRA). In a small percentage of children, it can cause eye inflammation, which may lead to cataracts, glaucoma, or loss of vision.

Louis, a tiny 3-year-old with a big smile, limped into my office. He loved to dance and was one of the favorites of my front office staff. He sang to them every visit (his rendition of Britney Spears's "Womanizer" had them in stitches).

Louis had arthritis. No one wants to see a child unable to run around the playground or play with his friends because of swollen, painful joints. This isn't supposed to happen until you get older. But Louis's knees were swollen like balloons; even his tiny toes were big and red. He had to wear sandals because shoes hurt his feet too much.

Louis was diagnosed with JRA at 6 months old, and his rheumatologist put him on methotrexate and naproxen. While this was saving his joints, it was killing his liver. Every month, Louis needed to have his liver enzymes tested to make sure that the drugs weren't damaging his liver to an excessive degree. (The doctors were fine with damaging it a little bit, just not excessively.)

When Louis came to see me, his mother simply wanted him healthy. "He's so little," she said. "I just want him to be able to live without pain."

I immediately put him on a three-tiered naturopathic approach:

1. Remove triggers of food allergies and food sensitivities from the diet.

2. Protect the liver from the methotrexate.

3. Stop the inflammation in the joints.

All arthritis, including JRA, involves inflammation, and once the inflammation is stopped so is the pain. Suppressing food allergies and food sensitivities reduces joint inflammation. Even adult patients who do this will have dramatic reductions in pain.

JRA is an autoimmune disease—one in which the immune system attacks the body—that may be triggered by a viral infection or IgA deficiency. A child's IgE and IgG antibodies to foods should be tested. Lyme disease should also be ruled out as a cause.

After Louis's mom used the elimination diet to determine that wheat was his enemy and gave him the anti-inflammatory supplements for his joints and the liver-repairing supplements for a while, Louis was able to get off of naproxen.

Another month passed and we wanted more, so I added an anti-inflammatory oil to apply topically. The swelling and redness decreased dramatically. We were also able to stop the methotrexate, the toxic liver drug. His liver enzymes normalized. We were all very excited. We held our breath, but the symptoms never returned. We were glad to give him the prescription drugs when he needed them, and we didn't wean him off the methotrexate until all of his lab work came back okay and his symptoms were gone.

Now, Louis is taking a karate class and a swim class and fighting with his new baby brother. It's been a year, and the arthritis is completely gone. No more drugs. Mom rubs on a little oil every night, and she cringes a little when he kicks in karate or falls, but Louis is on his way to having an arthritis pain-free life. If your child has JRA, don't stop giving him or her the prescribed medications on your own. Consult your physician to make sure the inflammation is gone and doesn't cause further joint damage.

Inflammation is at the heart of arthritis. The ability of fish oil to decrease this inflammation has often been studied. In a trial involving 23 children, a diet with increased omega-3 fatty acids decreased the use of ibuprofen by 17.3 percent, compared to a 6.5 percent decrease in the placebo group.

Another study showed that omega-3 fatty acid supplements in 16 JRA patients significantly decreased their blood levels of a substance called C-reactive protein, which indicates inflammation in the body.

## Natural Prescriptions*

| Vitamins/Supplements | |
|---|---|
| 5-MTHF 200 to 400 mcg daily | Vitamin C 500 to 1,000 mg daily |
| Calcium 1,000 mg daily | Vitamin D 1,000 to 4,000 IU daily |
| CoQ10 10 to 250 mg daily | Vitamin E 200 to 400 IU daily |
| Fish oil EPA 2 to 4 g daily | Zinc 10 to 20 mg daily |
| Selenium 20 to 200 mcg daily | |
| **Naturopathic Remedies** | |
| Castor oil applied topically to the joints daily | |

*Refer to the appendix at the back of the book for a comprehensive list of interactions and condition-based doses.*

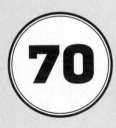

# 70 OSGOOD-SCHLATTER DISEASE

## COMMON SYMPTOMS

Occurrence in children who are physically active

Pain in the knee

Swelling below the kneecap

Does your preteen have knee pain? If so, take a close look and ask your child where the pain is located. Right on the kneecap, or below it? Feel your own kneecap, and then drop down an inch toward your feet. There's a bump at the top of the lower leg bone (the tibia) where the patellar tendon attaches the kneecap to the tibia. The four muscles on the front of the thigh, collectively called the quadriceps, pull on the kneecap, which pulls on the tibia at that bump. Growing children's leg bones have growth plates made of cartilage that will later harden into bone, so when an athletic kid's quads pull repeatedly on the tibia's growth plate at that bump below the knee, the patellar tendon can pull away from it. That's what causes the pain and swelling. Naturopathic prescriptions will help heal it more rapidly.

## Natural Prescriptions*

| Vitamins/Supplements | |
|---|---|
| Calcium 200 to 500 mg daily | Vitamin D 1,000 to 4,000 IU daily |
| Selenium 20 to 400 mcg daily | Vitamin E 200 to 400 IU daily |
| **Alternative Treatments** | |
| Physical therapy as directed by a physician. | |

*\* Refer to the appendix at the back of the book for a comprehensive list of interactions and condition-based doses.*

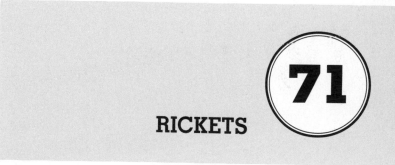

# RICKETS
# 71

## COMMON SYMPTOMS

Awkward gait

Bowlegs

Soft skull bones

Weak muscles

Rickets occurs when calcium and phosphate are taken from the growing bones because there's too little in the blood due to a severe, chronic deficiency of vitamin D. It can be caused by a dietary deficiency of calcium, phosphorus, or vitamin D, because vitamin D enables your body to use the calcium and phosphorus in food. Though uncommon, there has been a slight rise in the number of nutritional rickets cases in the US. This may be due to a decrease in sun exposure coupled with a reduced use of vitamin D–fortified foods. Children with darker skin create less vitamin D from sunshine than lighter-skinned children do. They are therefore at greater risk for rickets, as are children who are exclusively breast-fed. Breast milk does not contain sufficient vitamin D to prevent the disease in infants who don't get adequate sunlight, regardless of the mother's vitamin D level.

In 2007, I attended a vitamin D conference at the National Institutes of Health in Bethesda, Maryland. This conference set off a chain reaction across the country in the form of more research studies and a vitamin D awakening, and we are now learning about the benefits of this wonderful nutrient. The RDA for vitamin D was raised in 2010 to 600 IU, with the tolerable upper intake limit ranging from 2,500 to 4,000 IU for children of different ages (we make approximately 10,000 IU during a full day in the sun). When your child is taking high doses (more than 2,000 IU) of vitamin D, make sure your pediatrician is monitoring his or her vitamin D and calcium levels. Vitamin D has been a very popular subject the last few years, with various organizations claiming we should get more or less of it. New values were settled on by the Institute of Medicine in December 2010.

Bryson was 4 years old and had odd-looking bumps on all of his ribs, like a chain of beads going down each side of his chest. A surgeon suggested breaking each one of his 12 pairs of ribs (that's 24 total) and setting them with a full-body cast. Bryson's mother said no to these unnecessary surgeries.

Mother and son came to my office and we looked at the x-rays together. Bryson had rickets, a condition that was rarely seen 10 years ago but is now becoming more common. With kids playing video games all day long, they're not getting outside and playing in the sunshine. Without the sun, our bodies can't make vitamin D, which is essential for bone growth. I prescribed high-dose vitamin D, and Bryson's bones grew back together as if by magic, changing shape almost before in front of our eyes. After 6 months, you couldn't tell that anything had ever been wrong with him.

## Natural Prescriptions*

| Vitamins/Supplements |
| --- |
| Calcium 500 to 1,500 mg daily |
| Vitamin D 2,000 to 4,000 IU daily (If your child has been diagnosed with rickets, consult your physician for the appropriate dose.) |

| Alternative Treatments |
| --- |
| MODERATE SUN EXPOSURE DAILY:<br><br>Make sure your child regularly gets midday sun exposure (between 10 a.m. and 3 p.m.) in the late spring, summer, and early fall. Don't apply sunscreen. Be careful not to let the child get a sunburn. Fair-skinned children will need about 20 to 30 minutes in the sun, and children with darker skin may need 2 hours or more to produce enough vitamin D. If it is a sunny day, you may want to have your child go outside during the morning or evening hours, especially if he or she has dark skin and needs a longer period of exposure. |

*Refer to the appendix at the back of the book for a comprehensive list of interactions and condition-based doses.*

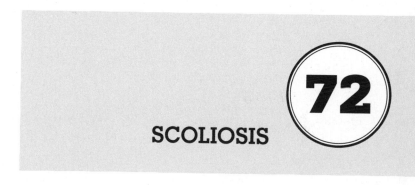

# SCOLIOSIS 72

## COMMON SYMPTOM

Lateral curvature of the spine

Scoliosis is lateral (to the side) curvature of the spine of more than 10 degrees. There are multiple causes, including genetics, connective tissue disorders, and having legs of different lengths. Adolescents with scoliosis have an increased risk of osteopenia and osteoporosis.

Every child should be checked for scoliosis. Usually the doctor will have your child bend forward and touch the toes while he or she feels for a curve in the spine. The spine naturally curves forward and back, but it should not curve from side to side. When it does, that is scoliosis.

Our bones support us. Muscles attach one bone to another to facilitate movement. Ligaments connect one bone to another to maintain stability. The spine is the only bony connection from the hips to the head. It looks like a stack of 33 blocks from the tailbone to the skull. If your child's muscles or connective tissues such as ligaments and tendons are weak, the tower of vertebrae becomes unstable. Naturopathic prescriptions that strengthen muscles and ligaments, along with corrective physical therapy, can help your child improve his or her scoliosis.

## Natural Prescriptions*

| Vitamins/Supplements | |
| --- | --- |
| Calcium 1,000 to 1,500 mg daily | Vitamin C 500 to 1,000 mg daily |
| Selenium 20 to 200 mcg daily | Zinc 10 to 20 mg daily |
| Tryptophan 1 to 5 g daily | |
| **Alternative Treatments** | |
| Physical therapy when needed | |
| Chiropractic manipulation when needed | |
| Orthotics (for children with unequal leg lengths) | |

*Refer to the appendix at the back of the book for a comprehensive list of interactions and condition-based doses.*

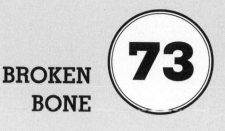

# BROKEN BONE 73

## COMMON SYMPTOMS

Broken bone visible or protruding through skin

Pain, swelling, and bruising at point of impact

Nothing spoils the summer for a child like a fracture that requires a cast. Itchy and hot, a cast keeps a child unhappy on the sidelines.

Kids are resilient, and they heal so much faster than adults do. We can accelerate the healing of broken bones even more by giving children the nutrients that bones are made of.

Researchers at the George Washington University School of Medicine and Health Sciences tested vitamin D levels in 17 African American children with forearm fractures and discovered that 59 percent of them were vitamin D insufficient. Although dark-skinned children are more likely than others to produce too little vitamin D, all children with broken bones should have their levels tested.

## Natural Prescriptions*

| Vitamins/Supplements | |
|---|---|
| Calcium 400 mg daily | Vitamin D 1,000 to 4,000 IU daily |
| Copper 2 mg daily | Vitamin $K_2$ 100 mcg daily |
| Magnesium 200 mg daily | Zinc 20 mg daily |
| Manganese 5 mg daily | |
| **Homeopathic Remedies** | |
| Homeopathic Arnica 30C, 5 pellets daily | |
| Homeopathic Symphytum 30C, 5 pellets daily | |

* Refer to the appendix at the back of the book for a comprehensive list of interactions and condition-based doses.

## Pulmonary

I remember the first child I ever saw who had asthma. She held on to her inhaler like a lifeline she couldn't live without, taking gasps from it whenever she felt she couldn't breathe. Tears started to well up in my eyes as I realized that this child might require this device for the rest of her life. There would be no playing outside with friends, going camping or hiking, or having a dog, all due to her asthma attacks. She had to live in a partial bubble, tethered to her inhaler to survive.

Meeting that child started me on my search for natural answers to breathing and lung problems. Asthma is the most common chronic disease in children, but I wanted to find answers for all of them, from simple bronchitis and croup to asthma and cystic fibrosis. Conventional medicine was offering a wonderful bandage, an inhaler that allowed a child to breathe, but there was no cure in sight, just a lifetime of inhaled steroids and bronchodilators. But asthma can be dangerous, and even deadly. Don't stop your child's medication before consulting your physician.

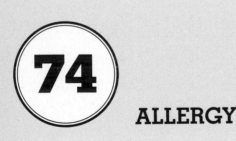

## ALLERGY

**COMMON SYMPTOMS**

| | |
|---|---|
| Congestion | Runny nose |
| Headache | Sneezing |
| Nasal discharge | Watery eyes |

Many of the children who walk into my office have allergies. Some come in with the typical runny noses and watery eyes. This usually occurs in the spring and fall, when so many particles of pollen are in the air from grasses, trees, and flowers. The immune system creates proteins called immunoglobin E (IgE), which are the antibody soldiers that attack allergens in your bloodstream and help to create the allergic symptoms that get rid of the offender. Other children walk in with red, itchy skin as a sign of their allergies. These children usually have this symptom all year long; it is commonly a result of allergies to foods, pets, mold, and dust mites.

Every child with allergies needs to be tested to determine the offender. Your allergist may have performed a skin test, in which he or she inserted tiny amounts of different allergens into the skin and waited for bumps to appear. Another option is a blood test that measures IgE levels to determine what the allergens are. Children who have seasonal allergies should be tested for reactions to pollens, trees, and grasses, whereas children who have yearlong allergies should be tested for foods, pets, molds, and dust mites.

Once we find the offending allergen, we need to help the child avoid it and also to retrain the immune system to accept the substance as a nonallergen. Conventional allergists do this sometimes through allergy shots. They periodically inject a very tiny amount of the allergen into the child until the immune system learns that this pollen or pet hair or food is not a bad allergen, but something the body should accept.

Naturopathic medicine achieves this exact same response, but with vitamins, supplements, and homeopathy. I always prefer to avoid shots and needles, so I give a diluted amount of an allergen orally until the immune system has been retrained and the child is no longer allergic.

## Natural Prescriptions*

| Vitamins/Supplements | |
| --- | --- |
| Bromelain 200 to 500 mg daily | |
| Flavonoids (such as rutin or quercetin) 200 to 400 mg divided into 2 or 3 doses daily<br>    Add flavonoids to your child's diet. Food sources of flavonoids include blackberries, blueberries, capers, cherries, dark chocolate, grapefruit, kale, lemons, onions, oranges, parsley, raspberries, thyme, black tea, and green tea. | |
| Quercetin 250 to 500 mg divided into 2 or 3 doses daily | Vitamin C 500 to 1,000 mg daily |
| **Naturopathic Remedies** | |
| *Euphrasia* (Eyebright) 50 to 200 mg daily | Stinging nettle leaf (*Urtica*), 1 percent silicic acid, 250 to 500 mg daily |
| *Scutellaria* (skullcap) 250 to 500 mg daily | Turmeric standardized extract 100 mg daily |
| **Homeopathic Remedies** | |
| Homeopathic nosode of the specific allergen | |

* Refer to the appendix at the back of the book for a comprehensive list of interactions and condition-based doses.

# 75

## ASTHMA

### COMMON SYMPTOMS

Chest and abdominal pain

Coughing

Trouble breathing

Wheezing

Asthma is an inflammatory airway disease that often limits a child's activities and keeps him or her attached to an inhaler. It's triggered by allergens, airborne irritants, sensitivity to particular foods and food additives, exercise, cold air, and stress.

Asthma is the most common chronic pulmonary disease in children. More than 7.1 million children (9.6 percent) in the US have it. Ten and a half million school days are missed because of asthma, and it is the third leading cause of hospitalization in children under 15.

More boys (11.3 percent) have asthma than girls (7.9 percent), and it's most prevalent in children with Puerto Rican ancestry (16.6 percent). The jet stream—the current of high-speed winds that drives global weather and therefore air pollution from west to east across continental America—likely contributes to more children in the Northeast having asthma (more than 9.8 percent, compared to approximately 7.2 percent on the West Coast).

Asthma attacks happen when the airways (the bronchial tubes) constrict and begin to secrete mucus. When the bronchial tubes narrow, only a tiny space remains for air to move in and out. The wheezing noise we hear is air trying to squeeze through the small space. Children panic when they can't get air into their lungs.

We spend $5.9 billion every year in the US on inhalers and other prescription treatments for asthma. It is important for your child to continue using his or her asthma medications—after all, asthma attacks can be fatal—but adding natural options will improve your child's health. A Harvard study analyzed 1,194 pairs of mothers and children and found that the children of mothers who had higher vitamin D intake during pregnancy had a lower risk of having two or more wheezing attacks before the age of 3. Another Harvard study looked at asthmatic children in Costa Rica. The lower the children's levels of vitamin D, the higher their blood markers of asthma severity.

The effects of fish oil on asthma prevention have also been studied. The children of mothers who took fish oil while they were pregnant had significantly lower risks of asthma and asthma that arises in response to an allergy than the children whose mothers did not take fish oil.

## Natural Prescriptions*

| Vitamins/Supplements | |
| --- | --- |
| For the mother throughout pregnancy:<br>Fish oil EPA + DHA 2 to 4 g daily | Vitamin C 1,000 mg daily |
| Magnesium 200 mg daily | Vitamin D 1,000 to 4,000 IU daily |
| Vitamin B$_6$ (pyridoxine) 1 to 20 mg daily | |
| **Naturopathic Remedies** | |
| *Cordyceps sinensis* 100 to 500 mg daily or tincture, 5:1 ratio, 30 drops 2 times daily | |

*\* Refer to the appendix at the back of the book for a comprehensive list of interactions and condition-based doses.*

# BRONCHIOLITIS (INFANT BRONCHITIS)  76

## COMMON SYMPTOMS

Cough

Crankiness

Fever

Runny nose

Usual occurrence in children 2 to 24 months old

Infant bronchitis, which is caused by the respiratory syncytial virus (RSV) virus, is the most common cause of severe lower respiratory tract infections in US children less than 1 year of age. It causes the bronchioles, the smallest airways in the lungs, to swell and fill with mucus, making it hard to breathe. Risk and incidence are higher in those born prematurely and those who have cardiopulmonary (heart and lung) disease. Those who contract bronchiolitis seem to have an increased risk of childhood asthma, although it isn't clear if it's a cause-and-effect relationship. RSV is spread via respiratory droplets in the air.

My best friend from college called me one day in a panic. He and his wife had had their first daughter 6 months before and she hadn't had any infectious diseases so far, just like most kids who are breast-fed. But she'd spiked a fever of 103°F, was coughing up lots of phlegm, and didn't want to eat. He didn't know what to do.

I could tell right away that she had bronchiolitis, and since it is a viral infection, antibiotics would be ineffective. Naturopathic remedies are powerful antiviral medicines. I advised my friend to provide his daughter with plenty of fluids and the right naturopathic remedies—and that they must go to the emergency room immediately if she experienced any difficulty breathing, Thankfully, it did not come to that, and she was better within a couple of days.

A study of preterm newborns with a very serious respiratory condition called bronchopulmonary dysplasia found that infants who had it had lower vitamin A levels than premature infants who didn't. It wasn't clear whether the deficiency was the cause or an effect of the condition, but the authors nevertheless suggested that the low vitamin A level might impair the lungs' healing in these babies. Children with bronchiolitis may also benefit from higher levels of Vitamin A.

## Natural Prescriptions*

| Vitamins/Supplements |
| --- |
| NAC 600 to 2,400 mg by mouth daily |
| Vitamin A 200,000 IU in 1 dose |

| Alternative Treatments |
| --- |
| WARMING SOCKS (to stimulate the immune system and reduce fever):<br>1. When your child is ready for bed or a nap, wet a pair of cotton socks with cold water.<br>2. Wring them out and put them on his or her feet.<br>3. Cover those socks with a pair of dry wool socks. |

*Refer to the appendix at the back of the book for a comprehensive list of interactions and condition-based doses.*

CROUP **77**

## COMMON SYMPTOMS

Cough that is worse at night      Stereotypical seal-bark cough

Fever

Croup, a common viral infection of the airways, is spread by respiratory droplets in the air or on surfaces, and it results in a cough that sounds like a seal barking. It normally occurs in children between 6 months and 3 years of age and is typically caused by human parainfluenza virus type 1 (HPV-1), though it can spur a simultaneous bacterial infection.

In the middle of a cold January night, my pager went off and woke me up. It was 1:00 a.m. I dialed the number and heard a woman's voice.

"Hi, Dr. Skowron, it's my daughter again. She can't stop coughing. It's hard for her to catch her breath. I've never heard her cough like this before. It's like . . . a seal at Sea World."

Croup causes swelling in the upper airway—the larynx, trachea, and sometimes the bronchi. The swelling makes it hard for the child to breathe, and that's what makes the cough sound like a seal barking. No other respiratory illness sounds like this.

Antibiotics don't help for this viral condition, but natural medicines cure it very quickly. Homeopathy also excels at treating croup. There are three specific remedies that should be given 2 hours apart.

## Croup Red Flags

You should call your pediatrician right away or take your child to the emergency room if he or she:

- Makes a whistling sound when inhaling
- Can't speak for lack of air

- Is struggling to breathe
- Has bluish lips or skin
- Is drooling and having trouble swallowing

## Natural Prescriptions*

| Vitamins/Supplements |
| --- |
| Immediately after diagnosis in children ages 6 months to 1 year: <br> Vitamin A 100,000 IU in 1 dose |
| Immediately after diagnosis in children over 1 year old: <br> Vitamin A 200,000 IU in 1 dose |
| Vitamin C 500 to 1,000 mg daily |
| Vitamin D 1,000 to 4,000 IU daily |
| Zinc 10 to 20 mg daily |
| **Naturopathic Remedies** |
| *Cordyceps sinensis* 100 to 500 mg daily or tincture, 5:1 ratio, 30 drops 2 times daily |
| **Homeopathic Remedies (Give 2 Hours Apart)** |
| Homeopathic Aconite 30C, 5 pellets 3 times daily |
| Homeopathic Hepar Sulphur 30C, 5 pellets 3 times daily |
| Homeopathic Spongia 30C, 5 pellets 3 times daily |

*Refer to the appendix at the back of the book for a comprehensive list of interactions and condition-based doses.*

# CYSTIC FIBROSIS

## COMMON SYMPTOMS

Cough

Foul-smelling stools

Recurrent lung infections

Slimy stools with mucus

Cystic fibrosis (CF) is a chronic genetic disease in which the body produces extremely thick mucus throughout the body. It is most common in Caucasians but can affect children of any ethnicity.

Although many body systems are affected by CF, the lungs and pancreas are most affected. CF shortens the life span because bacteria become established in the sticky mucus in the lungs that is difficult to cough up and cause repeated episodes of infection. Affected individuals also have poor digestion because the enzymes released by the pancreas to digest food in the small intestine are unable to work the way they should. These children are usually smaller than average and can also have failure to thrive.

While there is no cure for a genetic disease such as CF, there are natural remedies that can improve a child's quality of life, as well as lengthen his or her life span. The goal is to keep the mucus thin so it can move out of the body. Certain nutrients, along with a technique called postural drainage and percussion, will help your child the most.

In a study of N-acetylcysteine (NAC) in 52 patients with cystic fibrosis and chronic *Pseudomonas* infection, the participants were given either 200 mg of NAC three times a day or 400 mg twice a day. Most patients did not have any improvement in subjective symptoms or lung function test results, but those with the worst lung function did have a significant improvement in their test results.

## Natural Prescriptions*

| Vitamins/Supplements | |
| --- | --- |
| Coenzyme Q10 (CoQ10) 60 mg daily | NAC 200 to 800 mg 3 times daily |
| Digestive enzymes 2 capsules each meal | Zinc 10 to 20 mg daily |
| **Alternative Treatments** | |
| Postural drainage and percussion 1 to 3 times a day—Follow your physician's instructions for this technique. | |

*\* Refer to the appendix at the back of the book for a comprehensive list of interactions and condition-based doses.*

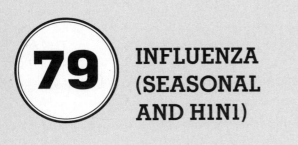

# 79 INFLUENZA (SEASONAL AND H1N1)

## COMMON SYMPTOMS

Cough

Diarrhea

Fever

Malaise

Nausea

Sore throat

Vomiting

Influenza is a viral infection that attacks the respiratory system, causing symptoms that include fever, headache, fatigue, dry cough, sore throat, and muscle aches. Nausea, vomiting, and diarrhea are more common in children than adults. The virus is transmitted via respiratory droplets in the air or on surfaces.

Every February, there's a line that goes out my office door: Patients march in like it's a July 4th parade. Once influenza gets into a school or day-care center, it spreads like wildfire. Then someone takes it home and it spreads through the family, sometimes several times, giving parents and kids multiple infections.

Seasonal influenza is caused by one particular group, type B, of human influenza viruses. Five to 20 percent of Americans have it every year, leading to 200,000 hospitalizations and 20,000 deaths. Most of these are in the elderly, but they can also occur in children. Swine flu is a unique strain of influenza virus called H1N1.

So what are we to do to treat or prevent a virus, for which antibiotics are ineffective? The Centers for Disease Control and Prevention (CDC) recommends that children who are at high risk for developing serious complications from influenza infection get a flu shot every year (see the list at www.cdc.gov/flu/about/disease/high_risk.htm), but natural remedies have helped patients in my practice. All of the parents in my practice choose to avoid the flu vaccine, because they know the truth about it. First, some are preserved with thimerosal, which contains brain-damaging mercury. While childhood vaccines no longer contain thimerosal and you can get thimerosal-free influenza vaccine, some formulations of the flu vaccine still have it. If you decide to have your child get the flu shot, make sure you request a thimerosal-free vaccine. You can't buy a mercury thermometer anymore because the mercury is too dangerous if the thermometer breaks and mercury vapor is released into the air, but the CDC states that it's still okay to inject it into a child as thimerosal in the flu vaccine every year. Mercury may also pass from a mother into a developing child before birth.

The other fact about the flu vaccine is that it's made based on last year's flu. Every year, the flu virus mutates and becomes something new. We don't know what it will look like, and scientists can't make a vaccine for something that is unknown. They pick the most virulent strains circulating and hope that they're right. But what I see is that the children who get the flu first in the season (October and November) are the ones who've received the vaccine. Patients in my practice rarely get influenza, because we prevent infection with natural anti-viral therapies. So many in vitro studies prove that natural remedies are the most effective at killing the influenza virus.

In a research study of 60 patients who took elderberry syrup or placebo for 5 days, the influenza symptoms of those taking the syrup went away an average of 4 days earlier, and those patients needed fewer rescue medications.

## Natural Prescriptions*

| Vitamins/Supplements | |
|---|---|
| Selenium 20 to 200 mcg daily | Vitamin D 1,000 to 4,000 IU daily |
| Vitamin A 200,000 IU in 1 dose | Vitamin E 200 to 400 IU daily |
| Vitamin C 500 mg 3 times daily | Zinc 5 mg every 2 hours, for a maximum of 20 mg daily |
| **Naturopathic Remedies** | |
| Elderberry syrup 1 tsp 2 times daily | |
| Licorice (*Glycyrrhiza*) root extract, 16 to 18 percent glycyrrhizin, 100 to 400 mg daily | |
| Siberian ginseng 250 to 1,000 mg daily | |
| **Homeopathic Remedies** | |
| Homeopathic Oscillococcinum, entire tube of pellets when symptoms arise | |

*\* Refer to the appendix at the back of the book for a comprehensive list of interactions and condition-based doses.*

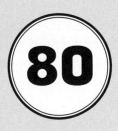

# 80

# PNEUMONIA

## COMMON SYMPTOMS

Bluish skin or lips
in severe cases

Breathing problems

Cough

Fever

Wheezing

Pneumonia is a lung inflammation commonly caused by infection with a virus, bacterium, or fungus or by inhaling a foreign object. Specific offenders include bacteria such as *Streptococcus* and *Staphylococcus* and viruses such as human influenza virus type B (Hib).

The agents that cause pneumonia aren't in the airways of the lungs but in the tiny air sacs of the lung, the alveoli. As far as symptoms go, pneumonia usually looks more serious than bronchiolitis, with the child having a higher fever and greater fatigue but a similar cough. Sometimes, however, pneumonia resembles a regular cold. Your pediatrician will order an x-ray to diagnose pneumonia. The pneumococcal and Hib vaccines are used to prevent cases of pneumonia.

A study of almost 2,500 children ages 6 to 30 months who were given a single high dose of vitamin A (100,000 mg for infants and 200,000 for the others) at the study's start showed that compared to those who got placebo, the group that was also given zinc daily (10 mg for infants and 20 mg for older children) had substantially fewer cases of pneumonia. Many studies using high-dose vitamin A are performed in countries where people are commonly deficient in it, so you should have your child's vitamin A level tested to ascertain if supplementing with it would be helpful.

## Natural Prescriptions*

| Vitamins/Supplements |
| --- |
| Fish oil EPA + DHA 2 to 4 g daily |
| Vitamin A 200,000 IU in 1 dose (if other family members or people your child has contact with have pneumonia, give your child 1 dose to prevent pneumonia; if pneumonia is suspected or diagnosed in your child, give him or her 1 dose on the first day of symptoms) |
| Zinc 10 to 20 mg daily |
| **Naturopathic Remedy** |
| Garlic 1 clove, minced, 2 times daily |

*Refer to the appendix at the back of the book for a comprehensive list of interactions and condition-based doses.*

# 81 SUDDEN INFANT DEATH SYNDROME

**COMMON SYMPTOM**

Sudden death while sleeping

Sudden infant death syndrome (SIDS) is the sudden and unexplained death, during sleep, of an apparently healthy infant. It is diagnosed when no other cause for the death can be identified.

SIDS occurs without warning, overturning a family with grief. Ninety percent of these deaths occur in infants who are younger than 6 months old. Most deaths occur in infants 2 to 4 months old. With approximately 2,500 infants dying yearly in the US with no apparent cause, we must do everything possible to prevent this. Since the American Academy of Pediatrics first suggested that infants be put to bed on their backs in 1992, SIDS cases have fallen dramatically—by 50 percent. Follow these guidelines to reduce the risk of SIDS for your infant.

## Prevention

- Place your baby on his or her back to sleep, even for naps. This is the number one way to reduce the risk of SIDS.

- Place the baby to sleep on a firm mattress or other firm surface covered with a fitted sheet. Do not put him or her down on soft surfaces such as pillows, blankets, sofas, and waterbeds.

- Keep soft objects such as toys and loose bedding (blankets, pillows, and so on) out of the sleeping area and away from the baby's face.

- Avoid overheating the baby during sleep. Dress him or her in light sleep clothes and keep the room at a temperature that's comfortable for adults.

- Do not smoke during pregnancy or afterward, or expose the baby to second-hand smoke. All increase the SIDS risk.

- Monitor tummy time. Awake time spent on the abdomen strengthens the head, neck, and shoulder muscles and improves coordination, but someone must be watching at all times.

- Avoid bed sharing. Sleeping in a bed with others—including other children—increases the risk of SIDS, especially in the first 2 or 3 months of life. The crib is the safest place.

- Consider giving a pacifier at sleep time, which may protect against SIDS. Don't force the baby to take it, though, and wait until he or she is 1 month old to use a pacifier if you are breast-feeding. Make sure the pacifier is clean to prevent infections. Use of pacifiers before the age of 5 is unlikely to cause long-term dental or orthodontic problems.

- Consider breast-feeding, which has a protective effect against SIDS. This may be because breast-fed infants can be more easily aroused than formula-fed children, as well as because breast milk prevents some upper respiratory infections that may make SIDS more likely to occur.

- Consult your pediatrician before buying any product that claims to reduce the risk of SIDS. Product testing may not have been done.

- Run a fan in the room when your baby is asleep. It may lower the risk of SIDS.

# Skin

One of the best examples of the power of naturopathic medicine is its effectiveness in treating skin conditions. What does conventional medicine commonly use to treat skin problems? Steroids. Put on some cream, and the skin problem goes away. Stop using the cream, and it may come back. When that happens, are we really curing anything? No, we're just shoving it under the rug, from where it's bound to return someday, instead of curing the problem.

Generally, a skin condition is a sign that something deeper in the body is amiss. When you have a piece of moldy fruit in your kitchen, the problem isn't only on the outside but also deep within the fruit. For example, if you've ever had a drug reaction, your skin may have itched or developed a rash. Drug reactions can also cause a change in skin pigment.

When your child has skin issues, we need to treat the problem that's causing them, so don't be surprised when the natural prescription focuses on treating the intestines and liver.

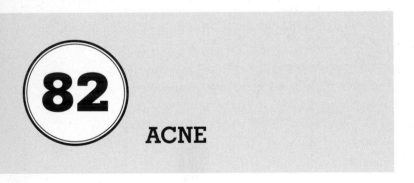

## 82

## ACNE

**COMMON SYMPTOMS**

Anxiety and embarrassment
over physical appearance

Red pustules on the face, back,
neck, shoulders, or chest

Acne is caused by increased production of skin cells in the follicles, which plugs them. Excess production of sebum—a fatty substance the skin secretes for lubrication and protection—is also involved, and often associated with elevated hormone production.

Mark walked into my office after calling to say he had an emergency. When you work with children and young people, you get accustomed to such dramatic pronouncements. The prom was scheduled for the next month, and he needed to get rid of a bad case of acne. Nothing had mattered more in Mark's entire 16 years of life. While acne is a rite of passage for most teenagers, some, like Mark, have it worse than others; it can even be so severe that it causes permanent scars. In fact, acne can make a good-looking young man like Mark feel like a pariah.

I told Mark: As without, so within. He needed to dedicate himself to cleaning his inside, and then his outside would match. I suggested the appropriate diet, some supplements to nourish the skin, and a natural face wash. He vowed to stick with this regimen.

A month later he called me. He had been chosen homecoming king! And it was the happiest night of his life—so far.

The Department of Nutrition at Harvard asked 4,000 teenage boys about their fat-free milk consumption and acne and found that those who drank the most rated their acne as the most severe of all the participants. The same group also looked at the reported diets during high school of more than 47,000 women who had also been diagnosed with severe acne during that time. Acne was most strongly associated with fat-free milk, but also linked to whole and low-fat milk and other dairy products, including instant breakfast drinks, sherbet, cottage cheese, and cream cheese.

Vitamin $B_3$ is one of the best vitamins for the skin when used topically. Research has shown that it is as effective as the antibiotic clindamycin for improving acne. Some patients want to do as much as they can to stop acne, especially to prevent severe scarring. This may include using a pharmaceutical treatment to go along with the natural interventions I suggest here.

## Natural Prescriptions*

| Diet | |
|---|---|
| Adopt a low-glycemic-load diet. | Eliminate other possible triggers (chocolate, nuts, eggs, fried foods, wheat) |
| Avoid dairy products. | Increase fiber. |
| Decrease sugar intake. | |
| **Vitamins/Supplements** | |
| Vitamin A 1,000 to 5,000 IU daily | |
| Vitamin B$_3$ 4 percent niacinamide wash applied topically daily | |
| Zinc 10 mg daily | |
| **Alternative Treatments** | |
| Washing your face with a mild soap and water nightly and after playing sports or sweating is often helpful. | |

*Refer to the appendix at the back of the book for a comprehensive list of interactions and condition-based doses.*

# 83 ALOPECIA (HAIR LOSS)

## COMMON SYMPTOMS

Complete baldness

Partial baldness

Hairs broken close to the roots

Hair loss in young children is rare. When it occurs, it may be patchy or diffuse.

Kids shouldn't be losing hair. If they are, we need to put on our Sherlock Holmes hats and figure out what is causing it. Take a close look at your child's hair. Is there any redness or peeling on the scalp where the hair has fallen out? This can be a sign of a skin infection such as ringworm (which is actually a fungus). Psoriasis can also affect a kid's scalp, so have him or her evaluated if there's a family history of this disorder.

If there's no redness on the scalp, check for short hairs, which may indicate that the child is tearing out his or her hair, a biologically based condition known as trichotillomania that may be related to obsessive-compulsive disorder.

If the hair is thinning, it may be a sign of something internal, such as hypothyroidism or extreme toxicity. Have your child's levels of thyroid hormones and heavy metals evaluated so you can locate the root of the problem.

## Natural Prescriptions*

| Vitamins/Supplements | |
|---|---|
| To stimulate hair growth: Vitamin C 500 to 1,000 mg daily | Vitamin D 1,000 to 4,000 IU daily |
| L-carnitine 500 to 1,000 mg daily | Zinc 20 mg daily |
| **Naturopathic Remedies** | |
| To treat dandruff, which may cause your child to scratch the scalp and break hairs: Selenium sulfide applied topically daily | |
| To treat a fungal infection of the scalp, which can cause hairs to break close to their roots: Tea tree oil, less than 7 percent cineole, applied topically daily for 2 weeks | |

*Refer to the appendix at the back of the book for a comprehensive list of interactions and condition-based doses.*

# 84

## BIRTHMARK

### COMMON SYMPTOMS

No itching or bleeding

No rapid changes in shape or size

Patch of brown, white, or another color on the skin

We're all born with some birthmarks, often known as "beauty marks" on girls. Most are harmless, but some may need to be surgically removed. Let's take a tour to help you identify them.

- **Acne Neonatorum:** This is an acne eruption in infants that rarely needs treatment. Breast-feeding mothers should have their hormone levels and food sensitivities evaluated since they might be contributing to the child's acne.

- **Café-Au-Lait Spot:** These light brown spots are the color of coffee with cream and are harmless.

- **Milia:** Tiny white dots on the cheeks and around the eyes, these are harmless and should be left alone. They are not baby acne.

- **Mole:** Moles are harmless flat, brown dots. Check them periodically, and if they match any of these descriptions, see your dermatologist.
  A. Asymmetry—The two halves different from each other
  B. Border—An irregular, scalloped, or indistinct border
  C. Color—Multiple colors; inconsistent color throughout, with shades of tan, brown, black, red, white, or blue
  D. Diameter—Larger than ¼ inch
  E. Evolving—Change in size, shape, or color or looks different from your other moles

- **Mongolian Spot:** A child may be born with a bluish spot or spots anywhere on the body, but most often it is on the lower back. This birthmark must be documented by your physician; on a trip to the emergency room, someone may mistake the birthmark for evidence that you disciplined your child too severely.

- **Port-Wine Stain:** A reddish, flat stain usually on the face, this is another type of harmless birthmark. However, if your child has this birthmark along with seizures, have him or her evaluated by your neurologist.

- **Strawberry Hemangioma:** Does it look like there's a strawberry or raspberry on your child's skin? These are very common and found in 10 percent of infants. They are not dangerous unless they are on a sensitive part of the body, especially the skin around the eye. They can also be sensitive on the buttocks if it is where a child sits on it. They usually go away within 5 years, and 90 percent of them are gone by age 12. Fish oil and organic berries can help shorten the healing time. Give your child 500 mg of fish oil and ¼ cup of organic berries daily.

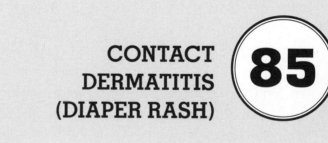

# CONTACT DERMATITIS (DIAPER RASH) 85

## COMMON SYMPTOMS

Localized rash

Pain or itching

Peeling

Diaper rash is a common condition in which inflamed skin appears as a red patchwork in the areas covered by a diaper. A type of contact dermatitis, these eruptions are due to irritants in the diaper or in the groin.

Here is a rundown of some possible causes:

- Common contact dermatitis irritants include vinyl in diapers, fragrances, dyes, plasticizers, bubble bath, harsh laundry soaps, and woolen or rough-weave fabrics.

- The child's own saliva can cause contact dermatitis around the mouth as well as on the hands and feet if the child is sucking on them.

- Certain toothpaste and mouthwash flavorings and additives, such as cinnamic aldehyde, sodium benzoate, and sodium lauryl sulfate, can irritate the mouth area.

- Glues and dyes used in the manufacture of shoes can produce a reaction on the tops of the toes and feet.

- Dyes used in clothing can cause rashes in areas where clothing rubs or where there is increased perspiration.

- Topical medications, such as neomycin ointment, can irritate the skin where they are applied.

- While dermatitis is typically only red, a *Candida* infection that develops because of the diaper rash will occasionally have white scales, and a *Staphylococcus* or other bacterial infection of the area will have pustules and crusty areas. Consult your pediatrician to see if an antifungal or antibiotic medication is needed.

A group of 309 children with minor skin injuries, diaper-area contact dermatitis, or inflamed skin in a limited area were treated with hamamelis ointment or dexpanthenol—vitamin $B_5$—ointment. Physicians and parents saw equal improvements with both ointments.

Everybody knows Preparation H and what it's used for. You may have some in your medicine cabinet, along with a bottle of witch hazel. Did you know they used to be the same? "Hamamelis" is the Latin name for the witch hazel genus of plants. The cream used to be a preparation of hamamelis, which was eventually shortened to Preparation H. Unfortunately, the modern cream includes many synthetic chemicals and no longer contains witch hazel (though the medicated wipes do). The natural stuff works best, so use that on hemorrhoids (but only the external ones).

## Natural Prescriptions*

### Naturopathic Remedies

Use one of these at a time to treat diaper rash, then switch to another if there is no improvement after 2 days.

A&D Ointment applied at every diaper change

Hamamelis ointment applied at every diaper change (pregnant women should avoid hamamelis.)

Honey, olive oil, and beeswax in equal proportions applied at every diaper change

Tocopherol acetate ointment applied at every diaper change

Vitamin B$_5$ (dexpanthenol) ointment applied at every diaper change

### Alternative Remedies

TO PREVENT DIAPER RASH:
1. Remove any irritants.
2. Change wet or soiled diapers right away.
3. Do not rub or scrub the skin; clean the diaper area with water and a soft washcloth or remove the stool by spraying the area with water from a squirt bottle.
4. Apply a thick layer of a protective ointment or cream, such as A&D Ointment.
5. Avoid using wipes that dry the skin.
6. Do not put diapers on too tight, especially overnight.

*Refer to the appendix at the back of the book for a comprehensive list of interactions and condition-based doses.*

# 86 ATOPIC DERMATITIS (ECZEMA)

## COMMON SYMPTOMS

Blistered and red skin

Itchy rash

Occurs first as scales or dry skin, then forms bumps that can grow together in a patch

Scaly skin

Usual occurrence in the elbow or knee folds or on the face

Eczema is an annoying, itchy inflammation of the skin that affects infants and young children alike.

A mother called me, frantic. Her children had eczema, and the creams weren't working anymore. She had been to dermatologists and allergists as well as kinesiologists and even psychics, but no one had been able to stop the itching.

She brought in her three children, and the song "Three Coins in the Fountain" popped into my head. Born one right after another, they sat on my table, boy, girl, boy, the youngest one with bright red hair. They were completely covered with eczema. It was so itchy that they couldn't stop themselves from scratching.

The skin on their feet, hands, arms, and legs was not only red and inflamed, but also had scratch marks and scabs all over from the constant scratching.

It was time to get serious; steroid creams from the dermatologist weren't working anymore. Neither were other creams she had tried. They had switched to all-natural soaps to no avail. Remember, with the skin, as without, so within.

The mother told me, "I feed them organic everything!" But the problem wasn't how the food was produced, it was the food itself.

I analyzed the children's food allergies and food sensitivities and found that they all were extremely allergic to foods, such as carrots and apples, that rarely cause immune reactions. These are usually healthy foods, but they caused skin rashes in these children.

I immediately placed them on an elimination diet based on their lab results. I gave them probiotics, fish oil, and vitamin D—all beneficial for the skin—to heal them from the inside. Within a week, the itching stopped. A week after that, the mother stopped giving them the steroids. A week after that, they looked like healthy kids again—no more rashes, no more itching, no more drugs. When you treat the core of the problem naturopathically, it always works.

A study showed that the infants of 474 pregnant women who had taken a *Lactobacillus* strain probiotic during the last month of pregnancy and until 6 months after childbirth if breast-feeding had a significantly reduced prevalence of eczema at 2 years old compared to those of women who took a placebo. The children also took the probiotic for the first 2 years of their lives.

What the pregnant mother eats is also important. A study of 2,641 2-year-old children revealed that if their mothers ate a lot of margarine and vegetable oils during the last 4 weeks of their pregnancies, their children's risk of eczema was higher than that of the children of mothers who ate a lot of fish.

To treat eczema, we combine gastrointestinal rehabilitation with nutrient supplementation. Note that children who have eczema often develop asthma or allergic rhinitis.

## Natural Prescriptions*

| Diet |
| --- |
| Anti-inflammatory diet (for breast-feeding mothers; vegetables, fruits, whole grains, and lean meats) |
| Hypoallergenic diet (avoid food additives and preservatives; eliminate sugar; emphasize fish and foods containing zinc, vitamins A, B, D, and E, and selenium) |
| **Vitamins/Supplements** |
| Fish oil EPA + DHA 1,000 to 4,000 mg daily |
| Probiotics 5 to 10 billion CFU daily (combination of *Lactobacillus* and *Bifidus* strains works best) |
| Vitamin D 1,000 to 4,000 IU daily |
| Zinc 10 to 20 mg daily |

* Refer to the appendix at the back of the book for a comprehensive list of interactions and condition-based doses.

# IMPETIGO

## COMMON SYMPTOMS

Honey-colored crusty patches on the skin

Possible itching

Rash

Impetigo is the most prevalent of all the pediatric bacterial skin infections, especially in children between the ages of 2 and 7, and it can spread quickly through families and schools. Staph or strep bacteria get into a little cut or abrasion and cause red lesions to develop on and around the mouth. These sores rupture, ooze, and then form a yellowish crust.

Impetigo is highly contagious, so physical contact with a sore must be kept to a minimum, and hands should be regularly washed.

Jimmy's mouth hurt. He was so embarrassed about how he looked that he didn't want to go to school. Yellow crusts oozing fluid were all around his lips. It hurt to touch them and when he moved his mouth.

He was allergic to most prescription antibiotics, so his mother wanted a naturopathic answer. Herbs are extremely powerful natural antibiotics. I put together a formulation of herbs that research has shown kills staph and strep. Methicillin-resistant *Staphylococcus aureus,* an antibiotic-resistant strain of bacteria, has been destroyed by garlic in laboratory tests.

Jimmy came back the next week and his impetigo was completely healed. He was so happy to be able to show his face again at school, and his mother was happy that he didn't have an allergic reaction to another antibiotic.

## Natural Prescriptions*

| Naturopathic Remedies |
| --- |
| Cinnamon oil applied topically 2 times daily |
| Garlic 1 or 2 cloves, minced, daily |
| Licorice (*Glycyrrhiza*) applied topically 2 times daily |
| St. John's wort (*Hypericum*) applied topically 2 times daily |

| Homeopathic Remedies |
| --- |
| Homeopathic Staphylococcinum 200C, 5 pellets in 1 dose |
| Homeopathic Streptococcinum 200C, 5 pellets in 1 dose |

*\* Refer to the appendix at the back of the book for a comprehensive list of interactions and condition-based doses.*

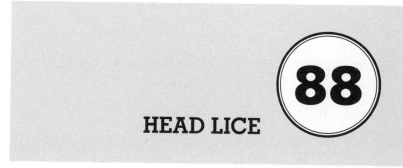

# HEAD LICE 88

## COMMON SYMPTOM

Itchy scalp, eyebrows,
and/or eyelashes

Head lice are parasitic insects that infest the scalp and, less commonly, the eyebrows and eyelashes. Nits are lice eggs that usually line the hair shaft about a quarter inch from the scalp.

Lice are spread by head-to-head contact and by shared items such as hats, scarves, brushes, towels, bedclothes, and headphones. Personal hygiene is not a factor in whether or not someone gets lice.

The easiest way to get rid of lice is to shave the child's head, and many parents do that in the summer. Without hair, there's no place for the insects to live. But if it's cold or you don't want to give your child a crew cut, there are a multitude of natural medicines that you can wash his or her hair with that will kill the insects.

## Natural Prescriptions*

| Naturopathic Remedies |
|---|
| Wash one of these undiluted fluids into the hair for a week, then change to another. Do not use them in children under the age of 10. Be careful not to get any oil into your child's eyes because it could harm them. |
|    Citronella oil 10 drops applied topically for 5 minutes daily |
|    Coconut oil 10 drops applied topically for 5 minutes daily |
|    Eucalyptus oil 10 drops applied topically for 5 minutes daily |
|    Lavender oil 10 drops applied topically for 5 minutes daily |
|    Noni, fresh fruit or bottled juice, ¼ cup applied topically for 5 minutes daily |
|    Tea tree oil, less than 7 percent cineole, applied topically for 5 minutes daily |

*Refer to the appendix at the back of the book for a comprehensive list of interactions and condition-based doses.*

# 89

# PSORIASIS

## COMMON SYMPTOM

Thick, scaly, itchy skin patches,
   usually on the elbows,
      knees, and scalp

Psoriasis is a common chronic inflammatory skin disease that is caused by an overactive type of white blood cell that attacks the skin. This spurs rapid production of new skin cells, so the dead skin builds up in thick, red patches with silvery scales that are often dry and painful.

Psoriasis has a strong genetic link. If one parent has it, his or her children have a 17 percent chance of having it, too. If both parents have it, their children's chances of developing it rise to 50 percent.

The rough plaques of psoriasis usually form on the elbows and knees on the outside of the bend. Don't confuse this with eczema, which appears on the backs of the knees and the fronts of the elbows, inside the bend.

In younger children, psoriasis may grow only on the scalp. Some kids with psoriasis are very sensitive to gluten, and in my practice I have seen such children improve after a year of not eating any products made with wheat, barley, or rye, including breads, bagels, cookies, crackers, pasta, pizza, and cereals. Celiac disease has no obvious symptoms in some affected children, but if the inflammation from the gluten intolerance is stopped, psoriasis may go into remission.

The best naturopathic therapy to treat a flare-up is a combination of vitamin D cream and, if the child is gluten-sensitive, a gluten-free diet; these should be tried before other remedies.

## Natural Prescriptions*

| Diet | |
|---|---|
| Gluten-free diet | |
| **Vitamins/Supplements** | |
| Fish oil EPA + DHA 1 to 2 g daily | Vitamin D cream 0.005 percent applied topically 3 times a day |
| Vitamin A 1,000 to 4,000 IU daily | |
| **Naturopathic Remedies** | |
| *Aloe vera* gel applied topically 3 times daily | |
| Oregon grape root (*Mahonia aquifolium*) 10 percent cream, applied topically 3 times daily | |

* Refer to the appendix at the back of the book for a comprehensive list of interactions and condition-based doses.

# 90 SEBORRHEIC DERMATITIS (CRADLE CAP)

## COMMON SYMPTOM

Crusted and oily yellow
scales on the scalp

Though not serious, cradle cap can cause thick crusting and yellow or white scales on the scalp or face. It is an inflammatory condition with an unknown cause, but it may involve the immune system reacting abnormally to a type of yeast growing in the sebum (natural oils) in the skin. It usually occurs in children under the age of 3.

You've probably seen a young child with this condition: His or her scalp and possibly the forehead has greasy, rough scaling that almost looks like a cap. This can be confused with psoriasis or a fungal infection, so make sure you get it diagnosed by your pediatrician. If it is cradle cap, naturopathic medicines will help clear it up quickly.

## Natural Prescriptions*

| Vitamins/Supplements | |
|---|---|
| Mineral oil applied topically daily | Selenium sulfide applied topically daily |
| **Homeopathic Remedies** | |
| Homeopathic Calc Carb 30C, 1 to 3 times daily | |
| **Alternative Treatments** | |
| Gentle brushing of the scalp 2 times daily | |

* Refer to the appendix at the back of the book for a comprehensive list of interactions and condition-based doses.

# TINEA (RINGWORM, ATHLETE'S FOOT, JOCK ITCH)

## 91

## COMMON SYMPTOMS

Patchy discoloration and scaling, usually in a ring pattern

Peeling skin

Yellow toenails

Tinea is a fungal infection that appears as circular red patches and other discolorations and is often itchy. It is common in young children and usually is called ringworm. Where on the body it occurs determines what specific type of tinea it is. Two very common examples are jock itch (tinea cruris), which occurs in the groin, and athlete's foot (tinea pedis), which affects the feet, especially between the toes.

Charlie came into my office with white, scaly circles all over his chest. His mother said the dermatologist had diagnosed him with eczema and given him steroids. But the creams weren't working. Was there a naturopathic prescription for eczema I could give them?

I told Charlie's mother that there were plenty of great natural medicines, but he had ringworm, not eczema.

"Ringworm? That's a fungus! How did he get a fungus?"

I told her that eczema and ringworm look very similar and patients commonly confuse them, but most health care providers can tell the difference quite easily, either by looking at it or doing a skin scraping. In different locations on the body, tinea looks slightly different. Ringworm lesions look like circles or ovals of scaling skin overlaying red circles. Athlete's foot causes cracking and peeling and discolored toenails. Jock itch also brings on red, peeling skin. Natural remedies can quickly and effectively kill the fungus without side effects.

## Natural Prescriptions*

| Naturopathic Remedies |
|---|
| Apply one of these to the affected area for a week, then switch to another one.<br>1. Garlic gel applied topically 2 times daily<br>2. Tea tree salve applied topically 2 times daily<br>3. Honey, olive oil, and beeswax mixed in equal proportions and applied topically 2 times daily |
| **Alternative Treatments** |
| Debridement, a medical procedure in which dead, damaged, and infected tissues are removed, is used to improve the healing potential of the surrounding tissues. In the case of tinea, debridement of the affected epidermal tissue (the outer layer of the skin) allows topical remedies greater contact with the area and reduces treatment time. |

*\* Refer to the appendix at the back of the book for a comprehensive list of interactions and condition-based doses.*

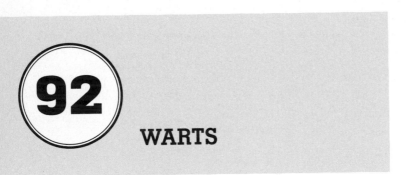

## 92

# WARTS

## COMMON SYMPTOM

Rough growths on or
in the hands or feet

Warts are small, rough, mainly painless skin growths that are generally harmless.

Warts appear on most children at some time in their lives. On most of the body, including the hands, they usually look like little cauliflowers growing up off the skin. The bottoms of the feet, however, grow warts of a different kind that are usually flat and grow inward instead of outward. If you look closely at either kind of wart, you can see that it is pushing the ridges of the fingerprint or footprint to the sides. This characteristic is what differentiates a wart from the similar-looking corn and callus.

Warts are caused by viruses (human papillomavirus, or HPV, and others) that live in the skin. Getting rid of the virus is easy with naturopathic prescriptions. Try applying duct tape over a wart every night before bed. In my practice, I've seen them go away within a month in children who have done this. You can also make a paste by dissolving an aspirin in a few drops of water, applying it to the wart, and covering it with a bandage twice daily. Among the standard conventional remedies is freezing the wart (called cryotherapy).

In a testament of the power of mind over matter, you can "buy" warts from children who are about 4 to 7 years old. Give your child a quarter and tell him he has to give you the wart while he's sleeping. Though it will seem quite magical when the wart disappears, it really just proves the power of the immune system and our subconscious control of it.

Use one of these remedies at a time to judge its effectiveness; if it doesn't seem to be working after a week or so, try a different one. When you find one that works, keep using it until the wart is gone.

## Natural Prescriptions*

| Vitamins/Supplements |
| --- |
| Vitamin B$_{12}$ 100 mcg injected into the wart (consult your naturopathic physician) |
| Vitamin D 0.005 percent lotion applied topically nightly |
| **Naturopathic Remedies** |
| Garlic gel applied topically nightly |
| Green tea 15 percent kunecatechins ointment applied topically nightly |
| Tea tree oil, less than 7 percent cineole, applied topically nightly |
| **Alternative Treatments** |
| Duct tape applied nightly. Do not use topical lotions and gels in conjunction with duct tape therapy. |

*Refer to the appendix at the back of the book for a comprehensive list of interactions and condition-based doses.*

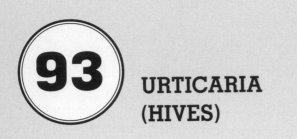

# 93

# URTICARIA (HIVES)

**COMMON SYMPTOM**

Red or white itchy patches

Hives often appear instantly when a child encounters an allergen. They commonly occur around the mouth when the allergen is eaten and can spread to other parts of the body. Hives vary in size from a small circle to multiple joined lesions the size of a plate. The allergens that most commonly cause hives are foods such as nuts (especially peanuts), chocolate, tomatoes, and milk; any medications, but especially antibiotics; and herbs. In some people, even cold or sunlight can cause hives.

Hives can be dangerous if the allergic reaction causes a swelling of the throat, wheezing, or breathing trouble. If this happens, use an EpiPen of epinephrine; administer antihistamines; and go to the emergency room. Antihistamines and cortisone are usually given in milder, nonemergency cases of hives, but naturopathic remedies work well.

## Natural Prescriptions*

| Vitamins/Supplements | |
|---|---|
| Quercetin 500 mg divided into 2 or 3 doses daily | |
| **Naturopathic Remedies** | |
| *Aloe vera* gel applied topically as needed | |
| **Homeopathic Remedies** | |
| Homeopathic Apis 30C, Homeopathic Histaminum 30C, and Homeopathic Urtica 30C | 5 pellets 3 times daily each |
| **Alternative Treatments** | |
| Oatmeal strained water and cornstarch, 1:1 ratio, applied topically—To make the oatmeal water, prepare very watery oatmeal, let stand for 2 hours, then strain out the oats. | |

* Refer to the appendix at the back of the book for a comprehensive list of interactions and condition-based doses.

Painful menstrual periods and urinary tract infections (UTIs) in children can be difficult for parents to handle. They seem like adult disorders, and suddenly they are happening to your kids!

While UTIs are relatively rare in children, abnormal menses are becoming increasingly common, possibly due to the endocrine-disrupting chemicals in our foods and environment. I've seen girls who got their periods at the age of 9! Naturopathic prescriptions are ideal for those families who want to avoid putting their daughters on birth control pills to control hormones.

# ENURESIS (BED-WETTING)

## COMMON SYMPTOM

Urinary incontinence, usually at night

Nighttime incontinence, or bed-wetting, is so common that it is rarely a concern unless it is still occurring when the child is 5 or older. Conditions that predispose a child to bed-wetting include diabetes, constipation, cystitis, urethral obstruction, hyperthyroidism, and stress.

Charlie was turning 10 years old that weekend, and he wanted to have a big birthday party with all of his friends. His mom wanted him to have a sleepover, but Charlie had hated them ever since he had started wetting the bed at night.

It had started a couple of years before. Anytime he got stressed, he'd wet the bed. If his friends came over, he was so fearful of wetting the bed that all the stress would make it happen.

Charlie's mom brought him in to find an answer because he was unable to hang out with his friends overnight. No sleepovers, no camping.

Bed-wetting in older children who have been potty trained can occur for several different reasons, but it shouldn't be a concern unless they're older than 5. Sometimes inflammation from food allergies and food sensitivities can cause a child to wet the bed.

One study involved 21 children who had, in addition to enuresis, food-induced migraine or hyperkinetic behavior disorder that responded to a change to a simple diet of only specific, limited meats, vegetables, and fruits. The bed-wetting stopped in 12 of these children, and it improved in 4 others. In 8 of the 12 and in the 4 who improved, one or more food triggers for the enuresis could be identified.

Other children have an imbalance in their nervous systems that prevents the bladder from holding the urine. Eliminating triggers in food-sensitive children and correcting the nervous system imbalance with the amino acid phenylalanine usually will help stop the bed-wetting, and it helped Charlie, too. He came back to see me a few weeks later with a smile on his face. He'd recently had six friends over for a sleepover. He'd been able to stay up late and join in the festivities without worrying about bed-wetting.

## Natural Prescriptions*

| Diet |
| --- |
| Oligoantigenic diet (including only fish, turkey, vegetables, fruits, and rice) |
| **Vitamins/Supplements** |
| Tryptophan 500 mg daily |
| **Homeopathic Remedies** |
| Homotoxicology: Detoxifying homeopathic remedies combined in a treatment known as homotoxicology were found in one study to be superior to placebo, though much less effective than treatment with desmopressin (dDAVP). Look for these combination detoxifying remedies from your homeopathic remedy source. |

* Refer to the appendix at the back of the book for a comprehensive list of interactions and condition-based doses.

# PREMENSTRUAL SYNDROME

## COMMON SYMPTOMS

| | |
|---|---|
| Abdominal cramps | Mood swings |
| Diarrhea | Nausea |
| Headache | |

Patty stormed into the office ahead of her mother. "I don't want to! How many times do I have to tell you!"

Patty's mother was obviously embarrassed by her daughter's behavior. She went on to explain that Patty had started her period about a year before and her premenstrual symptoms had grown increasingly worse. They had started calling her "PMS Patty." She was irritable and had horrible headaches and pelvic pain.

I reassured Patty that many women, both young and old, have these symptoms before their periods. These symptoms, which in severe cases is called premenstrual dysphoric disorder, can range from mood swings, headaches, and pain to weight gain, breast tenderness, acne, muscle pain, and severe depression. Dull or throbbing cramps that often occur just before or during menstruation are often caused by poor diet.

I told Patty that we are what we eat, and that she needed to change her diet to change who she was inside. Of course, the most important meal of the day is breakfast. Caffeine and alcohol should be avoided too, because they worsen symptoms. I told Patty that the more vegetarian foods she ate, including soy products, before her period, the better. These would improve her mood and pain. I gave her some fish oil and B vitamins as well.

When Patty and her mother came back a few months later, her mother was ecstatic. "You turned my PMS Patty into Princess Patty. Thank you!"

## Natural Prescriptions*

| Diet | |
|---|---|
| Eat breakfast; avoid alcohol and caffeine; eat soy foods. | |
| **Vitamins/Supplements** | |
| Calcium 800 to 2,000 mg daily | Vitamin B₁ 100 mg daily |
| Fish oil EPA + DHA 2 to 4 g daily | Vitamin B₆ 20 to 40 mg daily |
| Magnesium 100 to 200 mg daily | Vitamin D 1,000 to 4,000 IU daily |
| **Naturopathic Remedies** | |
| Fennel extract, liquid, 30 drops 2 times daily | |
| *Ginkgo biloba* leaf extract, 50:1 ratio, 24 percent ginkgo heterosides, 6 percent terpene lactones, 80 mg daily | |
| Saffron 60 mg daily | |
| Valerian root, 0.8 percent valerinic acid, 250 mg daily | |
| *Vitex* (chasteberry) fruit, 5 percent vitexin, 20 to 40 mg daily | |

*\* Refer to the appendix at the back of the book for a comprehensive list of interactions and condition-based doses.*

# 96

# MENORRHAGIA (ABNORMAL PERIODS)

## COMMON SYMPTOM

Short or long menstrual periods

Our world is filled with toxic endocrine disruptors such as xenoestrogens (environmental substances that either do the same things as or block the activities of natural estrogen) such as DDT, polychlorinated biphenyls (PCBs), bisphenol A, and phthalates.

Although there are other possible causes for girls' periods becoming heavier, lasting for longer, and beginning earlier than ever, in today's toxic society, endocrine disruptors very well may be playing a role. A typical cycle lasts between 21 and 35 days and includes 3 to 5 days of bleeding, but adolescent girls' cycles can be up to 45 days long. If your daughter's cycle is shorter or longer than the typical range or she has spotting between periods, talk to your pediatrician.

The conventional response to these symptoms is either to wait (many symptoms or abnormal cycles spontaneously resolve as girls get older) or to give birth control pills to control the hormones driving menstruation. Some new birth control pills result in only four—or even no—periods a year. While that may seem beneficial, in my opinion, this is not what nature intended. Our bodies were built and adapted to be the way they are for a reason. Trying to go against nature only leads to problems.

A pediatric gynecologist, family doctor, nurse practitioner, or physician's assistant should evaluate any girl who is having abnormal bleeding. However, if nothing wrong is discovered, natural remedies can bring balance to an abnormal cycle.

## Natural Prescriptions*

| Diet |
| --- |
| SEED ROTATION: <br><br> Certain seeds have beneficial oils and fibers that act similarly to hormones. While they do not contain any hormones, they have wonderful effects on the uterus and ovaries. The seeds must be ground and eaten fresh daily. They taste quite good on salads, in oatmeal, and in rice and quinoa. The grinding is necessary because our bodies cannot digest tiny seeds like flaxseeds and sesame seeds. <br><br> I have seen this seed rotation perform miracles. It has balanced abnormal periods, stopped spotting, and cured infertility in women who were trying to become pregnant. |
| First 2 weeks of a menstrual cycle (from the first day of bleeding to ovulation): <br> 1 Tbsp flaxseeds and 1 Tbsp pumpkin seeds |
| Second 2 weeks of a menstrual cycle (from ovulation to the first day of bleeding): <br> 1 Tbsp sesame seeds and 1 Tbsp sunflower seeds |

| Vitamins/Supplements | |
| --- | --- |
| Fish oil EPA + DHA 2 to 4 g daily | Pycnogenol 50 mg daily |

| Naturopathic Remedies |
| --- |
| *Vitex* (chasteberry) fruit, 5 percent vitexin, 20 to 40 mg daily |

* Refer to the appendix at the back of the book for a comprehensive list of interactions and condition-based doses.

# 97 URINARY TRACT INFECTION

## COMMON SYMPTOMS

Burning pain with urination

Fever, poor appetite, vomiting, or no symptoms in young children

Suddenly needing to run to the bathroom

Urinating small amounts, but more frequently

A urinary tract infection (UTI) is commonly caused by the bacterial strain *Escherichia coli*. The urinary system includes the kidneys, ureters, bladder, and urethra. A UTI can be serious if the kidneys become involved. UTIs are more common in women than men, and few children get them: only 8 percent of girls and 2 percent of boys will have one during childhood.

A child may have symptoms similar to those of a UTI if he or she gets an irritant, such as soap during a bath, in the urethra. Other children have vesicoureteral reflux, which is caused by a faulty valve between the ureter and the bladder. The valve lets urine flow backward from the bladder into the ureter and then to the kidney, where bacteria can grow in the retained urine. Other children get bacterial UTIs from sexual abuse. If your child has a UTI, talk to your pediatrician and discover the cause.

Most UTIs are treated effectively with antibiotics, but we can also treat them naturally in conjunction with conventional therapies and prevent future ones with simple remedies.

The best food for preventing UTIs is cranberries. I tell parents to get a bag of frozen cranberries and cook them in some water to make their own juice. Many cranberry juices sold in stores are diluted with other juices or have added sugar, which makes a UTI worse. Cranberry is also available as a supplement called D-mannose.

If your child is older and having intercourse, it is common for a UTI to occur with a new partner. Children who are having intercourse and have recurrent UTIs probably have a partner who is infected. Male sexual partners are normally asymptomatic carriers, and they must also be tested and treated if there is a history of UTI after intercourse. Because the symptoms of a UTI are the same as those of some sexually transmitted infections (STIs), sexually active children who are having symptoms should be tested for STIs as well as for bacteria in the urine.

## Natural Prescriptions*

| Diet | |
|---|---|
| Drink fresh juices, especially berry juices. | Consume fermented dairy products. |
| **Vitamins/Supplements** | |
| D-mannose 500 to 2,000 mg daily | *Lactobacillus* 100 billion CFU in 1 dose |
| **Naturopathic Remedies** | |
| Cranberry juice extract 100 mg 3 times daily | *Saccharomyces boulardii* 5 billion CFU daily |

*\* Refer to the appendix at the back of the book for a comprehensive list of interactions and condition-based doses.*

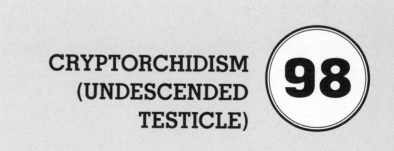

# CRYPTORCHIDISM (UNDESCENDED TESTICLE)

# 98

Was your son born with one or both testicles not in the scrotum? When a child is in the womb, the testicles grow inside the body, in almost the same place as the ovaries. Typically, they eventually drop down into the scrotum, but in some boys, they don't.

Your pediatrician should check your son's testicles during routine physical exams. They are tiny and feel like frozen peas when boys are young. Be gentle when feeling them, and make sure the room and your hands are warm.

A child with undescended testicles needs surgery to have it corrected. This can reduce the risk of infertility and cancer that is associated with this condition if it is not surgically corrected.

## Natural Prescriptions*

| Vitamins/Supplements | |
| --- | --- |
| Vitamin A 400 to 1,000 IU daily | Vitamin D 1,000 to 4,000 IU |

*Refer to the appendix at the back of the book for a comprehensive list of interactions and condition-based doses.*

## OBESITY  99

### COMMON SYMPTOMS

Breathlessness                        High body mass index

Difficulty doing daily activities     Lethargy

Childhood obesity is one of our nation's biggest health problems. The Centers for Disease Control and Prevention (CDC) states that 20 percent of US children ages 6 to 11 were obese in 2008. In the same year, 18 percent of kids ages 12 to 19 were obese. And obesity is now appearing earlier in life, affecting 10 percent of children ages 2 to 5. We have some of the largest children in the industrialized world.

Your child's body mass index (BMI) indicates whether he or she is overweight for his or her age and height. Your pediatrician can measure the BMI, or you can calculate it yourself at http://apps.nccd.cdc.gov/dnpabmi. Using the BMI and a growth chart, your doctor will determine your child's percentile—how he or she compares with other children of the same sex and age. For example, you might be told that your child is in the 80th percentile. This means that 80 percent of children of the same sex and age have lower BMIs. The CDC and considers children between the 85th and 94th percentiles overweight and children at or above the 95th percentile obese. However, BMI testing may not be 100 percent accurate, so talk to your naturopathic physician about your child's weight.

Obesity leads to heart disease, high cholesterol, gallstones, type 2 diabetes, high blood pressure, liver disease, and joint problems, not to mention social problems such as teasing and bullying, weight discrimination, and depression resulting from a negative body image.

As a parent, you are the answer. You must teach your children to eat healthfully by serving healthy foods at home. You need to exercise with them. You must be the example for them to follow. As the parent, your child looks to you and follows in your footsteps. Be the person you want your children to grow up and become.

If your child is overweight or obese, do *not* put him or her on a diet. Instead, serve healthy foods and an appropriate number of calories for the child's age, and let the child grow into the weight. It's important to teach children the habits of healthy eating that they should practice throughout life rather than introduce them to the habits of dieting and bingeing. Talk to your naturopathic physician about nutritional guidance and dietary planning. Also make sure to encourage daily exercise.

## Natural Prescriptions*

| Vitamins/Supplements | |
|---|---|
| Fish oil (with high DHA) 1 to 2 g daily | Pycnogenol 50 to 150 mg daily |
| Psyllium 6 g daily | Vitamin B$_3$ (niacin) 10 to 20 mg daily |
| **Naturopathic Remedies** | |
| Green tea (decaffeinated) 1 to 3 cups daily | Plant sterols 1.5 to 2.3 g daily |

*\* Refer to the appendix at the back of the book for a comprehensive list of interactions and condition-based doses.*

# FAILURE TO THRIVE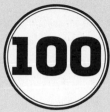

## COMMON SYMPTOMS

Delayed development of secondary sexual characteristics in adolescents

Delayed mental and social skills

Delayed physical skills (rolling over, sitting, standing, walking)

Height, weight, and head circumference below normal

This condition is diagnosed when a child fails to achieve the expected standards of growth.

Some children do not grow rapidly enough, and if they are 20 percent below the ideal weight for their height, they are diagnosed as having failure to thrive. Children should be checked by their pediatricians at the following ages to ensure that they are still developing: 1 month, 2 months, 4 months, 6 months, 9 months, 12 months, 15 months, 18 months, 24 months, 30 months, and 36 months, and then once a year.

If a child is not growing, it may be due to one of these reasons:

A serious health problem

Poor digestion and absorption

Poor metabolism

Poor nutrition

Some children may not be getting enough nutrients. If a breast-feeding mother has certain health problems or malnutrition, the child will not receive sufficient nutrition in the breast milk. Some parents may water down formula to make it last longer, and their infants will not grow quickly enough. Teenagers who are bulimic or anorexic can become so underweight that they fail to thrive.

Some children have a gastrointestinal disease, such as celiac disease or cystic fibrosis, that prevents them from absorbing enough calories and nutrients to grow, even if they're eating adequate food. The food goes in one end and out the other, and if your child is not growing and has smelly stools, ask your pediatrician to evaluate him or her.

Another cause of failure to thrive is a problem with metabolism, especially in cases of hyperthyroidism and some rare conditions. These children eat enough nutrients and calories and have adequate intestinal absorption, but either can't convert the calories into energy or burn them too quickly. Have a pediatric specialist diagnose and treat your child.

## Natural Prescriptions*

| Diet |
| --- |
| Avoid gluten if your child is sensitive to it. Have your naturopathic physician test your child for food sensitivities and allergies and recommend a dietary plan. |
| **Vitamins/Supplements** |
| Glutamine 250 mg/kg (2,500 mg for every 22 pounds) daily |
| Probiotics 10 to 20 billion CFU |

*Refer to the appendix at the back of the book for a comprehensive list of interactions and condition-based doses.*

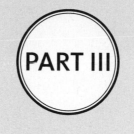

PART III

# BODY SYSTEM REMEDIES

# 5

# KEY FOODS AND NATUROPATHIC REMEDIES

**IF I COULD CREATE A WORLD ENTIRELY** from my imagination, it would be a utopia: birds singing, days of endless sunshine, and children running around happy and healthy. They would go to school, play with their friends, eat dinner with their families, and grow up to fulfill their purpose in life, helping others by creating, serving, entertaining, building a family—whatever brings joy to their hearts. In this world, no one would be chronically ill. A cold during the winter, a sniffle in the spring, but no children taking medicine for a lifetime.

Of course, we don't live in this world, but the reality is that we can live in it. Many of the diseases and conditions that affect adults today result entirely from choices made when they were younger about diet and physical activity level. We can help prevent heart disease, cancer, and other leading killers in adults by teaching our children healthy habits. The temptations of sugar, fat, and relaxing in front of our 42-inch LCD televisions are strong. Realize that your children will imitate what they see you do in the first 7 years of their lives. Together, we can change the world, one child at a time.

## Cardiovascular Recommendations

Most children with cardiovascular disease have a genetic condition or anatomical abnormality. However, with the increase in childhood obesity, more children have high blood pressure and high cholesterol than ever before, which can lead to an earlier onset of heart disease, perhaps even in early adulthood. There are a multitude of health conditions that can cause abnormal cholesterol and blood pressure in young people, so have your child evaluated by your pediatrician. If your child is overweight or obese, do not put him or her on a low-calorie diet. Start a healthy diet that provides an appropriate number of calories for the child's age. If you increase exercise, supplement appropriately, and visit a naturopathic physician who specializes in pediatrics, your child can become healthier for life.

| Diet |
| --- |
| MEDITERRANEAN DIET: |
| Fruits: 2 servings daily, plus more for snacks |
|     Apples, pears, and bananas daily |
| Low-fat protein (chicken, turkey, fish, nuts, or beans): Serve with every meal, especially breakfast. |
| Vegetables: 2 servings with every meal; steamed and dipped in extra virgin olive oil after cooking |
|     Cook with garlic and onions. |
| Whole grains: 1–2 servings daily |
|     Brown rice, quinoa, steel cut oats |
|     Avoid white-flour products, such as white bread, white-flour pasta, cookies, crackers, bagels. |
| Beverages |
|     Decaffeinated green tea—1 to 2 cups daily; steep in the sun ahead of time and refrigerate for iced green tea; sweeten with the amino acid glycine instead of sugar |
| **Vitamins/Supplements** |
| Arginine 750 mg daily |
| Coenzyme Q10 (CoQ10) 10 mg daily (for every 10 pounds of body weight) |
| Fish oil (mostly as docosahexaenoic acid [DHA]) 1 to 2 g daily |
| Folic acid 200 mcg daily |
| Magnesium 100 to 200 mg daily |

| |
|---|
| Psyllium 6 g daily (drink plenty of water with fiber) |
| Pycnogenol 50 to 100 mg daily |
| Vitamin $B_3$ (niacin) 2 to 30 mg daily (primarily for children with high cholesterol) |
| Vitamin $B_{12}$ 10 to 100 mcg daily |
| Vitamin E 200 to 400 IU daily |

# Eyes, Ears, Nose, and Throat Recommendations

Most conditions of the eyes, ears, nose, and throat in children are acute infections. The majority of these infections are viral and better treated with naturopathic remedies, but other conditions can be dangerous and should be treated with antibiotics. Ideally, your child's health should be safeguarded by a team of health care practitioners, including specialists in conventional medical treatment, surgery, and natural medicine, because the integrative approach permits using the treatment that is most appropriate.

| Diet |
|---|
| When a child is acutely ill and has a poor appetite, don't force him or her to eat, but make sure hydration is adequate. |
| Low-fat protein |
| Avoid cow's milk products (milk, cheese, yogurt, ice cream). |
| Vegetables |
|     Make homemade vegetable soups. |
|     Encourage eating garlic and onions, which have antimicrobial properties. |
| Fruits |
|     Puree in a blender or juicer for a tasty boost of antioxidants and vitamin C. |
| Whole grains |
| Beverages |
|     Avoid milk. |

| | |
|---|---|
| Drink plenty of water and hot tea. | |
| Drink echinacea and elderberry tea to stimulate the immune system. | |
| **Vitamins/Supplements** | |
| Bromelain 200 to 400 mg daily | |
| Fish oil (mostly eicosapentaenoic acid [EPA]) 1 to 4 g daily (more effective than DHA as an anti-inflammatory) | |
| NAC 100 to 600 mg daily | |
| Probiotics 10 billion CFU daily | |
| Vitamin A 100,000 IU in 1 dose | |
| Vitamin C 500 to 1,000 mg daily | |
| Vitamin D 1,000 to 4,000 IU daily | |
| Vitamin E 100 to 400 IU daily | |
| Zinc 10 to 20 mg daily | |
| **Naturopathic Remedies** | |
| Astragalus 100 to 500 mg daily | |
| *Echinacea purpurea* tincture, 1:2.5 ratio, 30 drops 2 times daily (for infections) | |
| Elderberry glycerite, 1:4 ratio, 30 drops 3 times daily (for infections) | |
| *Euphrasia* (Eyebright) 3X eyedrops daily (for eye infections) | |
| Garlic and mullein in olive oil eardrops daily (for ear conditions) | |
| Stinging nettle leaf (*Urtica*) 100 to 500 mg daily (for allergies) | |
| **Homeopathic Remedies** | |
| Homeopathic Arnica 30C + Homeopathic Phosphorus, 5 pellets of each every 2 hours for a nosebleed until it stops | |

# Gastrointestinal Recommendations

Problems with digestion are the second most prevalent types of conditions that I treat in children. Treatment of gastrointestinal (GI) conditions revolves around food more than that for any other condition. Since children are genetically and constitutionally different from each other, they all need different diets to be healthy. Some children shouldn't have dairy, while others should avoid gluten, soy, peanuts, or other items. If a child is having a gastrointestinal problem, test for food IgE allergies and food IgG sensitivities, or go through a modified elimination diet instead to identify the offending foods. This is another area where naturopathic remedies cure the disease, rather than merely masking symptoms.

| Diet |
| --- |
| Low-fat protein |
|    Lean meats |
|    Soy can cause problems in some children. |
|    Check food sensitivities and food allergies. |
| Vegetables: 3 servings per meal |
|    Fiber improves stomach pain and bowel function. |
|    Apple cider vinegar on vegetables stimulates digestion. |
|    Cabbage juice can be used to treat ulcers and ulcerative colitis. |
| Fruits |
|    Eat well-tolerated fruits daily. |
|    Bananas can constipate. |
|    Prunes can cause loose stools. |
|    Pineapples and papayas have natural digestive enzymes. |
| Whole grains |
|    Oatmeal made with steel cut oats and the herb slippery elm can soothe the stomach. |
|    Avoid wheat if your child is IgE or IgG reactive to it. |
| Beverages |
|    Avoid milk if your child is IgE or IgG reactive to it. |
|    Chamomile tea |

| Vitamins/Supplements |
| --- |
| Berberine 200 mg daily (for infectious diarrhea) |
| Butyrate 4 g daily |
| Calcium 500 to 1,000 mg daily (for diarrhea) |
| Digestive enzymes 1 or 2 capsules with each meal |
| Fish oil EPA + DHA 1 to 4 g daily |
| Glutamine 500 mg one to three times daily |
| L-carnitine 500 to 1,000 mg daily |
| Magnesium 100 to 200 mg daily (for constipation) |
| Melatonin 0.5 to 1.5 mg before bedtime (for gastrointestinal reflux disease) |
| Probiotics 10 to 20 billion CFU daily |
| Vitamin D 1,000 to 4,000 IU daily |
| Zinc 10 to 20 mg daily (for infectious diarrhea) |

| Naturopathic Remedies |
| --- |
| Castor oil rubbed clockwise on the belly before bedtime (for constipation) |
| Chamomile tea 3 cups daily |
| Deglycyrrhized licorice (DGL) daily—Determine the appropriate dose for your child by adjusting the recommended adult dose, found on the packaging. The recommended adult dosage of an herb is usually calculated for a 150-pound adult. Therefore, if your child weighs 50 pounds, give him or her $1/3$ of the adult dosage. Talk to your physician before giving your child licorice for more than 1 day. Never give licorice to an infant or toddler. |
| Fennel tea $1/4$ cup 3 times daily (for colic) |
| Olive leaf 200 mg daily (for infectious diarrhea) |

| Homeopathic Remedies |
| --- |
| Give your child one of these remedies for a week and if the symptoms don't improve, try a different one for a week.<br><br>1. Homeopathic Lycopodium 30C, 5 pellets daily<br>2. Homeopathic Arsenicum 30C, 5 pellets daily<br>3. Homeopathic Nux Vomica 30C, 5 pellets daily |

# Neurological Recommendations

The increasing prevalence of neurological conditions in our children is staggering. According to 2007 statistics on current autism spectrum disorder diagnoses as reported by parents, 1 in 91 children and 1 in 58 boys are now affected. Naturopathic remedies offer a viable solution for symptomatic improvement. We must evaluate your child's load of toxic chemicals, which affect the brain and nervous system more than other body systems. The children in my practice are filled with heavy metals such as arsenic and mercury along with pesticides, plastics, and chemicals inhaled from carpets and other places.

Remove all processed foods from the diet. They can trigger neurological problems.

| Diet |
| --- |
| Healthy-fat protein—Fish truly is brain food because of its high levels of beneficial essential fatty acids. Eat fish daily, always wild caught, never farm raised. Avoid or limit intake to 12 ounces weekly of fish that accumulate high levels of mercury in their bodies, such as King mackerel, Spanish mackerel, shark, swordfish, tilefish, tuna, grouper, marlin, and Orange roughy. |
|    Fresh, wild-caught salmon has low levels of mercury, but farmed salmon should be avoided because it has a high level of PCBs. |
|    Nuts and seeds are also good sources of healthy fats. Ever wonder why a walnut looks like a brain? Because it makes you smarter! |
| Vegetables: 2 servings with every meal |
| Fruits: 2–3 servings daily; great as snacks |
| Whole grains: 2 servings daily |
|    Avoid gluten if your child is sensitive to it. |
| Beverages |
|    Keep your child well hydrated. |
|    *Ginkgo biloba* tea |
|    Avoid dairy if your child is IgE or IgG allergic or sensitive to it. |
| **Vitamins/Supplements** |
|    Acetyl-L-carnitine 500 to 1,500 mg daily |
|    B-complex vitamin daily |

| |
|---|
| Coenzyme Q10 (CoQ10) 10 mg for every 10 pounds daily |
| Digestive enzymes 1 or 2 capsules with each meal |
| Fish oil (mostly DHA) 1 to 2 g daily (to improve brain function) |
| 5-hydroxytryptophan (5-HTP) 50 to 200 mg daily (have amino acid levels tested first) |
| Gamma-aminobutyric acid (GABA) 750 to 1,500 mg daily (for hyperactivity) |
| Magnesium 200 to 400 mg daily |
| Melatonin 0.5 to 1.5 mg before bedtime (for sleep problems) |
| Phenylalanine 500 to 1,000 mg daily (have amino acid levels tested first) |
| Probiotics 10 to 20 million CFU daily |
| Taurine 1,000 mg daily (for hyperactivity) |
| Vitamin B$_{12}$ 1,000 mcg daily |
| **Naturopathic Remedies** |
| Chamomile tea 1 cup 3 times daily |
| *Ginkgo biloba* leaf extract, 50:1 ratio, 24 percent ginkgo heterosides, 6 percent terpene lactones, 50 to 200 mg daily |
| Spectrum Awakening 3 scoops daily |

# Endocrine Recommendations

There are many different conditions that affect hormones. I've focused on the more common conditions of hypothyroidism and diabetes mellitus, skipping rare endocrine conditions that can also affect children. Visit a pediatric endocrinologist to get a correct diagnosis. Naturopathic therapy for endocrine conditions revolves around eating an appropriate diet. Make sure to structure meals and snacks so your child eats correctly.

| **Diet** |
|---|
| Foods for children with either type of diabetes should have a low glycemic index. |
| Vegetables |
| The fiber in vegetables slows down the intestines' absorption of sugar, which prevents the blood from being flooded with sugar. |

| | |
|---|---|
| | Vegetable snacks, such as cut-up carrots, celery sticks, cucumber slices, cherry tomatoes, etc., are better for children with diabetes than fruits are. |
| | Include seaweed for hypothyroidism (look for it at Asian food markets or in the Asian section of your grocery store). |
| Fruits | |
| | Although they're high in fructose , fruits provide important nutrients; serve a few a day with meals, but avoid those with the most fructose, such as raisins. |
| Whole grains | |
| | Brown rice, steel cut oats, quinoa, and other whole grains slow the absorption of sugar into the bloodstream. |
| | Put cassia cinnamon on oatmeal, rice, and other grains for children with type 2 diabetes. |
| Beverages | |
| | Avoid milk for children with type 1 diabetes. |
| | Chamomile tea |
| **Vitamins/Supplements** | |
| | Alpha-lipoic acid 100 mg daily |
| | Chromium 50 to 200 mcg daily |
| | Fish oil EPA + DHA 500 to 2,000 mg daily |
| | Magnesium 50 to 200 mg daily |
| | Selenium 20 to 200 mcg daily |
| | Tyrosine 500 mg daily (for hypothyroidism; avoid for hyperthyroidism) |
| | Vitamin C 250 to 1,000 mg daily |
| | Vitamin D 1,000 to 4,000 IU daily |
| | Vitamin E 100 to 400 IU daily |
| **Naturopathic Remedies** | |
| | Cassia cinnamon 250 to 500 mg 3 times daily |
| | Milk thistle 80 percent silymarin 200 to 500 mg daily |

# Exanthems (Viral Rashes) Recommendations

Skin rashes are common in children, and differentiating one from the other can be quite confusing. Viral rashes are at some point usually accompanied by a fever and cold symptoms, such as a sore throat, runny nose, or cough. Bacterial infections also have similar symptoms of fever, sore throat, and cough. Consult with your pediatrician any time your child develops a rash accompanied by these symptoms.

When children have a virus, it's best for them to fast and drink fluids. Don't force a child to eat if he or she has a fever; allow the body to concentrate on healing instead of digesting food.

| Diet |
| --- |
| Protein |
| Can be avoided during acute colds |
| Vegetables |
| Vegetable soups can be tolerated. Extra garlic and onions will help destroy the virus. |
| Fruits |
| Oranges and other citrus fruits have high levels of vitamin C that are beneficial during acute illness. |
| Whole grains |
| Can be avoided during acute colds |
| Beverages |
| Fresh juices (with no added sugar) are beneficial. Give plenty of fluids, because a child can become dehydrated during a fever. |
| **Vitamins/Supplements** |
| Vitamin A 100,000 to 200,000 IU in 1 dose |
| Vitamin C 500 to 1,000 mg daily |
| Vitamin D 1,000 to 4,000 IU daily |
| Zinc 10 to 20 mg daily, or 1 zinc lozenge every 1 to 2 hours during a cold |

| Naturopathic Remedies |
| --- |
| Astragalus 100 to 500 mg daily |
| *Echinacea purpurea* tincture, 1:2.5 ratio, 30 drops 2 times daily |
| Elderberry glycerite 1:4 ratio, 30 drops 3 times daily |
| Lemon balm 100 to 500 mg daily |
| Licorice (*Glycyrrhiza*) 100 to 500 mg daily |
| **Homeopathic Remedies** |
| Homeopathic Belladonna 30C, 5 pellets twice daily (for fever) |

# Musculoskeletal Recommendations

A growing child's bones and muscles are continually changing. During growth spurts, children become clumsy. Bumps and bruises are part of growing up. Children who don't get proper nutrition don't get the minerals that are so important in nourishing developing bones and muscles.

Daily exercise is essential, but easily forgotten in today's world. We should call it what it really is: playing. Get your kids to play outside, play sports, and play with you.

| Diet |
| --- |
| Low-fat protein |
| Lean protein is important for repairing muscles. |
| Eat the cartilage of organic poultry for nutrients that repair cartilage damage. |
| Eat the bones of sardines for nutrients that repair broken bones. |
| Vegetables |
| Dark green, leafy vegetables have minerals essential for bone construction. |
| Spinach is high in magnesium. |
| Collards, rhubarb, and spinach are high in calcium. |

| | |
|---|---|
| **Fruits** | |
| | Peaches, papayas, and strawberries are high in vitamin C. |
| **Whole grains** | |
| | Buckwheat flour and steel cut oats contain high levels of magnesium. |
| **Beverages** | |
| | If dairy foods are tolerated, organic dairy products are a great source of calcium for the bones. Make sure they are fortified with vitamin $D_3$, not vitamin $D_2$. |
| **Vitamins/Supplements** | |
| | Calcium 200 to 1,000 mg daily |
| | Coenzyme Q10 (CoQ10) 10 mg for every 10 pounds daily |
| | Fish oil EPA + DHA 1 to 2 g daily |
| | L-carnitine 500 to 1,000 mg daily |
| | Magnesium 100 to 200 mg daily |
| | Vitamin C 1,000 mg daily |
| | Vitamin D 1,000 to 4,000 IU daily |
| | Vitamin $K_2$ 100 mcg daily |
| | Zinc 10 to 20 mg daily |
| **Naturopathic Remedies** | |
| | Castor oil applied topically |
| | Menthol applied topically (do not use in children under the age of 10) |
| **Homeopathic Remedies** | |
| | Give your child one of these remedies for a week and if the symptoms don't improve, try a different one for a week.<br>1. Homeopathic Arnica 30C, 5 pellets daily<br>2. Homeopathic Symphytum 30C, 5 pellets daily |

# Pulmonary Recommendations

Every child gets colds and coughs during the year, and asthma is one of the most common chronic lung conditions in children. Regardless of the condition—bronchiolitis, respiratory syncytial virus infection, human parainfluenza virus infection, etc.—we need to make sure our children can breathe. Some of these pulmonary conditions are life threatening; consult your pediatrician when breathing problems arise. Naturopathic prescriptions that improve airflow and decrease mucus in the lungs should be given to all children in need of better breathing.

| **Diet** |
|---|
| Low-fat protein |
|     Lean meats should be eaten daily. |
| Vegetables |
|     Warming foods help open the lungs: garlic, onions, spicy foods, and horseradish. |
|     Eat red peppers and broccoli, which are high in vitamin C. |
| Fruits |
|     Eat foods high in vitamin C: peaches, papayas, strawberries. |
| Whole grains |
|     Daily servings of buckwheat and steel cut oats provide magnesium to keep airways relaxed and open. |
| Beverages |
|     Keep your child hydrated during colds. |
|     Stinging nettle tea can help during allergy season. |
| **Vitamins/Minerals** |
| Fish oil EPA + DHA 1 to 4 g daily |
| Flavonoids (such as rutin or quercetin) 200 to 400 mg divided into 2 or 3 doses daily |
| Magnesium 100 to 200 mg daily |
| NAC 100 to 600 mg daily |
| Quercetin 250 to 500 mg daily |
| Vitamin A 200,000 IU in 1 dose |
| Vitamin C 500 to 1,000 mg daily |

| |
|---|
| Vitamin D 1,000 to 4,000 IU daily |
| Zinc 10 to 20 mg daily |
| **Naturopathic Remedies** |
| Stinging nettle leaf 100 to 250 mg daily |
| **Homeopathic Remedies** |
| Homeopathic Oscillococcinum, entire tube when symptoms first appear |

# Skin Recommendations

As within, so without. When we look at our children itching and scratching, we can feel their pain. No one wants to see their children in the misery of constant itching. From as early as the first few days of life, eczema and other rashes can make daily life a trial.

If there are problems in the stomach and intestines, we commonly have problems with the skin as well. So don't be surprised when some of the best naturopathic prescriptions for skin conditions treat the gastrointestinal system.

| **Diet** |
|---|
| Low-fat protein |
|     Avoid any foods that are triggers, such as nuts or eggs. |
|     Sunflower seeds have high levels of vitamin E. |
| Vegetables |
|     Increase fiber with extra daily servings of vegetables. |
|     Tomatoes have high levels of vitamin E. |
|     Carrots, pumpkin, and sweet potatoes have high levels of vitamin A. |
| Fruits: Serve daily. |
| Whole grains |
|     Increase daily servings for important fiber. |
|     Avoid triggers, such as wheat. |

| Beverages |
| --- |
| Avoid triggers, such as dairy, especially for acne. |
| **Vitamins/Supplements** |
| Fish oil EPA + DHA 2 to 4 g daily |
| Probiotics 10 billion to 50 billion CFU daily |
| Selenium 100 to 200 mcg daily |
| Vitamin A 2,000 IU daily |
| Vitamin D 1,000 to 4,000 IU daily |
| Vitamin E 100 to 400 IU daily |
| Zinc 10 to 20 mg daily |
| **Naturopathic Remedies** |
| Eucalyptus oil applied topically daily |
| Tea tree salve applied topically daily (do not give it to children under the age of 10) |

# Urinary and Reproductive Recommendations

Premenstrual syndrome and urinary tract infections commonly affect teenage girls. Naturopathic treatments are a wonderful alternative to medications for controlling hormone levels. Do you really want to alter your child's hormones when she's first starting to create them? Estrogens and other endocrine-disrupting chemicals in our foods, water, and cosmetics may be behind some girls' having their first periods when they're as young as 9 years old. We need to balance this out naturally and prevent health problems for them in the future.

| Diet |
| --- |
| Low-fat protein |
| Certain seeds, including flaxseed, pumpkin, sesame, and sunflower, improve the regularity of menses. |

| |
|---|
| Pork has high levels of vitamin $B_1$. |
| Hummus is high in vitamin $B_6$. |
| Vegetables |
| Collards, rhubarb, and spinach have higher levels of calcium than milk. |
| Fruits |
| Cranberries should be eaten daily by children who often get UTIs. |
| Whole grains |
| Rice and steel cut oats have high levels of Vitamin $B_1$. |
| Beverages |
| Take a pack of frozen cranberries and boil them in a pot to make cranberry tea. |
| **Vitamins/Supplements** |
| Calcium 250 to 1,000 mg daily |
| Fish oil EPA + DHA 1 to 4 g daily |
| Magnesium 100 to 200 mg daily |
| Probiotics 10 to 50 billion CFU daily |
| Vitamin $B_1$ (thiamine) 20 to 100 mg daily |
| Vitamin $B_6$ 20 to 40 mg daily |
| **Naturopathic Remedies** |
| Cranberry fruit extract, 25:1 ratio, 500 mg 3 times daily |
| D-mannose 500 to 1,000 mg daily |
| *Ginkgo biloba* leaf extract, 50:1 ratio, 24 percent ginkgo heterosides, 6 percent terpene lactones, 50 to 200 mg daily |
| *Vitex* (chasteberry) fruit 5 percent vitexin 20 to 40 mg daily |
| **Homeopathic Remedies** |
| Homeopathic Sepia 30C, 5 pellets daily |

# — APPENDIX —

## Natural Remedies, Interactions, and Dosages

| NATURAL REMEDY/ POSSIBLE INTERACTIONS | DOSAGE | TREATS AND/OR PREVENTS |
|---|---|---|
| **Acetyl L-carnitine**<br>• May cause gastrointestinal upset. | 500–1,000 mg daily | • treats alopecia when stimulating hair growth |
| • May increase the frequency or severity of seizures in some patients. | 500–1,500 mg 3 times daily | • treats ADHD |
| | 500–2,000 mg daily | • treats Crohn's disease |
| **Aloe vera**<br>• May cause an allergic reaction.<br>• May affect the blood sugar level. Consult your physician before use if your child is taking a medication for diabetes.<br>• May not be taken by children who are taking a diuretic drug such as hydrochlorothiazide (HCTZ, Hydrodiuril, Microzide) or furosemide (Lasix).<br>• May not be taken by children who are taking digoxin (Lanoxin). | 750 mg daily for children over 10 years of age | • treats constipation |
| **Aloe vera gel**<br>• May cause an allergic reaction.<br>• May affect the blood sugar level. Consult your physician before use if your child is taking a medication for diabetes. | applied topically as needed | • treats urticaria |
| • May not be taken by children who are taking a diuretic drug such as hydrochlorothiazide (HCTZ, Hydrodiuril, Microzide) or furosemide (Lasix).<br>• May not be taken by children who are taking digoxin (Lanoxin). | applied topically 3 times daily | • treats psoriasis |

*(continued)*

| NATURAL REMEDY/ POSSIBLE INTERACTIONS | DOSAGE | TREATS AND/OR PREVENTS |
|---|---|---|
| **Alpha-lipoic acid (ALA)**<br>• May reduce the blood sugar level. If your child is taking a medication for diabetes or hypoglycemia, consult your physician before use.<br>• May reduce the thyroid hormone blood level, so consult your physician before use if your child is taking a medication for a thyroid condition. | 100 mg daily | • prevents pingueculae and pterygia<br>• treats complications of type 1 diabetes<br>• treats type 2 diabetes<br>• treats chicken pox |
| **Apple cider vinegar**<br>• May increase the side effects of digoxin (Lanoxin).<br>• May decrease potassium levels when taken with insulin or diuretic drugs such as furosemide (Lasix) and hydrochlorothiazide (HCTZ, HydroDiuril). | ¼ tsp before meals | • treats acid reflux |
| **L-arginine**<br>• Decreases blood pressure, so consult your physician before use if your child is taking a hypertension medication such as captopril (Capoten), amlodipine (Norvasc), hydrochlorothiazide (HydroDiuril), furosemide (Lasix), or others.<br>• Interacts with sildenafil (Viagra).<br>• Interacts with nitrates such as nitroglycerin and isosorbide.<br>• May increase the risk of a cold sore developing in children infected with the herpes simplex virus. | 1–2 g daily | • treats hypertension |
| **Artichoke leaf with 13 to 18 percent caffeoylquinic acids**<br>• There are no known drug interactions. | 200–500 mg daily | • treats IBS with diarrhea or alternating diarrhea and constipation |
| **Astragalus**<br>• May counteract the effects of immunosuppresant drugs such as cyclophosphamide (Cytoxan, Neosar) and corticosteroids like prednisone and cortisone. | 100–500 mg daily | • treats conditions of the eyes, ears, nose, and throat |

| NATURAL REMEDY/ POSSIBLE INTERACTIONS | DOSAGE | TREATS AND/OR PREVENTS |
|---|---|---|
| **Astragalus root tincture**<br>• May counteract the effects of immunosuppresant drugs such as cyclophosphamide (Cytoxan, Neosar) and corticosteroids like prednisone and cortisone. | 1:2 ratio, 30 drops 2 times daily | • prevents pharyngitis<br>• treats tonsillectomy |
| **B complex vitamin**<br>• Has multiple ingredients, any of which may have drug interactions. Consult your physician before use. | daily | • treats depression |
| **Baking soda**<br>• May increase the risk of developing kidney stones made of calcium.<br>• May increase the level of sodium in the blood.<br>• May cause edema in children with hypertension, heart failure, or liver disease. | ¼ tsp gargled or swallowed in water or formula 4 times a day | • treats oral candidiasis |
| **Berberine**<br>• May decrease the effectiveness of tetracycline antibiotics.<br>• May affect blood clotting. Consult your physician before use if your child is taking a blood thinner such as warfarin (Coumadin) or aspirin.<br>• May affect drugs that are metabolized by the liver. Consult your physician before giving your child berberine or goldenseal (from which berberine is derived) if he or she is taking any prescription or over-the-counter medicine. | 400 mg daily | • treats diarrhea caused by bacterial or viral gastroenteritis |
|  | 2 capsules 1–3 times daily | • treats gastroenteritis |
| **Berberine, echinacea, myrrh, and *Phytolacca* tincture**<br>• Berberine may decrease the effectiveness of tetracycline antibiotics.<br>• Berberine may affect blood clotting. Consult your physician before use if your child is taking a blood thinner such as warfarin (Coumadin) or aspirin. | 30 drops 3 times daily | • used to treat strep throat |

*(continued)*

| NATURAL REMEDY/ POSSIBLE INTERACTIONS | DOSAGE | TREATS AND/OR PREVENTS |
|---|---|---|
| **Berberine, echinacea, myrrh, and *Phytolacca* tincture *(cont.)*** <br><br> • Berberine may affect drugs that are metabolized by the liver. Consult your physician before giving your child berberine or goldenseal (from which berberine is derived) if he or she is taking any prescription or over-the-counter medicine. <br><br> • Echinacea strengthens the immune system and should be avoided if your child is taking an immunosuppressant medication. <br><br> • Echinacea may cause an allergic reaction in rare cases. <br><br> • Myrrh may lower blood sugar, so use it with caution if your child has diabetes. <br><br> • Myrrh may interact with warfarin (Coumadin) and related blood thinners. <br><br> • There are no known drug interactions to *Phytolacca*. | 30 drops 3 times daily *(cont.)* | • used to treat strep throat *(cont.)* |
| **Beta-glucan** <br><br> • May counteract the effects of immunosuppressant drugs such as azathioprine (Imuran), basiliximab (Simulect), cyclosporine (Neoral), daclizumab (Zenapax), mycophenolate (CellCept), prednisone (Deltasone), and others. | 50–100 mg daily | • treats fibromyalgia |
| | 500–1,000 mg daily | • treats rubella |
| **Black walnut hull tincture, 1:1 ratio** <br><br> • Pregnant and breast-feeding women should avoid black walnut supplements. <br><br> • Avoid if your child has liver or kidney disease or a gastrointestinal condition. <br><br> • Black walnut may interfere with the medications theophylline (Asmalix, Theodur, Uniphyl), codeine, ephedrine, and pseudoephedrine with iron. | 1 drop for each 10 pounds of weight in a glass of water 3 times daily (do not give to children with nut allergy) | • treats gastrointestinal candidiasis |

| NATURAL REMEDY/ POSSIBLE INTERACTIONS | DOSAGE | TREATS AND/OR PREVENTS |
|---|---|---|
| **Bromelain**<br><br>• Pregnant women should not take bromelain.<br>• Children with clotting disorders, hypertension, or liver or kidney disease should not take bromelain.<br>• May increase the absorption of antibiotics.<br>• May interfere with blood-thinning medications such as warfarin (Coumadin), clopidogrel (Plavix), and aspirin.<br>• May increase the sedative effect of drugs and herbs. | 80–320 mg daily | • treats rhinitis<br>• treats obstructive sleep apnea<br>• treats Crohn's disease |
| | 100–200 mg daily | • treats bruises |
| | 200–500 mg daily | • treats allergy |
| | 250–1,000 mg daily | • treats ulcerative colitis |
| | 400–800 mg daily | • treats sinusitis |
| **Butterbur**<br><br>• May interact with medications such as carbamazepine (Tegretol), phenobarbital, phenytoin (Dilantin), rifampin, rifabutin, and others.<br>• Pregnant or breast-feeding women should not use butterbur.<br>• People with liver disease should not use butterbur.<br>• People who have ragweed and related allergies should not use butterbur. | 50–150 mg daily | • treats migraine |
| **Butyrate**<br><br>• There are no known drug interactions. | 4 g daily | • treats Crohn's disease |
| | 500–1,000 mg daily | • treats ulcerative colitis |
| **Calcium**<br><br>• May interfere with absorption of alendronate (Fosamax).<br>• May not be taken at the same time as antacids that contain aluminum.<br>• May interfere with the effects of some kinds of hypertension medications, including atenolol (Tenormin), propranolol (Inderal LA), amlodipine (Norvasc), nifedipine (Procardia, Adalat), and related drugs. | 200–500 mg daily | • treats and prevents diarrhea<br>• treats and prevents Osgood-Schlatter disease |
| | 200–1,000 mg daily | • treats fibromyalgia |
| | 400 mg daily | • treats a broken bone |

*(continued)*

| NATURAL REMEDY/ POSSIBLE INTERACTIONS | DOSAGE | TREATS AND/OR PREVENTS |
|---|---|---|
| **Calcium** *(cont.)*<br>• High doses may cause a toxic reaction to digoxin, while a low blood level of calcium can make digoxin less effective.<br>• May interact with diuretic drugs.<br>• May not be taken with the antibiotic gentamicin because it may damage the kidneys.<br>• May interfere with the absorption of quinolone and tetracycline antibiotics.<br>• When taken at the same time as any other supplement or medication, calcium may decrease the other's absorption. | 500–1,000 mg daily | • treats and prevents rickets |
| | 800–2,000 mg daily | • prevents PMS |
| | 1,000 mg daily | • treats juvenile rheumatoid arthritis (JRA) |
| | 1,000–1,500 mg daily | • treats scoliosis |
| **Caprylic oil**<br>• There are no known drug interactions. | 250–500 mg daily | • treats gastrointestinal candidiasis |
| **Carotenoids, mixed**<br>• Certain medications, such as those for high cholesterol, obesity, gout, or gastric reflux, can decrease the absorption of carotenoids.<br>• Excess carotenoids can turn the skin yellow or orange. | 1,000–5,000 IU daily | • prevents rhinitis |
| **Castor oil**<br>• There are no known drug interactions as a topical therapy. | rubbed clockwise on the abdomen | • treats and prevents constipation |
| | applied topically to the joints daily | • treats JRA |
| **Chamomile**<br>• Should not be taken by people with ragweed and related allergies.<br>• May interfere with the effectiveness of birth control pills. | 100 mg daily | • treats ADHD |

| NATURAL REMEDY/ POSSIBLE INTERACTIONS | DOSAGE | TREATS AND/OR PREVENTS |
|---|---|---|
| **Chamomile** *(cont.)* <br><br> • May interfere with the metabolism of amitriptyline (Elavil), haloperidol (Haldol), ondansetron (Zofran), propranolol (Inderal), theophylline (Asmalix), verapamil (Calan), lovastatin (Mevacor), ketoconazole (Nizoral), itraconazole (Sporanax), fexofenadine (Allegra), triazolam (Halcion), and other drugs that are metabolized by the liver. <br><br> • May cause drowsiness and can add to the effect of sedatives, including alprazolam (Xanax), clonazepam (Klonopin), diazepam (Valium), lorazepam (Ativan), pentobarbital, phenobarbital, fentanyl, morphine, zolpidem (Ambien), and others. <br><br> • May alter the effect of chemotherapy. Consult your oncologist before use. <br><br> • May increase the effect of blood thinners. Consult your physician before use. | 100 mg daily *(cont.)* | • treats ADHD *(cont.)* |
| **Chamomile oil (topical)** <br><br> • Should not be taken by people with ragweed and related allergies. <br><br> • May interfere with the effectiveness of birth control pills. <br><br> • May interfere with the metabolism of amitriptyline (Elavil), haloperidol (Haldol), ondansetron (Zofran), propranolol (Inderal), theophylline (Asmalix), verapamil (Calan), lovastatin (Mevacor), ketoconazole (Nizoral), itraconazole (Sporanax), fexofenadine (Allegra), triazolam (Halcion), and other drugs that are metabolized by the liver. <br><br> • May cause drowsiness and can add to the effect of sedatives, including alprazolam (Xanax), clonazepam (Klonopin), diazepam (Valium), lorazepam (Ativan), pentobarbital, phenobarbital, fentanyl, morphine, zolpidem (Ambien), and others. | 3 times daily | • treats otitis media |

*(continued)*

| NATURAL REMEDY/ POSSIBLE INTERACTIONS | DOSAGE | TREATS AND/OR PREVENTS |
|---|---|---|
| **Chamomile oil (topical) *(cont.)***<br><br>• May alter the effect of chemotherapy. Consult your oncologist before use.<br><br>• May increase the effect of blood thinners. Consult your physician before use. | 3 times daily *(cont.)* | • treats otitis media *(cont.)* |
| **Chamomile tea**<br><br>• Should not be taken by people with ragweed and related allergies.<br><br>• May interfere with the effectiveness of birth control pills.<br><br>• May interfere with the metabolism of amitriptyline (Elavil), haloperidol (Haldol), ondansetron (Zofran), propranolol (Inderal), theophylline (Asmalix), verapamil (Calan), lovastatin (Mevacor), ketoconazole (Nizoral), itraconazole (Sporanax), fexofenadine (Allegra), triazolam (Halcion), and other drugs that are metabolized by the liver.<br><br>• May cause drowsiness and can add to the effect of sedatives, including alprazolam (Xanax), clonazepam (Klonopin), diazepam (Valium), lorazepam (Ativan), pentobarbital, phenobarbital, fentanyl, morphine, zolpidem (Ambien), and others.<br><br>• May alter the effect of chemotherapy. Consult your oncologist before use.<br><br>• May increase the effect of blood thinners. Consult your physician before use. | ¼ cup 3 times daily<br><br>1 cup before bedtime<br><br>2 cups daily | • treats colic<br><br>• treats insomnia<br><br>• treats ADHD |
| **Chamomile, fennel, and lemon balm oil**<br><br>• Buy the combination oil over the counter, or combine 2 to 3 drops of each oil yourself and give a total of 5 to 10 drops<br><br>• Chamomile should not be taken by people with ragweed and related allergies. | 5–10 drops | • treats colic |

| NATURAL REMEDY/ POSSIBLE INTERACTIONS | DOSAGE | TREATS AND/OR PREVENTS |
|---|---|---|
| **Chamomile, fennel, and lemon balm oil** *(cont.)*<br><br>• Chamomile may interfere with the effectiveness of birth control pills.<br><br>• Chamomile may interfere with the metabolism of amitriptyline (Elavil), haloperidol (Haldol), ondansetron (Zofran), propranolol (Indeal), theophylline (Asmalix), verapamil (Calan), lovastatin (Mevacor), ketoconazole (Nizoral), itraconazole, fexofenadine, triazolam (Halcion), and other drugs that are metabolized by the liver.<br><br>• Chamomile may cause drowsiness and can add to the effect of sedatives, including alprazolam (Xanax), clonazepam (Klonopin), diazepam (Valium), lorazepam (Ativan), pentobarbital, phenobarbital, fentanyl, morphine, zolpidem (Ambien), and others.<br><br>• Chamomile may alter the effect of chemotherapy. Consult your oncologist before use.<br><br>• Chamomile may increase the effect of blood thinners. Consult your physician before use.<br><br>• Fennel has no known drug interactions.<br><br>• Lemon balm has no known drug interactions, but it may cause an allergic reaction. | 5–10 drops *(cont.)* | • treats colic *(cont.)* |
| **Cherry bark**<br>• Can cause birth defects.<br><br>• Interacts with medications that are metabolized by the liver. Consult your physician before use.<br><br>• May increase the effectiveness of some medications for diabetes. Consult your physician before use. | 100–500 mg daily | • treats bronchitis |
| **Chlorophyll**<br>• There are no known drug interactions | 5–20 mg daily | • treats acute pancreatitis |

*(continued)*

| NATURAL REMEDY/ POSSIBLE INTERACTIONS | DOSAGE | TREATS AND/OR PREVENTS |
|---|---|---|
| Chromium | 50–200 mcg daily | • treats type 1 diabetes<br>• treats type 2 diabetes |
| Cinnamon, cassia<br><br>• May decrease blood sugar. If your child takes a diabetes medication, consult your physician before use.<br><br>• May cause liver damage if your child also takes another medication that may cause liver damage, such as acetaminophen (Tylenol), erythromycin (Erythrocin), or statin cholesterol drugs. | 1–2 g ($\frac{1}{3}$–$\frac{2}{3}$ tsp) 3 times daily | • treats type 2 diabetes |
| Cinnamon oil<br><br>• May decrease blood sugar. If your child takes a diabetes medication, consult your physician before use.<br><br>• May cause liver damage if your child also takes another medication that may cause liver damage, such as acetaminophen (Tylenol), erythromycin (Erythrocin), or statin cholesterol drugs. | applied topically 2 times daily | • treats impetigo |
| Citronella oil<br><br>• Pregnant or breast-feeding women should avoid citronella oil.<br><br>• May casue skin irritation.<br><br>• Can severely irritate the lungs if inhaled.<br><br>• May cause death when ingested. | 10 drops applied topically for 5 minutes daily | • treats head lice |
| Coconut oil<br><br>• There are no known drug interactions. | 10 drops applied topically for 5 minutes daily | • treats head lice |
| Coenzyme Q10 (CoQ10)<br><br>• May alter the effects of chemotherapy drugs. Consult your oncologist before use.<br><br>• May enhance the effect of antihypertensive medications such as diltiazem (Cardizem), metoprolol (Lopressor, Toprol), enalapril (Vasotec), and nitroglycerin. | 10–20 mg for every 22 pounds daily | • treats chicken pox |
| | 10–250 mg | • treats JRA |
| | 60 mg daily | • treats cystic fibrosis |

| NATURAL REMEDY/ POSSIBLE INTERACTIONS | DOSAGE | TREATS AND/OR PREVENTS |
|---|---|---|
| **Coenzyme Q10 (CoQ10)** *(cont.)*<br>• May decrease the effects of blood-thinning medications such as warfarin (Coumadin) and clopidogrel (Plavix). | 100 mg daily | • treats fibromyalgia |
| | 100–300 mg daily | • treats migraine |
| **Copper**<br>• Should be avoided by children taking birth control pills or estrogen.<br>• Enhances the effects of NSAIDs.<br>• May decrease blood sugar. Consult your physician before use if your child is taking medications for diabetes. | 500–1,000 mcg daily | • treats herpes type 1 sores |
| | 200–2,000 mcg daily | • prevents tonsillectomy |
| | 200 mg daily | • treats a broken bone |
| **Cordyceps sinensis** | 100–500 mg daily or tincture, 5:1 ratio, 30 drops 2 times daily | • treats asthma<br>• treats croup |
| **Cranberry juice extract**<br>• May interfere with blood-thinning medications such as warfarin (Coumadin). Consult your physician before use. | 100 mg 3 times daily | • treats and prevents UTI |
| **Curcumin**<br>• Turmeric (from which curcumin is derived) thins the blood and can interfere with warfarin (Coumadin), aspirin, or clopidogrel (Plavix). Consult your physician before use.<br>• May interfere with drugs that reduce stomach acid, such as ranitidine (Zantac), famotidine (Pepcid), Esomeprazole (Nexium), and lansoprazole (Prevacid).<br>• May enhance the effects of drugs used to treat diabetes. Consult your physician before use. | 500–1,000 mg daily | • treats ulcerative colitis |
| **D-mannose**<br>• D-mannose may affect blood sugar control for children with diabetes.<br>• There are no known drug interactions. | 500–1,000 mg daily | • treats UTI |

*(continued)*

| NATURAL REMEDY/ POSSIBLE INTERACTIONS | DOSAGE | TREATS AND/OR PREVENTS |
|---|---|---|
| **Deglycyrrhizinated licorice (DGL)**<br>• There are no known drug interactions for DGL, but those for licorice may apply (glycyrrhizin is the active ingredient in licorice).<br>• May decrease the effectiveness of warfarin (Coumadin).<br>• May increase blood pressure. Avoid it if your child is taking an antihypertensive medication.<br>• May increase the toxicity of digoxin (Lanoxin).<br>• May increase the effectiveness of steroid medications.<br>• May affect the blood sugar level. Consult your physician if your child is taking a medication for diabetes.<br>• May increase potassium loss in combination with laxatives.<br>• May increase the effects of MAOI antidepressants, which include selegiline (Eldepryl, Zelapar), isocarboxazid (Marplan), and phenelzine (Nardil). | 300 mg 3 times daily<br><br>Determine the appropriate dose for your child by adjusting the recommended adult dose, found on the packaging. The recommended adult dose of an herb is usually calculated for a 150-pound adult. Therefore, if your child weighs 50 pounds, give him or her $\frac{1}{3}$ of the adult dosage. Talk to your physician before giving your child licorice for more than 1 day. Never give licorice to an infant or toddler. | • GERD/reflux/heartburn |
| **Digestive enzymes**<br>• Should not be taken with the medications acarbose (Precose) or miglitol (Glyset). | 1 or 2 capsules with each meal | • treats autism<br>• treats and prevents abdominal pain caused by parasites, viruses, ulcers, bacteria, and fungi<br>• prevents celiac disease flare-ups<br>• treats all forms of IBS<br>• treats chicken pox<br>• treats cystic fibrosis |
| *Echinacea purpurea* **tincture**<br>• Strengthens the immune system and should be avoided if your child is taking an immunosuppressant medication.<br>• May cause an allergic reaction in rare cases. | 1:2.5 ratio, 1 tsp 3 times daily | • treats labyrinthitis |

| NATURAL REMEDY/ POSSIBLE INTERACTIONS | DOSAGE | TREATS AND/OR PREVENTS |
|---|---|---|
| **Elderberry glycerite**<br><br>• Should not be used by pregnant or breast-feeding women.<br><br>• May increase the effect of diuretics, which include hydrochlorothiazide and furosemide (Lasix).<br><br>• May lower blood sugar levels, so consult your physician before giving it to your child if he or she is taking medications for diabetes.<br><br>• May interact with chemotherapy drugs. Consult your oncologist before use.<br><br>• Can act as a laxative and shouldn't be used with other laxatives.<br><br>• May reduce the blood level of theophylline (TheoDur).<br><br>• Stimulates the immune system and should be avoided when taking immunosuppressants such as prednisone. | 1:4 ratio, 30 drops 3 times daily | • treats pharyngitis early in its course |
| | 1:4 ratio, 30 drops 3 times daily | • treats pharyngitis |
| | 1 tsp 2 times daily | • treats flu |
| **Essential amino acid combination**<br><br>• Contains multiple ingredients, any of which may interact with certain medications. Consult your physician before use. | 500–2,000 mg daily | • treats autism |
| **Eucalyptus oil**<br><br>• Do not give to children under the age of 10.<br><br>• Like tea tree oil, can be caustic if applied undiluted.<br><br>• Topical eucalyptus enhances the absorption of topical 5-fluorouracil.<br><br>• May increase the elimination of medications, including pentobarbital and amphetamine.<br><br>• May affect drugs that are metabolized by the liver. Consult your physician before use. | 10 drops applied topically for 5 minutes daily | • treats head lice |

*(continued)*

| NATURAL REMEDY/ POSSIBLE INTERACTIONS | DOSAGE | TREATS AND/OR PREVENTS |
|---|---|---|
| *Euphrasia* (Eyebright)<br><br>• There are no known drug interactions. | 50 to 200 mg daily | • treats allergy |
| | 3X eyedrops 1 to 5 times daily | • treats a black eye |
| Fennel extract, liquid<br><br>• There are no known drug interactions. | 30 drops 2 times daily | • treats PMS symptoms |
| Fennel oil<br><br>• There are no known drug interactions. | 5–10 drops | • treats colic |
| Fennel tea<br><br>• There are no known interactions, but it may cause an allergic reaction. | 3 cups daily | • treats colic |
| Feverfew<br><br>• Children under the age of 2 should not be given feverfew.<br><br>• Pregnant or breast-feeding women should not take feverfew.<br><br>• May alter clotting, so consult your physician before use if your child has a bleeding disorder or is taking a blood-thinning medication such as warfarin (Coumadin) or aspirin. | 20–100 mg daily | • treats migraine |
| Fiber<br><br>• May decrease the effectiveness of tricyclic antidepressants, such as amitriptyline (Elavil) and imipramine (Tofranil).<br><br>• Reduces the absorption of many medications. Take medications at least 1 hour before or 2 to 4 hours after taking a fiber supplement. | 5–15 g, 3 times daily with plenty of water | • treats IBS<br>• treats diarrhea<br>• treats Crohn's disease |
| Fish oil EPA + DHA<br><br>• Should be used cautiously in children who have bleeding disorders because it can increase the risk of bleeding. Fish oil should not be taken by children who are taking blood thinners such as warfarin (Coumadin) or aspirin. | 1 g daily | • treats sinusitis |
| | 1–2 g daily | • improves heart function<br>• treats psoriasis |
| | 1–4 g daily | • treats otitis media<br>• treats eczema |

| NATURAL REMEDY/ POSSIBLE INTERACTIONS | DOSAGE | TREATS AND/OR PREVENTS |
|---|---|---|
| **Fish oil EPA + DHA** *(cont.)*<br><br>• Some fish oil brands contain toxins, including heavy metals, polychlorinated biphenyls (PCBs), and dioxins. Buy only brands produced by reputable manufacturers and that have been filtered or purified.<br><br>• May increase the blood sugar level and should be used cautiously in children taking a medication for diabetes, such as glipizide (Glucotrol), glyburide (Micronase, Diabeta), glucophage (Metformin), or insulin. | 2–4 g daily | • treats and prevents ADHD<br>• treats autism<br>• treats depression<br>• treats migraine<br>• treats epilepsy<br>• treats JRA<br>• taken throughout pregnancy to prevents asthma<br>• treats pneumonia<br>• prevents PMS<br>• used throughout the cycle to prevent epimenorrhagia (abnormal period) |
| | 3 g daily | • treats Crohn's disease<br>• treats ulcerative colitis |
| | 4 g daily | • treats acute pancreatitis |
| | 500–1,000 mg daily | • treats fibromyalgia |
| | 500–2,000 mg daily | • treats type 1 diabetes |
| **Fish oil (with high DHA)** | 1–2 g daily | • treats obesity |
| **5-hydroxytryptophan (5-HTP)**<br><br>• Interacts with antidepressant medications. Get your physician's approval before use if your child is taking an antidepressant.<br><br>• May cause a serious skin problem in children taking carbidopa (Lodosyn).<br><br>• Should be avoided when taking the pain medication tramadol (Ultram, Ultracet).<br><br>• Should be avoided when taking a triptan migraine medication such as sumatriptan (Imitrex) or zolmitriptan (Zomig). | 50–100 mg daily | • treats depression<br>• treats insomnia |

*(continued)*

| NATURAL REMEDY/ POSSIBLE INTERACTIONS | DOSAGE | TREATS AND/OR PREVENTS |
|---|---|---|
| **Flavonoids (such as rutin or quercetin)**<br><br>• May enhance the effect of blood thinners such as warfarin (Coumadin), clopidogrel (Plavix), and aspirin. Consult your physician before use. | 200–400 mg divided into 2 or 3 doses daily | • treats and prevents allergy |
| • May affect chemotherapy drugs. Consult your oncologist before use.<br><br>• May cause corticosteroids, which include prednisone and cortisone, to stay in the body longer.<br><br>• May inhibit the absorption of cyclosporine. | 250–500 mg divided into 2 or 3 doses daily | • prevents nosebleed |
| **Folic acid or 5-methyltetrahydrofolate (5-MTHF)**<br><br>• Interferes with the absorption of the antibiotic tetracycline. | 200–400 mcg daily | • for children taking methotrexate; treats JRA<br><br>• treats and prevents megaloblastic anemia |
| • Interacts with medications for seizures such as fosphenytoin (Cerebyx), phenobarbital (Luminal), phenytoin (Dilantin), and primidone (Mysoline).<br><br>• May decrease the effectiveness of methotrexate (MTX, Rheumatrex).<br><br>• May decrease the effectiveness of pyrimethamine (Daraprim). | 400–1,000 mcg daily | • treats hernias |
| **Gamma-aminobutyric acid (GABA)**<br><br>• Should be used with caution if your child is taking an antianxiety medication, such as lorazepam (Ativan). | 750 mg before bedtime | • treats insomnia |
| | 750–1,500 mg daily | • treats autism<br>• treats epilepsy |
| *Ganoderma lucidum* (a medicinal mushroom also called reishi mushroom) 4 percent triterpenes, 10 percent polysaccharides<br><br>• May increase the risk of bleeding. Avoid it if your child is taking a blood-thinning medication such as warfarin (Coumadin). | 100–500 mg daily | • treats chicken pox |

| NATURAL REMEDY/ POSSIBLE INTERACTIONS | DOSAGE | TREATS AND/OR PREVENTS |
|---|---|---|
| *Ganoderma lucidum* (a medicinal mushroom also called reishi mushroom) **4 percent triterpenes, 10 percent polysaccharides** *(cont.)*<br><br>• Lowers blood pressure and may increase the effect of blood pressure medications.<br><br>• May increase the activity of the immune system and decrease the effectiveness of immunosuppressive drugs.<br><br>• May interact with chemotherapy. Consult your oncologist before use. | 100–500 mg daily *(cont.)* | • treats chicken pox *(cont.)* |
| **Garlic**<br><br>• May exaggerate the effects of the clot-inhibiting medications indomethacin (Indocid, Indocin), dipyridamole (Permole, Persantine), clopidogrel (Plavix), and aspirin. Consult your physician before use.<br><br>• May increase the risk of bleeding. If your child is taking a blood thinner such as warfarin (Coumadin), heparin, or aspirin, consult your physician before use.<br><br>• May reduce the blood level of protease inhibitors such as indinavir (Crixivan), ritonavir (Norvir), and saquinavir (Fortovase, Invirase). Consult your physician before use. | 250–500 mg daily | • treats gastrointestinal candidiasis |
| **Garlic cream or gel**<br><br>• May exaggerate the effects of the clot-inhibiting medications indomethacin (Indocid, Indocin), dipyridamole (Permole, Persantine), clopidogrel (Plavix), and aspirin. Consult your physician before use.<br><br>• May increase the risk of bleeding. If your child is taking a blood thinner such as warfarin (Coumadin), heparin, or aspirin, consult your physician before use. | applied topically nightly | • treats otitis externa<br>• treats warts |

*(continued)*

| NATURAL REMEDY/ POSSIBLE INTERACTIONS | DOSAGE | TREATS AND/OR PREVENTS |
|---|---|---|
| **Garlic cream or gel** *(cont.)*<br>• May reduce the blood level of protease inhibitors such as indinavir (Crixivan), ritonavir (Norvir), and saquinavir (Fortovase, Invirase). Consult your physician before use.<br>• There are no known interactions as a topical therapy, but it may cause an allergic reaction. | applied topically 2 times daily | • treats fungal infections |
| **Garlic extract (topical)**<br>• May exaggerate the effects of the clot-inhibiting medications indomethacin (Indocid, Indocin), dipyridamole (Permole, Persantine), clopidogrel (Plavix), and aspirin. Consult your physician before use.<br>• May increase the risk of bleeding. If your child is taking a blood thinner such as warfarin (Coumadin), heparin, or aspirin, consult your physician before use.<br>• May reduce the blood level of protease inhibitors such as indinavir (Crixivan), ritonavir (Norvir), and saquinavir (Fortovase, Invirase). Consult your physician before use. | applied topically 3 times daily | • treats otitis externa |
| **Garlic in food**<br>• May exaggerate the effects of the clot-inhibiting medications indomethacin (Indocid, Indocin), dipyridamole (Permole, Persantine), clopidogrel (Plavix), and aspirin. Consult your physician before use. | 1 clove, minced, 2 times daily | • treats pneumonia |
| • May increase the risk of bleeding. If your child is taking a blood thinner such as warfarin (Coumadin), heparin, or aspirin, consult your physician before use. | 1 to 2 cloves, minced, daily | • treats impetigo |
| • May reduce the blood level of protease inhibitors such as indinavir (Crixivan), ritonavir (Norvir), and saquinavir (Fortovase, Invirase). Consult your physician before use. | 1 to 3 cloves, minced, daily | • treats labyrinthitis<br>• treats pharyngitis<br>• treats strep throat<br>• treats abdominal pain<br>• treats gastroenteritis<br>• treats gastrointestinal candidiasis |

| NATURAL REMEDY/ POSSIBLE INTERACTIONS | DOSAGE | TREATS AND/OR PREVENTS |
|---|---|---|
| **Garlic oil eardrops**<br><br>• Have your pediatrician check for eardrum perforation before putting anything in the ear canal.<br><br>• May exaggerate the effects of the clot-inhibiting medications indomethacin (Indocid, Indocin), dipyridamole (Permole, Persantine), clopidogrel (Plavix), and aspirin. Consult your physician before use.<br><br>• May increase the risk of bleeding. If your child is taking a blood thinner such as warfarin (Coumadin), heparin, or aspirin, consult your physician before use.<br><br>• May reduce the blood level of protease inhibitors such as indinavir (Crixivan), ritonavir (Norvir), and saquinavir (Fortovase, Invirase). Consult your physician before use. | daily | • treats ear conditions |
| **Garlic paste**<br><br>• May exaggerate the effects of the clot-inhibiting medications indomethacin (Indocid, Indocin), dipyridamole (Permole, Persantine), clopidogrel (Plavix), and aspirin. Consult your physician before use.<br><br>• May increase the risk of bleeding. If your child is taking a blood thinner such as warfarin (Coumadin), heparin, or aspirin, consult your physician before use.<br><br>• May reduce the blood level of protease inhibitors such as indinavir (Crixivan), ritonavir (Norvir), and saquinavir (Fortovase, Invirase). Consult your physician before use. | applied topically 2 times daily | • treats oral candidiasis |
| **Garlic and mullein in olive oil eardrops**<br><br>• Have your pediatrician check for eardrum perforation before putting anything in the ear canal. | 3 times daily | • treats otitis media |

*(continued)*

| NATURAL REMEDY/ POSSIBLE INTERACTIONS | DOSAGE | TREATS AND/OR PREVENTS |
|---|---|---|
| **Garlic and mullein in olive oil eardrops** *(cont.)*<br><br>• May exaggerate the effects of the clot-inhibiting medications indomethacin (Indocid, Indocin), dipyridamole (Permole, Persantine), clopidogrel (Plavix), and aspirin. Consult your physician before use.<br><br>• May increase the risk of bleeding. If your child is taking a blood thinner such as warfarin (Coumadin), heparin, or aspirin, consult your physician before use.<br><br>• May reduce the blood level of protease inhibitors such as indinavir (Crixivan), ritonavir (Norvir), and saquinavir (Fortovase, Invirase). Consult your physician before use.<br><br>• No known interactions as a topical therapy, but it may cause an allergic reaction. | 3 times daily *(cont.)* | • treats otitis media *(cont.)* |
| **Gentian violet**<br><br>• There are no known drug interactions. | applied topically 2 times daily | • treats oral candidiasis |
| **Ginkgo biloba**<br><br>• Can reduce the effectiveness of seizure medications such as carbamazepine (Tegretol) and valproic acid (Depakote).<br><br>• May increase the risk of serotonin syndrome when taken with a selective serotonin reuptake inhibitor (SSRI) such as fluoxetine (Prozac), paroxetine (Paxil), or sertraline (Zoloft).<br><br>• May increase the effects of MAOI antidepressants, such as phenelzine (Nardil).<br><br>• May interfere with medications taken for high blood pressure. Ask your physician before use.<br><br>• May thin the blood. Consult your physician before giving your child ginkgo if he or she is taking a blood thinner such as aspirin, warfarin (Coumadin), or heparin. | 100–200 mg daily | • treats PMS symptoms |

| NATURAL REMEDY/ POSSIBLE INTERACTIONS | DOSAGE | TREATS AND/OR PREVENTS |
|---|---|---|
| **Ginkgo biloba (cont.)**<br><br>• May alter the insulin level. Do not use it if your child has diabetes. | | |
| **Ginkgo biloba leaf extract, 50:1 ratio, 24 percent ginkgo heterosides, 6 percent terpene lactones**<br><br>• Can reduce the effectiveness of seizure medications such as carbamazepine (Tegretol) and valproic acid (Depakote).<br><br>• May increase the risk of serotonin syndrome when taken with a selective serotonin reuptake inhibitor (SSRI) such as fluoxetine (Prozac), paroxetine (Paxil), or sertraline (Zoloft). | 50–200 mg daily | • treats ADHD |
| • May increase the effects of MAOI antidepressants, such as phenelzine (Nardil).<br><br>• May interfere with medications taken for high blood pressure. Ask your physician before use.<br><br>• May thin the blood. Consult your physician before giving your child ginkgo if he or she is taking a blood thinner such as aspirin, warfarin (Coumadin), or heparin.<br><br>• May alter the insulin level. Do not use it if your child has diabetes. | 80 mg daily | • treats PMS symptoms |
| **Ginkgo biloba 3X eyedrops**<br><br>• Can reduce the effectiveness of seizure medications such as carbamazepine (Tegretol) and valproic acid (Depakote).<br><br>• May increase the risk of serotonin syndrome when taken with a selective serotonin reuptake inhibitor (SSRI) such as fluoxetine (Prozac), paroxetine (Paxil), or sertraline (Zoloft).<br><br>• May increase the effects of MAOI antidepressants, such as phenelzine (Nardil). | 5 drops 1–5 times a day | • treats allergic conjunctivitis |

*(continued)*

| NATURAL REMEDY/ POSSIBLE INTERACTIONS | DOSAGE | TREATS AND/OR PREVENTS |
|---|---|---|
| *Ginkgo biloba* **3X eyedrops (cont.)**<br><br>• May interfere with medications taken for high blood pressure. Ask your physician before use.<br><br>• May thin the blood. Consult your physician before giving your child ginkgo if he or she is taking a blood thinner such as aspirin, warfarin (Coumadin), or heparin.<br><br>• May alter the insulin level. Do not use it if your child has diabetes. | 5 drops 1–5 times a day (*cont.*) | • treats allergic conjunctivitis (*cont.*) |
| **Glutamine**<br><br>• May interact with cancer therapies. Consult your oncologist before use.<br><br>• May increase the blood-thinning effect of warfarin (Coumadin).<br><br>• May affect chemotherapy. Consult your oncologist.<br><br>• May interact with acetaminophen (Tylenol). | 250 mg/kg daily (2,500 mg for every 22 pounds) | • treats failure to thrive |
|  | 0.3 g/kg daily (3 g for every 22 pounds) | • treats diarrhea<br>• treats acute pancreatitis |
|  | 500 mg 1–3 times daily | • treats eardrum perforation<br>• treats abdominal pain caused by an ulcer<br>• treats peptic ulcer |
|  | 5,000 mg daily | • treats Crohn's disease |
| **Glycosaminoglycans (these include dermatan sulfate, heparin, and others; Emerson Ecologics' Better Veins is a good supplement to try)**<br><br>• May interfere with medications that dissolve blood clots or slow their formation, such as alteplase (Activase), streptokinase (Streptase), clopidogrel (Plavix), and warfarin (Coumadin). | 200–500 mg daily | • treats Osgood-Schlatter disease |
| **Goldenseal (*Hydrastis canadensis*)**<br><br>• Pregnant or breast-feeding women should not use goldenseal.<br><br>• Consult your physician before giving your child goldenseal if he or she has hypertension or liver or heart disease. | 5 drops used with nasal lavage | • treats sinusitis |

| NATURAL REMEDY/<br>POSSIBLE INTERACTIONS | DOSAGE | TREATS AND/OR<br>PREVENTS |
|---|---|---|
| **Goldenseal (*Hydrastis canadensis*) (*cont.*)**<br><br>• May decrease the effectiveness of tetracycline antibiotics.<br><br>• May affect blood clotting, so consult your physician if your child is taking a blood thinner such as warfarin (Coumadin) or aspirin.<br><br>• May affect drugs that are metabolized by the liver. Consult your physician before giving your child goldenseal (or berberine, the active ingredient in goldenseal) if he or she is taking any prescription or over-the-counter medicine. | 5 drops used with nasal lavage (*cont.*) | • treats sinusitis (*cont.*) |
| **Green tea (decaffeinated)**<br><br>• May inhibit the effects of adenosine, a medication given for irregular heart rhythms.<br><br>• The caffeine in green tea may reduce the effect of benzodiazepines such as lorazepam (Ativan) and diazepam (Valium).<br><br>• Caffeine may increase blood pressure, especially in people taking propranolol (Inderal) or metoprolol (Lopressor, Toprol).<br><br>• Should not be used by people taking the blood thinners warfarin (Coumadin) or aspirin. | 1–2 cups daily | • treats and prevents hypercholesterolemia |
| • May interact with chemotherapy drugs. Consult your oncologist before using.<br><br>• May reduce the effects of the antipsychotic clozapine (Clozaril, Fazaclo).<br><br>• May increase the side effects of ephedrine.<br><br>• Lowers the blood level of lithium.<br><br>• May increase blood pressure to a dangerous level when taken with a monoamine oxidase inhibitor, such as tranylcypromine (Parnate) and phenelzine (Nardil). | 1–3 cups daily | • treats and prevents obesity |

*(continued)*

| NATURAL REMEDY/ POSSIBLE INTERACTIONS | DOSAGE | TREATS AND/OR PREVENTS |
|---|---|---|
| **Green tea (decaffeinated)** *(cont.)*<br><br>• Oral contraceptives (birth control pills) can prolong the time caffeine stays in the body and increase its side effects.<br><br>• Caffeine and phenylpropan-olamine (an ingredient in many cough and cold medications and weight-loss products) can cause mania and a dangerous increase in blood pressure. | | |
| **Green tea, 15 percent kunecatechins ointment** | applied topically nightly | • treats warts |
| **Gymnema, 75 percent gymnemic acids**<br><br>• May lower blood sugar and may interact with medications for diabetes or insulin. Consult your physician before use. | 100 mg 2 times daily | • treats type 2 diabetes |
| **Honey**<br><br>• Do not give honey to children younger than 2 years old.<br><br>• Avoid honey if your child has pollen allergies. | 1 Tbsp daily | • treats rubella |
| **Honey, olive oil, and beeswax in equal proportions**<br><br>• Avoid honey if your child has pollen allergies.<br><br>• Olive oil may decrease blood sugar. Monitor your child's blood sugar level carefully if he or she is taking a medication for diabetes.<br><br>• Beeswax has no known drug interactions. | applied at every diaper change | • treats diaper rash |
| | mixed in equal proportions and applied topically 2 times daily | • treats fungal infections |
| **Hyperimmune bovine colostrum**<br><br>• There are no known drug interactions. | 500–1,000 mg 3 times daily | • treats diarrhea |

| NATURAL REMEDY/ POSSIBLE INTERACTIONS | DOSAGE | TREATS AND/OR PREVENTS |
|---|---|---|
| **Iodine**<br>• An iodide is a form of iodine, and it can be combined with another substance, such as potassium to make potassium iodide. Any iodide used together with an antithyroid medication such as propylthiouracil may have increased hypothyroid effects.<br>• Potassium iodide and lithium (Eskalith, Lithobid) may cause hypothyroidism.<br>• Potassium iodide may decrease the blood-thinning effects of warfarin (Coumadin). | 50–900 mcg daily | • treats hypothyroidism |
| **Iron**<br>• Commonly causes constipation.<br>• Should be avoided by people who have hemochromatosis.<br>• Should not be taken with allopurinol (Zyloprim), a medicine for gout.<br>• Iron and nonsteroidal anti-inflammatory drugs taken together may cause stomach upset.<br>• Decreases the absorption of tetracycline antibiotics, including minocycline (Minocin) and doxycycline (Vibramycin). | 7–10 mg daily | • improves surgical outcomes |
| • Decreases the absorption of the antibiotics ciprofloxacin (Cipro), norfloxacin (Noroxin), and levofloxacin (Levaquin).<br>• Decreases the absorption of bisphosphonates, which treat osteoporosis. They include alendronate (Fosamax), risedronate (Actonel), and others.<br>• Decreases the absorption of angiotensin-converting enzyme (ACE) inibitors that treat hypertension, such as captopril (Capoten), enalapril (Vasotec), and lisinopril (Zestril, Prinivil). | 10–40 mg daily | • treats whooping cough |

*(continued)*

| NATURAL REMEDY/ POSSIBLE INTERACTIONS | DOSAGE | TREATS AND/OR PREVENTS |
|---|---|---|
| **Iron** *(cont.)*<br>• Decreases the blood levels of carbidopa and levodopa.<br>• May decrease the effectiveness of levothyroxine (Armour Thyroid, Synthroid). | | |
| **Lactobacillus**<br>• Shouldn't be used by kids who have short-gut syndrome or weakened immune systems.<br>• May cause temporary stomach upset.<br>• Speed up the metabolism of the ulcerative colitis drug sulfasalazine (Azulfidine). | 4–20 billion CFU daily | • treats and prevents constipation |
| | 10–20 billion CFU daily | • prevents Kawasaki syndrome<br>• treats rhinitis<br>• treats and prevents colic<br>• treats and prevents abdominal pain caused by parasites, viruses, ulcers, bacteria, and fungi<br>• treats celiac disease<br>• treats all forms of IBS<br>• treats gastrointestinal candidiasis<br>• treats acute pancreatitis<br>• treats ulcerative colitis |
| | 10–20 billion CFU 4 times daily | • treats oral candidiasis |
| | 20–40 billion CFU daily | • treats and prevents diarrhea<br>• treats autism |
| | 100 billion CFU in 1 dose | • treats UTI |
| **Lavender oil**<br>• May cause breast development in boys.<br>• May cause an allergic reaction.<br>• May cause nausea, vomiting, headache, and chills.<br>• May increase the effects of narcotic pain relievers and of sedative and antianxiety drugs. Consult your physician before use. | 10 drops applied topically for 5 minutes daily | • treats head lice |

| NATURAL REMEDY/ POSSIBLE INTERACTIONS | DOSAGE | TREATS AND/OR PREVENTS |
|---|---|---|
| **Lemon balm**<br>• There are no known drug interactions, but it may cause an allergic reaction. | 100–500 mg daily | • treats rubella<br>• treats roseola<br>• treats fifth disease<br>• treats mumps<br>• treats shingles |
| **Lemon balm tincture, 1:5 ratio**<br>• There are no known drug interactions, but it may cause an allergic reaction. | 1 tsp 3 times daily | • treats labyrinthitis |
| **Lemon juice**<br>• There are no known drug interactions. | 1 Tbsp diluted in 8 oz of water and applied topically, gargled, or swallowed 2 times daily | • treats oral candidiasis |
| **Lemongrass**<br>• There are no known drug interactions. | infusion applied topically or gargled 2 times daily | • treats oral candidiasis |
| **Licorice (*Glycyrrhiza*)**<br>• May decrease the effectiveness of warfarin (Coumadin).<br>• May increase blood pressure. Avoid it if your child is taking an antihypertensive medication.<br>• May increase the toxicity of digoxin (Lanoxin).<br>• May increase the effectiveness of steroid medications.<br>• May affect the blood sugar level. Consult your physician if your child is taking a medication for diabetes.<br>• May increase potassium loss in combination with laxatives.<br>• May increase the effects of MAOI antidepressants, which include selegiline (Eldepryl, Zelapar), isocarboxazid (Marplan), and phenelzine (Nardil).<br>• Should be avoided if your child is taking oral contraceptives (birth control pills). | 100–500 mg daily | • treats roseola |
| | 100–400 mg daily, using root extract, 16–18 percent glycyrrhizin | • treats flu |
| | applied topically 2 times daily | • treats impetigo |

*(continued)*

| NATURAL REMEDY/ POSSIBLE INTERACTIONS | DOSAGE | TREATS AND/OR PREVENTS |
|---|---|---|
| **Lysine**<br>• There are no known drug interactions. | 1,000 mg daily | • prevents herpes type 1 sores |
| | 1,000–3,000 mg daily | • treats herpes type 1 sores |
| **Magnesium**<br>• Children who have heart or kidney disease should not supplement with magnesium.<br>• May decrease the absorption of antibiotics and should be taken 1 hour before or 2 hours after taking ciprofloxacin (Cipro), moxifloxacin (Avelox), tetracycline (Sumycin), doxycycline (Vibramycin), or minocycline (Minocin).<br>• May increase the risk of side effects from calcium channel blockers in pregnant girls. They should avoid it if they are taking nifedipine (Procardia), amlodipine (Norvasc), diltiazem (Cardizem), felodipine (Plendil), or verapamil (Calan).<br>• May increase the absorption of medications for diabetes, especially glipizide (Glucatrol) and glyburide (Micronase). Talk to your doctor before use if your child is taking a diabetes medication.<br>• Antacids that contain magnesium may reduce the effectiveness of levothyroxine (Levothroid, Synthroid).<br>• May interfere with the absorption of osteoporosis medications such as alendronate (Fosamax).<br>• Can cause diarrhea or abdominal discomfort. | 6 mg/kg (60 mg for every 22 pounds) daily | • treats ADHD |
| | 50–350 mg daily | • prevents tonsillectomy<br>• treats insomnia |
| | 100–200 mg daily | • treats type 2 diabetes<br>• treats PMS symptoms |
| | 100–250 mg daily | • treats constipation |
| | 100–400 mg daily | • treats type 1 diabetes |
| | 200 mg daily | • treats depression<br>• treats bruxism<br>• treats fibromyalgia<br>• treats a broken bone<br>• treats asthma |
| | 200–400 mg daily | • treats tension headache |
| **Manganese**<br>• May cause side effects if your child is taking an antipsychotic medication such as haloperidol (Haldol). | 5 mg daily | • treats migraine<br>• treats tension headache |

| NATURAL REMEDY/ POSSIBLE INTERACTIONS | DOSAGE | TREATS AND/OR PREVENTS |
|---|---|---|
| **Manganese (cont.)**<br><br>• If your child is taking the antibiotic tetracycline, have him or her take the manganese at least 1 hour before or 2 hours after taking the antibiotic. | 5 mg daily (cont.) | • treats migraine (cont.)<br>• treats tension headache (cont.) |
| **Melatonin**<br><br>• May cause seizures at dosages of more than 0.3 mg.<br>• May decrease the effects of antidepressants. | 0.3–3 mg before bedtime | • treats insomnia |
| • May make blood pressure medications related to clonidine (Catapres) and methoxamine (Vasoxyl) less effective.<br>• May increase the risk of bleeding and should be used with care if your child is taking a blood thinner such as warfarin (Coumadin). | 1–3 mg daily | • treats stess and anxiety |
| • May prevent immunosuppressive medications and steroids from working. Avoid it if your child is taking a medication that inhibits the immune system. | 3 mg daily | • treats IBS with diarrhea or alternating diarrhea and constipation<br>• treats tension headache |
| **Menthol**<br><br>• Do not use in children under the age of 10.<br>• There are no known drug interactions as a topical therapy. | applied topically | • treats bumps and bruises of bones and muscles |
| **Milk thistle, 80 percent silymarin**<br><br>• Don't take milk thistle with antipsychotic medications such as chlorpromazine (Thorazine) and promethazine (Phenergan), phenytoin (Dilantin), or the anesthetic halothane. | 200 mg daily | • treats type 1 diabetes<br>• treats type 2 diabetes |

*(continued)*

| NATURAL REMEDY/ POSSIBLE INTERACTIONS | DOSAGE | TREATS AND/OR PREVENTS |
|---|---|---|
| **Milk thistle, 80 percent silymarin** *(cont.)*<br><br>• May interfere with drugs metabolized by the liver, including allergy medications such as fexofenadine (Allegra), statin cholesterol medications such as lovastatin (Mevacor), antianxiety drugs such as alprazolam (Xanax) and diazepam (Valium), blood thinners such as clopidogrel (Plavix) and warfarin (Coumadin), and chemotherapy drugs. Consult your physician before use if your child is taking a medicine that is processed by the liver. | 200 mg daily *(cont.)* | • treats type 1 diabetes *(cont.)*<br>• treats type 2 diabetes *(cont.)* |
| **Mineral oil**<br><br>• Mineral oil may interact with blood thinners such as warfarin (Coumadin) and oral contraceptives. Consult your physician before use. | applied topically daily | • treats cradle cap |
| **Multivitamin**<br><br>• Multivitamins and prenatal multivitamins contain multiple ingredients, any of which may interact with certain medications. Consult your physician before use. | 1 daily | • prevents sinusitis<br>• treats hernias |
| **N-acetylcysteine (NAC)**<br>• May increase the effect of ACE inhibitors used to treat hypertension, such as lisinopril (Prinivil).<br>• May strengthen the effects of immunosuppressive medications such as prednisone (Deltasone).<br>• May reduce the effects of cisplastin and doxorubicin. Consult your physician before use.<br>• May increase the effects and risk of side effects with the chest pain medications nitroglycerin and isosorbide (Isordil).<br>• Topical preparations of NAC may increase the effect of topical antifungal medications. | 100–600 mg by mouth daily | • treats sinusitis<br>• treats postnasal drip |
| | 600–1,800 mg daily | • treats and prevents G6PD events |
| | 600–2,400 mg daily | • treats bronchiolitis |
| | 200–800 mg 3 times daily | • treats cystic fibrosis |

| NATURAL REMEDY/ POSSIBLE INTERACTIONS | DOSAGE | TREATS AND/OR PREVENTS |
|---|---|---|
| **N-acetyl glucosamine**<br><br>• May change your child's need for medications for diabetes. Consult your physician before use.<br><br>• May increase the blood-thinning effect of warfarin (Coumadin).<br><br>• May affect chemotherapy. Consult your oncologist.<br><br>• May interact with acetaminophen (Tylenol). | 3–6 g daily | • treats Crohn's disease |
| **Noni, fresh fruit or bottled juice**<br><br>• Should not be used in children who have kidney disease.<br><br>• May affect liver function. Do not use it if your child has liver problems.<br><br>• May interact with blood thinners such as warfarin (Coumadin). Consult your physician before use. | ¼ cup applied topically for 5 minutes daily | • treats head lice |
| **Olive leaf**<br><br>• May enhance the effects of medications for diabetes. Consult your physician before use.<br><br>• May enhance the effect of hypertension medications. Consult your physician before use. | 250–1,000 mg daily | • treats gastroenteritis<br>• treats gastrointestinal candidiasis |
| **Oregon grape root (*Mahonia aquifolium*), 10 percent cream**<br><br>• Do not use Oregon grape for newborns.<br><br>• Pregnant and breast-feeding women should avoid Oregon grape.<br><br>• May cause an allergic reaction.<br><br>• May decrease the metabolism of medications processed by the liver, such as cyclosporine (Neoral, Sandimmune), lovastatin (Mevacor), clarithromycin (Biaxin), triazolam (Halcion), and many others. Consult your physician before use if your child is taking any medication. | applied topically 3 times daily | • treats psoriasis |

*(continued)*

| NATURAL REMEDY/ POSSIBLE INTERACTIONS | DOSAGE | TREATS AND/OR PREVENTS |
|---|---|---|
| *Panax (Asian) ginseng* root extract, 13 percent ginsenosides<br><br>• May lower blood sugar. Consult your physician before use if your child is taking a medication for diabetes.<br><br>• May delay blood clotting. Consult your physician before use if your child is taking a blood thinner such as warfarin (Coumadin), clopidogrel (Plavix), or aspirin. | 200 mg daily | • treats ADHD<br><br>• treats type 2 diabetes |
| **Passionflower tea**<br><br>• May enhance the effects of sedative medications.<br><br>• May increase the risk of bleeding. Consult your physician before use if your child is taking a blood thinner such as warfarin (Coumadin), clopidogrel (Plavix), or aspirin.<br><br>• May increase the therapeutic and side effects of MAOI antidepressants such as phenelzine (Nardil) and isocarboxazid (Marplan). | 1 cup 2 times daily | • treats stess and anxiety |
| **Pectin**<br><br>• There are no known drug interactions, affecting children. | 25–100 mg daily | • used to treat colic |
| **Peppermint oil**<br><br>• May increase the cyclosporine level in the body.<br><br>• May lower blood sugar. Consult your physician before use if your child is taking a medication for diabetes.<br><br>• May lower blood pressure. Consult your physician before use if your child is taking a medication for hypertension. | 1 enteric-coated capsule 3 times daily | • treats IBS |
| **Phenylalanine**<br><br>• May cause anxiety and hyperactivity. | 100 mg daily for every 10 pounds of body weight | • treats ADHD<br><br>• treats depression |

| NATURAL REMEDY/ POSSIBLE INTERACTIONS | DOSAGE | TREATS AND/OR PREVENTS |
|---|---|---|
| **Phenylalanine** *(cont.)*<br><br>• Should not be taken by people who have phenylketonuria.<br>• Should be avoided if your child takes an MAOI medication such as phenelzine (Nardil) or selegiline (Eldepryl, Zelapar).<br>• May reduce the absorption of baclofen (Lioresal).<br>• May reduce the effect of levodopa (Sinemet).<br>• May worsen the side effects of antiseizure medications, including phenytoin (Dilantin) and valproic acid (Depakene, Depakote). | 500 mg daily | • treats bed-wetting |
| | 500–1,000 mg + tyrosine 500 to 1,000 mg daily | • treats bruxism |
| **Phosphatidylserine**<br><br>• May decrease the effects of atropine, scopolamine, antihistamines, and antidepressants. | 100–250 mg daily | • treats stess and anxiety |
| **Plant sterols**<br><br>• There are no known drug interactions. | 1.5–2.3 g daily | • treats obesity |
| | 2–2.5 g daily | • treats hypercholesterolemia |
| **Prenatal multivitamin**<br><br>• Multivitamins and prenatal multivitamins contain multiple ingredients, any of which may interact with certain medications. Consult your physician before use. | 1 daily for pregnant women | • protects unborn from congenital heart defects |
| **Probiotics**<br><br>• Shouldn't be used by kids who have short-gut syndrome or weakened immune systems.<br>• May cause temporary stomach upset.<br>• Speeds up the metabolism of the ulcerative colitis drug sulfasalazine (Azulfidine). | 2–10 billion CFU daily | • treats rhinitis |
| | 5–10 billion CFU daily (combination of *Lactobacillus* and *Bifidus* strains works best) | • treats eczema<br>• treats and prevents colic |
| | 10–20 billion CFU daily | • treats failure to thrive |

*(continued)*

| NATURAL REMEDY/ POSSIBLE INTERACTIONS | DOSAGE | TREATS AND/OR PREVENTS |
|---|---|---|
| **Psyllium**<br><br>• Can inhibit the effects of tricyclic antidepressants, including amitriptyline (Elavil), doxepin (Sinequan), and imipramine (Tofranil).<br><br>• May decrease the absorption of carbamazapine (Tegretol), which is taken for seizures.<br><br>• May lower blood sugar. Consult your physician before use if your child is taking a medication for diabetes.<br><br>• May decrease the absorption of digoxin (Lanoxin), which is derived from the herb foxglove and treats heart disease.<br><br>• May lower the blood level of lithium, and the two should be taken at least 2 hours apart. | 6 g daily | • treats and prevents hypercholesterolemia<br><br>• treats obesity |
| **Pycnogenol**<br><br>• May increase the activity of the immune system and decrease the effectiveness of immunosuppressive drugs. | 50–150 mg daily | • treats and prevents G6PD events<br><br>• used throughout the cycle to prevent epimenorrhagia (abnormal period)<br><br>• treats obesity |
| **Quercetin**<br><br>• May enhance the effect of blood thinners such as warfarin (Coumadin), clopidogrel (Plavix), and aspirin. Consult your physician before use.<br><br>• May affect chemotherapy drugs. Consult your oncologist before use.<br><br>• May cause corticosteroids, which include prednisone and cortisone, to stay in the body longer.<br><br>• May inhibit the absorption of cyclosporine. | 200–400 mg divided into 2 or 3 doses daily | • treats rhinitis |
| | 250–500 mg divided into 2 or 3 doses daily | • treats and prevents allergy |
| | 500 mg divided into 2 or 3 doses daily | • treats urticaria |
| *Rhodiola rosea*<br><br>• There are no known drug interactions. | 100 mg daily | • treats stess and anxiety |

| NATURAL REMEDY/ POSSIBLE INTERACTIONS | DOSAGE | TREATS AND/OR PREVENTS |
|---|---|---|
| *Saccharomyces boulardii*<br>• A fungus that should not be taken by children who are allergic to yeast.<br>• Shouldn't be used by kids who have short-gut syndrome or weakened immune systems.<br>• May cause temporary stomach upset.<br>• Speeds up the metabolism of the ulcerative colitis drug sulfasalazine (Azulfidine). | 5 billion CFU daily | • prevents UTI |
| *Saffron*<br>• Should be avoided if your child has bipolar disorder.<br>• There are no known drug interactions. | 60 mg daily | • treats PMS symptoms |
| *Salvia miltiorrhizae composita*<br>• There are no known drug interactions. | 200 mg/kg daily (2 g for every 22 pounds of body weight) | • improves surgical outcomes |
| *Salvia officinalis,* 15 percent spray<br>• There are no known drug interactions, but it may cause an allergic reaction. | every 2 hours | • treats pharyngitis |
| *Scutellaria* (skullcap)<br>• Can increase the effects of sedatives such as phenytoin (Dilantin), alprazolam (Xanax), zolpidem (Ambien), amitriptyline (Elavil), and others.<br>• May decrease blood sugar. Consult your physician before use if your child is taking a medication for diabetes. | 250–500 mg daily | • treats allergy |
| Selenium<br>• May increase the risk of bleeding when taken with clopidogrel (Plavix), warfarin (Coumadin), heparin, or aspirin. | 20–200 mcg daily | • treats hypothyroidism<br>• treats JRA<br>• treats scoliosis<br>• treats flu |

*(continued)*

| NATURAL REMEDY/ POSSIBLE INTERACTIONS | DOSAGE | TREATS AND/OR PREVENTS |
|---|---|---|
| **Selenium** *(cont.)*<br>• May make barbiturates, such as butabarbital (Butisol), mephabarbital (Mebaral), phenobarbital (Nembutal), and secobarbital (Seconal), act for a longer time.<br>• May interfere with chemotherapy drugs. Consult your oncologist before use.<br>• May reduce the effectiveness of cholesterol-lowering medicines such as atorvastatin (Lipitor), fluvastatin (Lescol), lovastatin (Mevacor), prevastatin (Pravachol), and simvastatin (Zocor). | 20–400 mcg daily | • treats and prevents Osgood-Schlatter disease |
| | 45–200 mcg daily for 7 days before surgery | • improves surgical outcomes<br>• prevents pingueculae and pterygia<br>• treats otitis media |
| | 50–200 mcg daily | • treats chicken pox |
| **Selenium sulfide**<br>• May increase the risk of bleeding when taken with clopidogrel (Plavix), warfarin (Coumadin), heparin, or aspirin.<br>• May make barbiturates, such as butabarbital (Butisol), mephabarbital (Mebaral), phenobarbital (Nembutal), and secobarbital (Seconal), act for a longer time.<br>• May interfere with chemotherapy drugs. Consult your oncologist before use.<br>• May reduce the effectiveness of cholesterol-lowering medicines such as atorvastatin (Lipitor), fluvastatin (Lescol), lovastatin (Mevacor), prevastatin (Pravachol), and simvastatin (Zocor). | applied topically daily | • treats dandruff, which may cause your child to scratch the scalp and break hairs<br>• treats cradle cap |
| **Senna**<br>• Should not be taken by children who are taking the medication digoxin (Lanoxin).<br>• Should not be taken by children who are taking the blood thinner warfarin (Coumadin).<br>• Should not be taken by children who are taking a diuretic drug. | 4 g daily for children older than 10 years of age | • treats constipation |

| NATURAL REMEDY/ POSSIBLE INTERACTIONS | DOSAGE | TREATS AND/OR PREVENTS |
|---|---|---|
| **Siberian ginseng**<br>• May increase the amount of digoxin in the blood.<br>• May interact with blood-thinning medications such as warfarin (Coumadin), heparin, and aspirin.<br>• May enhance the effects of sedative medications. | 500 mg daily | • treats stess and anxiety |
|  | 250–1,000 mg daily | • treats flu |
| **Spectrum Awakening—Ingredients: vitamin B$_6$ (pyridoxal-5-phosphate), folic acid, vitamin B$_{12}$, methylcobalamin, vitamin E, biotin, magnesium glycinate, zinc glyinate, selenium, molybdenum, taurine, L-theanine, trimethylglycine, L-lysine, 5-HTP**<br>• Contains multiple ingredients, all of which may interact with certain medications. Consult your physician before use. | ¼ tsp 3 times daily | • treats autism |
| **St. John's wort (_Hypericum_)**<br>• Interacts with many medications, increasing the activity of some and decreasing that of others. Consult your physician before use if your child is taking any medication. | applied topically 2 times daily | • treats impetigo |
| **Stinging nettle leaf (_Urtica_), 1 percent silicic acid**<br>• Pregnant women should not use stinging nettle; it may increase the likelihood of miscarriage.<br>• May interfere with blood thinners such as warfarin (Coumadin), heparin, and aspirin.<br>• May interfere with blood pressure medications.<br>• Acts as a diuretic, so it may increase the effects of furosemide (Lasix) and hydrochlorothiazide. Consult your physician if your child is taking a diuretic medication. | 250–500 mg daily | • treats allergies |

*(continued)*

| NATURAL REMEDY/ POSSIBLE INTERACTIONS | DOSAGE | TREATS AND/OR PREVENTS |
|---|---|---|
| **Stinging nettle leaf (*Urtica*), 1 percent silicic acid (*cont.*)**<br><br>• Decreases blood sugar, so consult your physician before giving it to your child if he or she has diabetes.<br><br>• May enhance the effect of NSAIDs. Consult your physician before use. | 250–500 mg daily (*cont.*) | • treats allergies (*cont.*) |
| **Taurine**<br><br>• May decrease excretion of lithium (Eskalith, Lithobid). | 1,000 mg before bedtime | • treats insomnia |
| | 500 mg 3 times daily | • treats epilepsy |
| **Tea tree oil, less than 7 percent cineole**<br><br>• May cause skin irritation or an allergic reaction in some children. | applied topically daily for 2 weeks | • treats alopecia when stimulating hair growth<br>• treats fungal infections |
| | applied topically for 5 minutes daily | • treats head lice |
| | applied topically nightly | • treats warts |
| **Theanine**<br><br>• May decrease blood pressure and interfere with medications for hypertension.<br><br>• May interfere with stimulant medications. | 100–500 mg + GABA 750 mg daily | • treats bruxism |
| **Thyme**<br><br>• May increase the effects of drugs that slow blood clotting, such as ibuprofen, naproxen, enoxaparin (Lovenox), and warfarin (Coumadin). | 100–500 mg daily | • treats bronchitis |
| **Tocopherols, mixed (one of which is vitamin E)**<br><br>• Interferes with the absorption of tricyclic antidepressants such as desipramine (Norpramin).<br><br>• Inhibits the absorption of antipsychotic medications such as chlorpromazine (Thorazine).<br><br>• Thins the blood; care should be taken when also taking blood thinners or aspirin. Consult your physician before use. | 100–400 IU daily | • prevents rhinitis |

| NATURAL REMEDY/ POSSIBLE INTERACTIONS | DOSAGE | TREATS AND/OR PREVENTS |
|---|---|---|
| **Tocopherols, mixed (one of which is vitamin E)** *(cont.)*<br><br>• Inhibits the absorption of beta-blockers such as propranolol (Inderal) that treat hypertension.<br><br>• Vitamin E may reduce the effectiveness of chemotherapy. Consult your oncologist before use. | 100–400 IU daily *(cont.)* | • prevents rhinitis *(cont.)* |
| **Tocopherol acetate ointment**<br><br>• Vitamin E interferes with the absorption of tricyclic antidepressants such as desipramine (Norpramin).<br><br>• Vitamin E inhibits the absorption of antipsychotic medications such as chlorpromazine (Thorazine).<br><br>• Vitamin E thins the blood, and care should be taken when your child is also taking blood thinners or aspirin. Consult your physician before use.<br><br>• Vitamin E inhibits the absorption of beta-blockers such as propranolol (Inderal), which treats hypertension.<br><br>• Vitamin E may reduce the effectiveness of chemotherapy drugs. Consult your oncologist before use. | applied at every diaper change | • treats diaper rash |
| **Tormentil**<br><br>• There are no known drug interactions. | 1–3 g daily | • treats ulcerative colitis |
| **Tryptophan**<br><br>• Interacts with sibutramine (Meridia) and may cause a very serious reaction. Do not use them together.<br><br>• Interacts with sodium oxybate (Xyrem) and may cause a very serious reaction. Do not use them together. | 1–5 g daily | • treats IBS with diarrhea or alternating diarrhea and constipation<br>• treats scoliosis |
| | 500 mg daily | • treats bed-wetting |

*(continued)*

| NATURAL REMEDY/<br>POSSIBLE INTERACTIONS | DOSAGE | TREATS AND/OR<br>PREVENTS |
|---|---|---|
| **Tryptophan** *(cont.)*<br><br>• Interacts with MAOI antidepressants and may cause a possibly fatal reaction. Do not use MAOIs within 2 weeks before, during, or 2 weeks after taking tryptophan.<br><br>• Should be used with care when your child is taking levodopa (Sinemet), a triptan, an SSRI or tricyclic antidepressant, or St. John's wort.<br><br>• Should be used cautiously if your child is taking a medication that causes drowsiness. | 1,000 mg daily | • treats autism |
| **Turmeric standardized extract**<br><br>• Thins the blood and can interfere with warfarin (Coumadin), aspirin, and clopidogrel (Plavix). Consult your physician before use.<br><br>• May interfere with drugs that reduce stomach acid, such as ranitidine (Zantac), famotidine (Pepcid), esomeprazole (Nexium), and lansoprazole (Prevacid).<br><br>• May enhance the effects of drugs used to treat diabetes. Consult your physician before use. | 100 mg daily<br><br>400–600 mg daily | • treats allergy<br><br>• treats obstructive sleep apnea<br>• treats Crohn's disease |
| **Tyrosine**<br><br>• People who get migraine headaches should avoid tyrosine.<br><br>• Should not be given if your child takes an MAOI medication such as phenelzine (Nardil) or selegiline (Eldepryl, Zelapar).<br><br>• Should not be taken with synthetic thyroid hormones. | 500–1,500 mg daily | • treats ADHD<br>• treats hypothyroidism |
| **Valerian**<br><br>• Consult your physician before using valerian for more than 1 month.<br><br>• May increase the effects of sedative medications. | 500 mg daily | • treats stess and anxiety |

| NATURAL REMEDY/<br>POSSIBLE INTERACTIONS | DOSAGE | TREATS AND/OR<br>PREVENTS |
|---|---|---|
| **Valerian** *(cont.)*<br><br>• May interact with antihistamines, statins, antifungal medications, and other drugs that are processed by the liver.<br><br>• May increase the effects of anesthesia. | Valerian root, 0.8 percent valerinic acid, 250 mg daily | • treats PMS symptoms |
| **Valerian tea**<br><br>• Consult your physician before using valerian for more than 1 month.<br><br>• May increase the effects of sedative medications.<br><br>• May interact with antihistamines, statins, antifungal medications, and other drugs that are processed by the liver.<br><br>• May increase the effects of anesthesia. | 1 cup before bedtime | • treats insomnia |
| **Vitamin A**<br><br>• Supplementation beyond the amount included in prenatal multivitamins should be avoided by pregnant women.<br><br>• People with liver disease who are taking vitamin A must be monitored by their doctors.<br><br>• Doses of vitamin A of more than 40,000 IU daily combined with tetracylcine antibiotics, including demeclocycline (Declomycin) and minocycline (Minocin), may increase the pressure of the fluid surrounding the brain.<br><br>• Long-term use of vitamin A may thin the blood. Consult your physician if your child is taking a blood thinner such as warfarin (Coumadin), aspirin, or heparin.<br><br>• May increase the action of certain chemotherapy drugs. Consult your oncologist before use. | 1,000 IU daily | • prevents pingueculae or pterygia |
| | 100,000 IU in 1 dose | • treats otitis media<br>• treats labyrinthitis<br>• treats pharyngitis<br>• reduces swelling after tonsillectomy<br>• treats bronchiolitis<br>• treats herpes type 1 sores<br>In children ages 6 months to 1 year—immediately after diagnosis or when symptoms appear for:<br>• croup<br>• fifth disease<br>• mononucleosis<br>• mumps<br>• roseola<br>• rubella<br>• shingles |

*(continued)*

| NATURAL REMEDY/ POSSIBLE INTERACTIONS | DOSAGE | TREATS AND/OR PREVENTS |
|---|---|---|
| **Vitamin A** *(cont.)*<br><br>• There are no known drug interactions as a topical therapy. | 200,000 IU in 1 dose | *(cont.)*<br><br>• treats gastroenteritis<br><br>• treats hypothyroidism<br><br>• treats flu<br><br>In children older than 1 year—immediately after diagnosis or when symptoms appear for:<br><br>• chicken pox<br><br>• croup<br><br>• fifth disease<br><br>• mononucleosis<br><br>• mumps<br><br>• roseola<br><br>• rubella<br><br>• shingles |
| | if other family members or people your child has contact with have pneumonia, give your child 1 dose to prevent pneumonia; if pneumonia is suspected or diagnosed in your child, give him or her 1 dose on the first day of symptoms | • treats and prevents pneumonia |
| | 400–1,000 IU daily | • prevents cryptorchidism (undescended testicle) when taken by the father before conception |
| | 1,000–4,000 IU daily | • treats psoriasis |
| | 1,000–5,000 IU daily | • treats and prevents acne |
| | 2,000 IU daily | • treats autism |
| | 100,000 IU in 1 dose followed 4 weeks later by 100,000 IU in 1 dose | • treats measles— immediately after diagnosis or when symptoms appear in children ages 6 to 12 months |

| NATURAL REMEDY/ POSSIBLE INTERACTIONS | DOSAGE | TREATS AND/OR PREVENTS |
|---|---|---|
| **Vitamin A** *(cont.)* | 200,000 IU in 1 dose followed 4 weeks later by 200,000 IU in 1 dose | • treats measles—immediately after diagnosis or when symptoms appear in children more than 1 year old |
| | A&D Ointment applied at every diaper change | • treats diaper rash |
| **Vitamin B₁ (thiamine)**<br>• Very high doses may cause stomach upset, but these dosages will not. | 5–10 mg daily | • prevents tonsillectomy |
| | 100 mg daily | • treats PMS symptoms |
| **Vitamin B₂ (riboflavin)**<br>• Inhibits the abosorption of tetracycline antibiotics, so take them at different times of the day.<br>• May interact with cancer medications. Consult your oncologist before use.<br>• Riboflavin at doses of more than 10 mg may increase the risk of eye damage from the sun. Have your child wear sunglasses when taking this dosage. | 10–20 mg daily | • prevents tonsillectomy |
| | 40 mg daily | • treats migraine |
| **Vitamin B₃ (niacin)**<br>• A high dose of niacin can cause flushing. In my experience, the niacinamide form of niacin is most likely to cause it.<br>• Niacin in very high doses has caused liver damage and stomach ulcers.<br>• Should be avoided if your child has gout.<br>• May decrease the absorption of the antibiotic tetracycline.<br>• May increase the effect of blood thinners such as warfarin (Coumadin) and clopidogrel (Plavix)<br>• May increase the effect of alpha-blockers taken for hypertension, including tamsulosin (Flomax) and doxazosin (Cardura). | 5–20 mg daily | • treats hypercholes-terolemia |
| | 2–30 mg daily | • treats type 1 diabetes |
| | 4 percent niacinamide wash applied topically daily | • treats acne |
| | 10–20 mg daily | • treats obesity |

*(continued)*

| NATURAL REMEDY/ POSSIBLE INTERACTIONS | DOSAGE | TREATS AND/OR PREVENTS |
|---|---|---|
| **Vitamin B$_3$ (niacin)** *(cont.)*<br>• May interfere with the effects of cholesterol-lowering medications, so they should be taken at different times of the day.<br>• May raise blood sugar. Consult your doctor before use if your child is taking a medication for diabetes. | | |
| **Vitamin B$_5$ (pantothenic acid)**<br>• Lessens the absorption of the antibiotic tetracycline. | 2 mg daily | • treats stess and anxiety |
| **Vitamin B$_5$ (dexpanthenol)**<br>• Should not be used for children who have hemophilia. | ointment applied at every diaper change | • treats diaper rash |
| **Vitamin B$_6$ (pyridoxine)**<br>• Refer to the page 30.<br>• Interferes with the absorption of the antibiotic tetracycline.<br>• Reduces the effect of levodopa (Sinemet).<br>• Reduces the effect of seizure medication phenytoin (Dilantin). | 0.6 mg/kg daily (6 mg for every 22 pounds of body weight) | • treats ADHD<br>• treats autism |
| | 1– 20 mg daily | • treats asthma |
| | 20–40 mg | • treats PMS symptoms |
| **Vitamin B$_{12}$**<br>• Interferes with the absorption of the antibiotic tetracycline. | 1,000 mcg daily for 3 to 6 weeks | • treats and prevents megaloblastic anemia<br>• treats autism |
| | 100 mcg injected into the wart | • treats warts |
| | 5–10 mcg daily for 2–3 months | • treats megaloblastic anemia (giant red blood cells) |
| **Vitamin B-complex**<br>• Has multiple ingredients, any of which may have drug inter-actions. Consult your physician before use. | daily | • treats depression |

| NATURAL REMEDY/ POSSIBLE INTERACTIONS | DOSAGE | TREATS AND/OR PREVENTS |
|---|---|---|
| **Vitamin C**<br><br>• Excess vitamin C can cause diarrhea.<br><br>• Increases the absorption of some forms of iron. Patients with hemochromatosis should not take vitamin C supplements.<br><br>• High doses of vitamin C may make your child's body hold on longer to aspirin, acetaminophen (Tylenol), and other nonsteroidal anti-inflammtory drugs.<br><br>• Can increase the absorbtion of aluminum from medications that contain aluminum, such as the antacids Maalox and Gaviscon.<br><br>• May interfere with chemotherapy drugs. Consult your oncologist before use.<br><br>• Nitrate medications for heart disease may interact with vitamin C. Consult your physician before use.<br><br>• Can raise the estrogen level in girls taking oral contraceptives (birth control pills).<br><br>• Slightly lowers the blood level of protease inhibitors such as indinavir (Crixivan).<br><br>• Increases the absorption of tetracycline and similar antibiotics such as minocycline (Minocin) and doxycycline (Vibramycin).<br><br>• Rare reports indicate that high-dose vitamin C may interfere with blood thinners. While a dose of 1,000 mg daily does not cause this, consult your physician before use. | 100–1,000 mg daily | • treats or prevents herpes type 1 sores |
| | 250–1,000 mg daily | • treats type 1 diabetes |
| | 250–2,000 mg daily | • improve surgical outcomes<br>• treats Kawasaki syndrome |
| | 500–2,000 mg daily | • treats otitis media<br>• prevents nosebleed<br>• treats pharyngitis<br>• prevents tonsillectomy<br>• treats ulcerative colitis<br>• treats stess and anxiety |
| | 500–1,000 mg daily | • treats rhinitis<br>• treats roseola<br>• treats fifth disease<br>• treats chicken pox<br>• treats mononucleosis<br>• treats JRA<br>• prevents pinguecula and pterygium<br>• treats scoliosis<br>• treats and prevents allergy<br>• treats croup<br>• treats alopecia when stimulating hair growth |
| | 500 mg daily | • prevents bruises |
| | 500 mg 3 times daily | • treats flu |
| | 1,000 mg daily | • treats asthma |
| **Vitamin D**<br><br>• May reduce the abosrption of atorvastatin (Lipitor). Consult your physician before use. | 400–4,000 IU daily | • treats type 2 diabetes |
| | 600–4,000 IU daily | • treats type 1 diabetes |

*(continued)*

| NATURAL REMEDY/ POSSIBLE INTERACTIONS | DOSAGE | TREATS AND/OR PREVENTS |
|---|---|---|
| **Vitamin D** *(cont.)*<br><br>• May interfere with calcium channel blockers, which include nifedipine (Procardia), verapamil (Calan), and amlodipine (Norvasc).<br><br>• May increase the likelihood of having a toxic reaction to digoxin (Lanoxin). Consult your physician before use.<br><br>• There are no known drug interactions as a topical therapy. | 1,000–4,000 IU daily for 1 week | • treats otitis media<br>• treats pharyngitis<br>• treats ulcerative colitis<br>• treats mononucleosis<br>• treats JRA<br>• treats and prevents Osgood-Schlatter disease<br>• treats a broken bone<br>• treats asthma<br>• treats croup<br>• treats alopecia when stimulating hair growth<br>• treats eczema<br>• prevents PMS<br>• prevents cryptorchidism (undescended testicle) when taken by the father before conception |
| | 1,000–5,000 IU daily | • treats Crohn's disease |
| | 2,000–4,000 IU daily | • prevents rickets; if your child has been diagnosed with rickets, consult your physician for the appropriate dosing. |
| | A&D Ointment applied at every diaper change | • treats diaper rash |
| **Vitamin D cream**<br><br>• May reduce the abosrption of atorvastatin (Lipitor). Consult your physician before use.<br><br>• May interfere with calcium channel blockers, which include nifedipine (Procardia), verapamil (Calan), and amlodipine (Norvasc).<br><br>• May increase the likelihood of having a toxic reaction to digoxin (Lanoxin). Consult your physician before use. | 0.005 percent applied topically 3 times a day | • treats psoriasis |
| | 0.005 percent lotion applied topically nightly | • treats warts |

| NATURAL REMEDY/ POSSIBLE INTERACTIONS | DOSAGE | TREATS AND/OR PREVENTS |
|---|---|---|
| **Vitamin E**<br><br>• Interferes with the absorption of tricyclic antidepressants such as desipramine (Norpramin).<br><br>• Inhibits the absorption of antipsychotic medications such as chlorpromazine (Thorazine).<br><br>• Thins the blood and care should be taken when your child is also taking blood thinners or aspirin. Consult your physician before use.<br><br>• Inhibits the absorption of beta-blockers such as propranolol (Inderal), which are treats hypertension.<br><br>• May reduce the effectiveness of chemotherapy drugs. Consult your oncologist before use. | 100–400 IU daily | • treats type 1 diabetes |
|  | 200–400 IU daily | • treats and prevents G6PD events<br>• treats Kawasaki syndrome<br>• prevents pingueculae and pterygia<br>• treats labyrinthitis<br>• treats autism<br>• treats chicken pox<br>• treats herpes type 1 sores<br>• treats JRA<br>• treats Osgood-Schlatter disease<br>• treats flu |
|  | 100–400 IU daily | • treats pharyngitis<br>• prevents tonsillectomy |
| **Vitamin K$_2$**<br><br>• Should be avoided by children with G6PD deficiency.<br><br>• Interferes with some blood-thinning medications. Consult your physician before use if your child is taking a blood thinner such as warfarin (Coumadin) or heparin. | 100 mcg daily | • treats a broken bone |
| ***Vitex* (chasteberry), 5 percent vitexin**<br><br>• May affect hormone levels and should be used by women who are taking birth control pills or who have a hormone-sensitive condition only under the supervision of a physician.<br><br>• May affect dopamine levels and should be avoided if your child is taking medications that affect dopamine, such as some antipsychotics and Parkinson's disease medications.<br><br>• May cause gastrointestinal upset, rash, or dizziness. | 20–40 mg daily | • prevents PMS<br>• prevents epimenorrhagia (abnormal period) |

*(continued)*

| NATURAL REMEDY/ POSSIBLE INTERACTIONS | DOSAGE | TREATS AND/OR PREVENTS |
|---|---|---|
| *Withania* (also called ashwagandha)<br><br>• May increase the effect of barbituate medications.<br><br>• Pregnant women should avoid *Withania*.<br><br>• May reduce the effect of immunosuppressive medications. | 500–1,000 mg daily | • treats whooping cough |
| Zinc—short term<br><br>• Do not give your child zinc if he or she is taking amiloride (Midamor).<br><br>• May decrease the absorption of antibiotics, including ciprofloxacin (Cipro), tetracycline, and related antibiotics.<br><br>• May affect chemotherapy drugs. Consult your oncologist before use.<br><br>• Avoid zinc if your child is taking immunosuppressant drugs.<br><br>• Can reduce the absorption of NSAIDs. | 10–20 mg daily | • treats pharyngitis<br>• treats diarrhea<br>• treats gastroenteritis<br>• treats chicken pox<br>• treats croup<br>• treats cystic fibrosis<br>• treats and prevents pneumonia |
| | 20 mg daily | • treats a broken bone |
| Zinc—long term<br><br>• When your child is getting zinc over the long term, always give him or her 1 mg copper for every 10 mg zinc.<br><br>• Do not give your child zinc if he or she is taking amiloride (Midamor).<br><br>• May decrease the absorption of antibiotics, including ciprofloxacin (Cipro), tetracycline, and related antibiotics.<br><br>• May affect chemotherapy drugs. Consult your oncologist before use.<br><br>• Avoid zinc if your child is taking immunosuppresant drugs.<br><br>• Can reduce the absorption of NSAIDs.<br><br>• Copper supplements should be avoided by children taking birth control pills or estrogen.<br><br>• Copper enhances the effects of NSAIDs. | 10 mg daily | • treats fibromyalgia<br>• treats acne |
| | 5–20 mg daily | • prevents tonsillectomy<br>• treats type 2 diabetes |
| | 5 mg every 2 hours, for a maximum of 20 mg daily | • treats flu |
| | 10–20 mg daily | • treats ADHD |
| | 10–20 mg daily plus topical cream daily | • treats herpes type 1 sores |
| | 20 mg daily | • treats alopecia when stimulating hair growth |

# Homeopathic Remedies* and Dosages

| NATURAL REMEDY/ POSSIBLE INTERACTIONS | DOSAGE | TREATS AND/OR PREVENTS |
|---|---|---|
| Homeopathic Aconite 30C | 5 pellets before bed daily | • treats night terrors |
| | 5 pellets 3 times daily | • treats croup |
| Homeopathic Apis 30C | 5 pellets 3 times daily | • treats urticaria |
| Homeopathic Arnica 30C | 5 pellets daily | • improves surgical outcomes<br>• treats bruises<br>• treats a broken bone |
| Homeopathic Arnica 30C + Homeopathic Phosphorus 30C | 5 pellets of each every 2 hours | • treats a nosebleed until it stops |
| Homeopathic Arsenicum 30C | 5 pellets daily | • treats gastrointestinal conditions |
| Homeopathic Arundo Mauritanica 30C | 5 pellets daily | • treats rhinitis |
| Homeopathic Belladonna 30C | 5 pellets 3 times daily | • treats fever |
| Homeopathic Calcarea Carbonica 30C | 1–3 times daily | • treats cradle cap |
| | 5 pellets daily | • treats rhinitis |
| Homeopathic Chamomilla 30C | 5 pellets before bedtime daily | • treats night terrors |
| Homeopathic Hepar Sulphur 30C | 5 pellets 3 times daily | • treats croup |
| Homeopathic Histaminum 30C | 5 pellets 3 times daily | • treats urticaria |
| Homeopathic Hypericum 30C | 5 pellets 3 times daily | • treats chicken pox |
| Homeopathic Ignatia Amara 30C | 5 pellets twice daily | • treats depression |
| Homeopathic Lycopodium 30C | 5 pellets daily | • treats gastrointestinal conditions |
| Homeopathic Medorrhinum 30C | 5 pellets daily | • treats rhinitis |
| Homeopathic Natrum Muriaticum 30C | 5 pellets daily | • treats rhinitis |
| | 5 pellets 2 times daily | • treats depression |

*(continued)*

* Homeopathic remedies are not known to interact with conventional medications.

| NATURAL REMEDY/ POSSIBLE INTERACTIONS | DOSAGE | TREATS AND/OR PREVENTS |
|---|---|---|
| Homeopathic Nosode | 5 pellets daily | • treats allergy |
| Homeopathic Nux Vomica 30C | 5 pellets daily | • treats gastrointestinal conditions |
| Homeopathic Oscillococcinum | entire tube of pellets when symptoms arise | • treats flu |
| Homeopathic Phosphoricum Acidum 30C | 5 pellets daily | • treats rhinitis |
| Homeopathic Phosphorus 30C | 5 pellets before bed daily | • treats night terrors |
| | 5 pellets daily | • treats rhinitis |
| Homeopathic Phosphorus 200C | 5 pellets as needed | • treats nosebleed |
| Homeopathic Pulsatilla Nigricans 30C | 5 pellets daily | • treats rhinitis |
| Homeopathic Sepia 30C | 5 pellets daily | • treats UTI<br>• treats rhinitis |
| Homeopathic Spongia 30C | 5 pellets 3 times daily | • treats croup |
| Homeopathic Staphylococcinum 200C | 5 pellets in 1 dose | • treats impetigo |
| Homeopathic Streptococcinum 200C | 5 pellets in 1 dose | • treats impetigo |
| Homeopathic Sulphur 30C | 5 pellets daily | • treats rhinitis |
| Homeopathic Symphytum 30C | 5 pellets daily before bedtime | • treats eardrum perforation |
| | 5 pellets daily | • treats a broken bone<br>• treats bumps and bruises of bones and muscles |
| Homeopathic Thuja Occidentalis 30C | 5 pellets daily | • treats rhinitis |
| Homeopathic Tuberculinum 30C | 5 pellets daily | • treats rhinitis |
| | 5 pellets once a week | • treats eardrum perforation |
| Homeopathic Urtica | 5 pellets 3 times daily | • treats urticaria |

# — NATUROPATHIC TESTING — FOR YOUR CHILD

Testing is available at **www.100NaturalRemedies.com.**

Your pediatrician probably was taught about only a few laboratory tests, common ones that screen for infection or problems with cholesterol, sugar, or thyroid hormone levels. He or she probably wasn't educated about functional lab tests. There is a wealth of information you can learn from these naturopathic tests, including your child's vitamin, mineral, and protein statuses; toxicity load; and immune reactions to certain foods. These tests are available from a myriad of laboratories, and some are covered by health insurance while others are not. The question that should be asked about any lab test is whether it will generate information that can reveal an answer to a health problem or guide treatment. Remember that all tests have a margin of error, meaning that sometimes they show things that aren't there, miss things that are there, or otherwise fall short of what we want most—accuracy. Here is a list of the naturopathic tests you can use to help your child.

## Food Sensitivity (IgG) and Food Allergy (IgE) Testing

Antibodies are created by the immune system to fight invaders. These antibodies, also called immunoglobulins (abbreviated "Ig"), have names such as IgG, IgM, IgA, and IgE. When a child has a food allergy, the body produces many copies of a unique IgE antibody that create an allergic reaction whenever he or she eats that food. When there is a bacterial infection, the immune system produces copies of a unique IgG antibody that attack the bacteria and cause inflammation. When a child has a food sensitivity, his or her body produces an IgG antibody to the food that attacks it and causes symptoms in the gastrointestinal, nervous, and musculoskeletal systems.

Testing can be performed to look for both immune system reactions. Blood work for IgE antibodies shows us what foods a child is currently allergic to or at risk for developing an allergy to. Blood work for IgG antibodies shows us a child's food sensitivities, which cause the same kinds of symptoms as food allergies but are sometimes outgrown as the immune system matures. Unfortunately, neither of these blood tests reveals food intolerances, which involve a genetic inability to digest a particular food and normally cause fast-arising symptoms in the stomach and intestines. Suspected food intolerances can be confirmed by avoiding the food to see if the symptoms disappear.

## Who Needs These Tests?

### NEUROLOGICAL COMPLAINTS

Anxiety

Attention deficit
 hyperactivity disorder
 (ADHD)

Autism

Depression

Epilepsy

Headaches

Migraines

Seizures

### GASTROINTESTINAL COMPLAINTS

Abdominal pain

Acid reflux

Colic

Constipation

Diarrhea

Gastroesophageal reflux
 disease (GERD)

Heartburn

Inflammatory bowel disease
 (Crohn's disease,
 ulcerative colitis)

Irritable bowel syndrome (IBS)

### MUSCULOSKELETAL CONDITIONS

Arthritis

Fibromyalgia

Joint pain

Muscle pain

### OTHER

Recurrent ear infections

# Organic Acid Testing

Our bodies and cells possess an intricate set of enzymes and processes that convert food into energy. It's quite miraculous how eating a vegetable or a piece of fish produces a form of energy that allows our hearts to beat and our lungs to breathe. During the process of converting food into energy, substances called organic acids are created. Organic acid testing identifies specific nutrient deficiencies so you can make sure your child has all the vitamins and minerals needed for generating an abundance of energy.

## Who Needs This Test?

### NEUROLOGICAL COMPLAINTS

| | |
|---|---|
| ADHD | High blood sugar |
| Autism | Insomnia |
| Depression | Low blood sugar |
| Endocrine complaints | |

### OTHER

| | |
|---|---|
| Chronic fatigue | Weight gain |

# Amino Acid Testing

Amino acids are the building blocks of protein. We need protein for every cell in our bodies. It builds strong bones and muscles. Amino acids also create neurotransmitters and the antibodies that are essential for immune system function. If children are not eating a healthy diet, they may not be getting enough protein to nourish their bodies or enough vitamins and minerals to convert amino acids into protein.

## Who Needs This Test?

### NEUROLOGICAL COMPLAINTS

| | |
|---|---|
| ADHD | Epilepsy |
| Anxiety | Headache |
| Autism | Migraine |
| Depression | Seizure |

### OTHER

| | |
|---|---|
| Chronic fatigue | Weight loss |
| Frequent viral and/or bacterial infections | |

# Stool Testing

There is a wealth of information in what we normally flush down the toilet every day. Naturopathic stool testing is superior to standard stool tests. The newest technology for discovering organisms (bacteria causing food poisoning, the fungus *Candida*, viruses, parasites) is called polymerase chain reaction (PCR) testing. It looks at the DNA in the stool rather than looking for the organisms themselves under a microscope, as has been done for many years.

Different stool tests are available, some of which use the new technology and some the old. No test result is 100 percent accurate, with some including organisms that grew while in transit to the lab and others missing organisms that are there. The tests usually also analyze your child's digestive capabilities by looking for food that passed through the gastrointestinal tract undigested.

With one sample, we can answer the following questions:

Is your child digesting protein, fats, and carbohydrates?

Is your child absorbing protein, fats, and carbohydrates?

Are probiotics working?

Is your child's digestive tract infected with the bacterium *Helicobacter pylori*, with *Candida*, with parasites?

Does your child have bad gastrointestinal bacteria that are drug resistant?

Does your child have gastrointestinal inflammation?

Is your child bleeding inside the digestive tract?

Are there certain bacteria that are keeping your child overweight?

Once bad organisms are found, the test uses sensitivity testing to analyze which naturopathic prescription will most effectively clear them from your child's system.

Different labs specialize in different tests, but even if a lab offers a test, it doesn't mean it is an expert in performing it. Be sure to choose a reputable lab recommended by your physician.

## Who Needs This Test?

### NEUROLOGICAL COMPLAINTS

| | |
|---|---|
| ADHD | Autism |

### GASTROINTESTINAL COMPLAINTS

| | |
|---|---|
| Abdominal pain | GERD |
| Acid reflux | Heartburn |
| Colic | IBS |
| Constipation | Inflammatory bowel disease (Crohn's disease, ulcerative colitis) |
| Diarrhea | |

### OTHER

| | |
|---|---|
| Weight gain | Weight loss |

# Toxicity Testing

We live in a toxic world. Go to www.ScoreCard.org to discover the levels of toxins where you live. They're in the air, the food, the water, the toys, and almost anything that's manufactured. Because we can't live in plastic bubbles (plastics can be toxic, too!), our bodies remove toxins on a daily basis. Some children cannot remove them fast enough for genetic reasons, or maybe they frequently eat fish containing high levels of mercury, such as canned tuna, causing the amount of mercury in their bodies to build up. Testing them helps us understand if toxins are causing health problems.

Toxins can be analyzed in hair, blood, urine, and stool samples, but certain toxins are better analyzed using one kind of sample rather than another. A complete toxin analysis may require multiple samples. Consult a specialist in toxicity to have the best assessment for your child.

## Who Needs This Test?

### NEUROLOGICAL COMPLAINTS

| | |
|---|---|
| ADHD | Headaches |
| Anxiety | Insomnia |
| Autism | Migraines |
| Depression | Seizures |
| Epilepsy | |

### OTHER

| | |
|---|---|
| Auto-immune diseases | Chronic fatigue |
| | Cancer |

# — RECOMMENDED READING —

## ALLERGIES

Randolph, Theron G. *An Alternative Approach to Allergies: The New Field of Clinical Ecology Unravels the Environmental Causes of Mental and Physical Ills.* New York: Harper Perennial, 1990.

Weintraub, Skye. *Allergies and Holistic Healing.* Salt Lake City: Woodland Publishing, 1997.

## ATTENTION-DEFICIT/HYPERACTIVITY DISORDER

Berne, Samuel A. *Without Ritalin: A Natural Approach to ADD.* Chicago: Keats, 2002.

Hoffer, Abram. *Healing Children's Attention and Behavior Disorders.* Toronto: CCNM Press, 2004.

Jacobelli, Frank and Lynn A. Watson. *ADD/ADHD Drug Free: Natural Alternatives and Practical Exercises to Help Your Child Focus.* New York: American Management Association, 2008.

Zimmerman, Marcia. *The ADD Nutrition Solution: A Drug Free Thirty-Day Plan.* New York: Holt, 1999.

## DIABETES MELLITUS

Murray, Michael T. and Michael R. Lyon. *How to Prevent and Treat Diabetes with Natural Medicine.* New York: Riverhead Books, 2003.

## DIGESTION AND INTESTINAL DISORDERS

Larimore, Walt, Sherri Flynt, and Steve Halliday. *Supersized Kids: How to Rescue Your Child from the Obesity Threat.* Brentwood, TN: Center Street, 2005.

Scala, James. *The New Eating Right for a Bad Gut: The Complete Nutritional Guide to Ileitis, Colitis, Crohn's Disease, and Inflammatory Bowel Disease.* New York: Plume, 2000.

## HEART HEALTH

Ornish, Dean. *Dr. Dean Ornish's Program for Reversing Heart Disease: The Only System Scientifically Proven to Reverse Heart Disease without Drugs or Surgery.* New York: Random House, 1990.

## HERBAL MEDICINE AND HOMEOPATHY

Castleman, Michael. *The Healing Herbs.* Emmaus, PA: Rodale Press, 1991.

Castro, Miranda. *The Complete Homeopathy Handbook: A Guide to Everyday Health Care.* New York: St. Martin's Press, 1991.

Chevallier, Andrew. *Natural Health Encyclopedia of Herbal Medicine: The Definitive Reference to 550 Herbs and Remedies for Common Ailments.* New York: DK, 2000.

Culpeper, Nicholas. *Culpeper's Complete Herbal.* Ware, UK: Wordsworth Editions, 1998.

Dooley, Timothy R. *Homeopathy Beyond Flat Earth Medicine.* 2nd edition. San Diego: Timing Publications, 2002.

Fiedler, Christie. *The Complete Idiot's Guide to Natural Remedies.* New York: Alpha Books, 2009.

Gladstar, Rosemary. *Rosemary Gladstar's Herbal Recipes for Vibrant Health: 175 Teas, Tonics, Oils, Salves, Tinctures, and Other Natural Remedies for the Entire Family.* North Adams, MA: Storey, 2008.

Hayfield, Robin. *Homeopathy for Common Ailments.* Berkeley, CA: Frog, 1993.

Helfferich, Michael and Walther Hohenester. *Homeopathy: Self-Healing Handbook.* New York: Sterling, 1999.

Kent, James Tyler. *Lectures on Homeopathic Philosophy.* Berkeley, CA: North Atlantic Books, 1993.

Lipp, Frank. *Healing Herbs.* London: Thorsons, 2004.

Lockie, Andrew. *The Family Guide to Homeopathy: Symptoms and Solutions.* New York: Prentice Hall, 1991.

Lust, John B. *The Herb Book: The Complete and Authoritative Guide to More Than 500 Herbs.* Charlotte, NC: Beneficial Books, 2001.

Murray, Michael T. *Natural Alternatives to Over-the-Counter and Prescription Drugs.* New York: W. Morrow, 1994.

Papon, R. Donald. *Homeopathy Made Simple: A Quick Reference Guide.* Charlottesville, VA: Hampton Roads, 1999.

Sankaran, Rajan. *The Soul of Remedies.* Mumbai: Homeopathic Medical Publishers, 1997.

Shelton, Jay. *Homeopathy: How It Really Works.* Amherst, NY: Prometheus Books, 2004.

Tierra, Michael. *The Way of Herbs.* New York: Pocket Books, 1998.

Tilgner, Sharol. *Herbal Medicine: From the Heart of the Earth.* Creswell, OR: Wise Acres, 1999.

Ullman, Dana. *Discovering Homeopathy: Medicine for the 21st Century.* Berkeley, CA: North Atlantic Books, 1988.

Vithoulkas, George. *The Science of Homeopathy.* New Delhi: B. Jain, 1993.

Wood, Matthew. *The Book of Herbal Wisdom: Using Plants as Medicines.* Berkeley, CA: North Atlantic Books, 1997.

## NATUROPATHY AND NATURAL MEDICINE

Bricklin, Mark. *Rodale's Encyclopedia of Natural Home Remedies: Hundreds of Simple Healing Techniques for Everyday Illness and Emergencies.* Emmaus, PA: Rodale Press, 1982.

Burton Goldberg Group. *Alternative Medicine: The Definitive Guide.* Puyallup, WA: Future Medicine, 1993.

Dunn, Jon. *The Family Guide to Naturopathic Medicine.* CA: Naturopathic Health Care, 2010.

Levy, Thomas E. *Optimal Nutrition for Optimal Health.* Chicago: Keats, 2001.

Murray, Michael T. *Doctor Murray's Total Body Tune-Up: Slow Down the Aging Process, Keep Your System Running Smoothly, Help Your Body Heal Itself—for Life!* New York: Bantam, 2000.

Murray, Michael T. and Joseph Pizzorno. *Encyclopedia of Natural Medicine.* Revised 2nd edition. New York: Three Rivers Press, 1997.

Pizzorno, Joseph and Michael T. Murray, editors. *Textbook of Natural Medicine, Volumes 1 and 2*. 3rd edition. St. Louis: Churchill Livingston Elsevier, 2006.

Prousky, Jonathan. *Principles and Practices of Naturopathic Clinical Nutrition*. Toronto: CCNM Press, 2008.

Skowron, Jared M. *Fundamentals of Naturopathic Pediatrics*. Toronto: CCNM Press, 2009.

Smith, Fraser. *An Introduction to Principles and Practice of Naturopathic Medicine*. Toronto: CCNM Press, 2008.

Stengler, Mark. *The Natural Physician's Healing Therapies: Proven Remedies Medical Doctors Don't Know*. New York: Prentice Hall, 2010.

Thiel, Robert J. *Naturopathy for the 21st Century: Combining Old and New*. Warsaw, IN: W. Whitman, 2001.

Weil, Andrew. *Natural Health, Natural Medicine: The Complete Guide to Wellness and Self-Care for Optimum Health*. Boston: Houghton Mifflin, 2004.

Weil, Andrew. *Spontaneous Healing*. New York: Knopf, 1995.

Williams, Jude C. *Nature's Gentle Cures: Safe and Effective Healing Therapies*. New York: Sterling, 1997.

## NUTRITION AND DIET

Chopra, Deepak. *Perfect Health*. New York: Harmony Books, 1991.

Gussow, Joan Dye. *This Organic Life*. White River Junction, VT: Chelsea Green, 2002.

Haas, Elton and Buck Levin. *Staying Healthy with Nutrition: The Complete Guide to Diet and Nutritional Medicine*. Berkeley, CA: Celestial Arts, 2006.

Kendall-Reed, Penny and Stephen Reed. *The New Naturopathic Diet*. Toronto: CCNM Press, 2004.

Lappé, Frances Moore. *Diet for a Small Planet*. New York: Ballantine, 1991.

Pitchford, Paul. *Healing with Whole Foods*. Berkeley, CA: North Atlantic Books, 2002.

Robbins, John. *Diet for a New America*. Walpole, NH: Stillpoint, 1987.

Steinman, David. *Diet for a Poisoned Planet*. New York: Thunder's Mouth Press, 2007.

Wood, Rebecca. *The New Whole Foods Encyclopedia: A Comprehensive Resource for Health Eating*. New York: Penguin, 2010.

Wright, Jonathan V. *Guide to Healing with Nutrition*. New Canaan, CT: Keats, 1990.

## PARENTING AND CHILDREN'S HEALTH

Bove, Mary. *An Encyclopedia of Natural Healing for Children and Infants*. 2nd edition. Chicago: Keats, 2001.

Candee, Andrea. *Gentle Healing for Baby and Child: A Parent's Guide*. New York: Pocket Books, 2001.

Conkling, Winifred. *Natural Healing for Children: An Essential Handbook for Parents*. New York: St. Martin's Press, 1997.

Feder, Lauren. *Natural Baby and Childcare: Practical Medical Advice and Holistic Wisdom for Raising Healthy Children*. New York: Healthy Living Books, 2006.

Likowski Duncan, Alice. *Your Healthy Child: A Guide to Natural Health Care*. Neskowin, OR: Sanicula Press, 1995.

Marker, Susan and Linda F. Palmer. *What Your Pediatrician Doesn't Know Can Hurt Your Child: A More Natural Approach to Parenting.* Dallas: BenBella Books, 2010.

Romm, Aviva Jill. *Naturally Healthy Babies and Children: A Commonsense Guide to Herbal Remedies, Nutrition, and Health.* Berkeley, CA: Celestial Arts, 2003.

Ross, Julia. *The Mood Cure.* New York: Viking, 2002.

Scott, Julian. *Natural Medicine for Children.* New York: Avon Books, 1990.

Sears, Robert W. *The Vaccine Book: Making the Right Decision for Your Child.* New York: Little, Brown, 2007.

Sears, William, Martha Sears, Robert Sears, and James Sears. *The Baby Book: Everything You Need to Know About Your Baby from Birth to Age Two.* Boston: Little, Brown, 2003.

Stengler, Mark and Angela Stengler. *Your Vital Child: A Natural Healing Guide for Caring Parents.* Emmaus, PA: Rodale Press, 2001.

Ullman, Dana. *Homeopathic Medicine for Children and Infants.* New York: J.P. Tarcher, 1992.

Vann, Lizzie. *Organic Baby and Toddler Cookbook.* New York: Dorling Kindersley, 2000.

White, Linda B. and Sunny Mavor. *Kids, Herbs and Health.* Loveland, CO: Interweave Press, 1998.

Wilson, Sarah. *Natural Health for Kids: Complementary Treatments for More Than 50 Ailments.* London: Hamlyn, 2006.

## TOXINS

Leviton, Richard. *The Healthy Living Space: 70 Practical Ways to Detoxify the Body and Home.* Newburyport, MA: Hampton Roads, 2001.

Magaziner, Allan, Linda Bonvie, and Anthony Zolezzi. *Chemical-Free Kids: How to Safeguard Your Child's Diet and Environment.* New York: Twin Streams, 2003.

Siegel-Maier, Karyn. *The Naturally Clean House: 100 Safe and Easy Herbal Formulas for Nontoxic Cleansers.* Pownal, VT: Storey, 1999.

## VITAMINS AND SUPPLEMENTS

Balch, James F. and Mark Stengler. *Prescription for Natural Cures.* Hoboken, NJ: Wiley, 2004.

Balch, James, Mark Stengler, and Robin Young Balch. *Prescription for Drug Alternatives: All-Natural Options for Better Health without the Side Effects.* Hoboken, NJ: Wiley 2008.

Bratman, Stephen and Andrea Girman, editors. *Mosby's Handbook of Herbs and Supplements and Their Therapeutic Uses.* St. Louis: Mosby, 2002.

Braverman, Eric and Carl C. Pfeifer. *The Healing Nutrients Within.* Chicago: Keats Publishing, 1987.

Challem, Jack, editor. *User's Guide to Nutritional Supplements.* Laguna Beach, CA: Basic Health, 2003.

Combs, Gerald F. *The Vitamins: Fundamental Aspects in Nutrition and Health.* Burlington, MA: Elsevier, 2008.

Gottlieb, Bill. *Alternative Cures: More Than 1,000 of the Most Effective Natural Home Remedies.* New York: Ballantine, 2008.

Graedon, Joe and Teresa Graedon. *The People's Pharmacy Guide to Home and Herbal Remedies.* New York: St. Martin's Press, 2002.

Griffith, H. Winter. *Vitamins, Herbs, Minerals and Supplements: The Complete Guide.* New York: Fisher Books, 1998.

Haas, Elson M.. *Staying Healthy with Nutrition.* Berkeley, CA: Celestial Arts, 1992.

Hoffer, Abram and Jonathan Prousky. *Naturopathic Nutrition: A Guide to Nutrient-Rich Food and Nutritional Supplements for Optimum Health.* Toronto: CCNM Press, 2006.

Kalbacken, Joan. *Vitamins and Minerals.* Danbury, CT: Children's Press, 1998.

Kalyn, Wayne. *The Healing Power of Vitamins, Minerals, and Herbs.* New York: Reader's Digest, 1999.

Lieberman, Shari and Nancy Bruning. *The Real Vitamin and Mineral Book: The Definitive Guide to Designing Your Personal Supplement Program. 4th edition.* New York: Avery, 2007.

Lowe, Carl. *The Complete Vitamin Book.* New York: Berkley Books, 1994.

Mindell, Earl. *Earl Mindell's New Herb Bible.* New York: Fireside, 2000.

Mindell, Earl. *Earl Mindell's New Vitamin Bible.* New York: Grand Central, 2011.

Minich, Deanna M. *Quantum Supplements: A Total Health and Wellness Makeover with Vitamins, Minerals, and Herbs.* Newburyport, MA: Conari Press, 2010.

Murray, Michael T. *Encyclopedia of Nutritional Supplements.* Roseville, CA: Prima, 1996.

*Prevention* Magazine Editors. *The Complete Book of Vitamins and Minerals for Health.* Emmaus, PA: Rodale, 1988.

Rose, Sarah. *Vitamins and Minerals.* London: Hamlyn, 2003.

Royston, Angela. *Vitamins and Minerals for a Healthy Body.* Portsmouth, NH: Heinemann, 2003.

Schrier, E.W., editor. *Reader's Digest Guide to Drugs and Supplements: Vitamins, Minerals, and Herbs.* Pleasantville, NY: Reader's Digest, 2002.

Sharon, Michael. *Nutrient A-Z: A User's Guide to Foods, Herbs, Vitamins, Minerals and Supplements.* London: Carleton, 2009.

Sullivan, Karen. *Illustrated Elements of Vitamins and Minerals.* Salisbury, UK: Element, 2002.

Talbott, Shawn M. *A Guide to Understanding Dietary Supplements.* New York: Routledge, 2003.

# — ENDNOTES —

## INTRODUCTION

Task Force on Drug Importation. *Report on Prescription Drug Importation.* Hyattsville, MD: US Department of Health and Human Services, 2004.

World Health Organization. *World Health Statistics 2010.* Geneva: World Health Organization, 2010.

Centers for Disease Control and Prevention. Healthy Youth! Health Topics: Asthma. June 3, 2010. www.cdc.gov/HealthyYouth/asthma.

Kogan MD, Blumberg SJ, Schieve LA, et al. Prevalence of parent-reported diagnosis of autism spectrum disorder among children in the US, 2007. *Pediatrics* 2009; 124(5):1395–1403.

Centers for Disease Control and Prevention. Increasing prevalence of parent-reported attention-deficit/hyperactivity disorder among children—United States, 2003 and 2007. *Morbidity and Mortality Weekly Report* 2010; 59(44):1439–1443.

US Department of Health and Human Services. *Summary Health Statistics for U.S. Children: National Health Interview Survey, 2009.* Vital and Health Statistics Series 10, Number 247. Hyattsville, MD: US Department of Health and Human Services, 2010.

Nahin RL, Barnes PM, Stussman BJ, Bloom B. *Costs of complementary and alternative medicine (CAM) and frequency of visits to CAM practitioners: United States, 2007.* National Health Statistics Reports, No. 18. Hyattsville, MD: National Center for Health Statistics, 2009.

## PART I: NATURAL SOLUTIONS FOR YOUR KIDS

### CHAPTER 1

Boris M, Mandel FS. Foods and additives are common causes of the attention deficit hyperactive disorder in children. *Annals of Allergy* May 1994; 72(5):462–468.

[No authors listed.] Artificial food colouring and hyperactivity symptoms in children. *Prescrire International* 2009; 18(103):215.

Howard AL, Robinson M, Smith GJ, et al. ADHD is associated with a "Western" dietary pattern in adolescents. *Journal of Attention Disorders* 2010 Jul 14 doi: 10.1177/1087054710365990. [epub ahead of print]

Oddy WH, Robinson M, Ambrosini GL, et al. The association between dietary patterns and mental health in early adolescence. *Preventive Medicine* 2009; 49(1):39–44.

Pelsser LM, Buitelaar JK. [Favorable effect of a standard elimination diet on the behavior of young children with attention deficit hyperactivity disorder (ADHD): a pilot study]. *Nederlands Tijdschrift Geneeskunde* 2002; 146(52):2543–2547. [Dutch]

Kochan Z, Karbowska J, Babicz-Zielinska E. [Dietary trans-fatty acids and metabolic syndrome]. *Postepy Higieny i Medycyny Doswiadczelnej (Online)* 2010; 64:650–658. [Polish]

Webber LS, Srinivasan SR, Wattigney WA, Berenson GS. Tracking of serum and lipids and lipoproteins from childhood to adulthood: The Bogalusa Heart Study. *American Journal of Epidemiology* 1991; 33(9):884–899.

Dennison BA, Rockwell HL, Baker SL. Excess fruit juice consumption by preschool-aged children is associated with short stature and obesity. *Pediatrics* 1997; 99(1):15–22.


## CHAPTER 2

Davis A. *Let's Have Healthy Children*. New York: Harcourt Brace Jovanovich, 1972.

Stevens LJ, Kuczek T, Burgess T, et al. Dietary sensitivities and ADHD symptoms: Thirty-five years of research. *Clinical Pediatrics* 2011; 50(4):279–293.

Pelsser LM, Frankena K, Buitelaar JK, Rommelse NN. Effects of food on physical and sleep complaints in children with ADHD: A randomised controlled pilot study. *European Journal of Pediatrics* 2010; 169(9):1129–1138.

Pelsser LM, Frankena K, Toorman J, et al. A randomised controlled trial into the effects of food on ADHD. *European Child and Adolescent Psychiatry* 2009; 18(1):12–19.


## CHAPTER 3

Gonzalez S. Mind Disrupted: How Toxic Chemicals May Change How We Think and Who We Are. Learning and Developmental Disabilities Initiative, 2010. www.minddisrupted.org/documents/Mind%20Disrupted%20report.pdf.

Perera FP, Tang D, Tu YH, et al. Biomarkers in maternal and newborn blood indicate heightened fetal susceptibility to procarcinogenic DNA damage. *Environmental Health Perspectives* 2004; 112(10)1133–1136.

Marks AR, Harley K, Bradman A, et al. Organophosphate pesticide exposure and attention in young Mexican-American children: The CHAMACOS study. *Environmental Health Perspectives* 2010; 118(12):1768–1774.

Bouchard MF, Bellinger DC, Wright RO, Weisskopf MG. Attention-deficit/hyperactivity disorder and urinary metabolites of organophosphate pesticides. *Pediatrics* 2010; 125(6):e1270–e1277.

Roberts EM, English PB, Grether JK, et al. Maternal residence near agricultural pesticide applications and autism spectrum disorders among children in the California Central Valley. *Environmental Health Perspectives* 2007; 115(10):1482–1489.

Sutton R. Teen girls' body burden of hormone-altering cosmetics chemicals: Adolescent exposures to cosmetic chemicals of concern. Environmental Working Group, September 2008. www.ewg.org/reports/teens.

National Institute of Environmental Health Sciences. *Issues and Challenges in Environmental Health*. National Institutes of Health Publication #87–861. Research Triangle Park, NC: US Department of Health and Human Services, 1987.

Marks, Amy et al. ADHD Linked to Prenatal Pesticide Exposure. *Environmental Health Perspectives* August 2010.

Eskenazi B, Marks AR, Bradman A, et al. Organophosphate pesticide exposure and neurodevelopment in young Mexican-American children. *Environmental Health Perspectives* 2007; 115(5):792–798.

Rauh VA, Garfinkel R, Perera FP, et al. Impact of prenatal chlorpyrifos exposure on neurodevelopment in the first 3 years of life among inner-city children. *Pediatrics* 2006; 118(6):e1845–e1859.

Fortes C, Mastroeni, S, Boffetta P, et al. Reliability of self-reported household pesticide use. *European Journal of Cancer Prevention* 2009; 18(5):404–406.

Boers D, Portengen L, Bueno-de-Mesquita HB, et al. Cause-specific mortality of Dutch chlorophenoxy herbicide manufacturing workers. *Occupational and Environmental Medicine* 2010; 67(1):24–31.

## PART II: TOP 100 PEDIATRIC HEALTH CONDITIONS AND SAFE, NATURAL SOLUTIONS

### CHAPTER 4

Mokdad AH, Marks JS, Stroup DF, Gerberding JL. Actual causes of death in the United States, 2000. *The Journal of the American Medical Association* 2004; 291(10):1238–1245.

### (1) HYPERTENSION (HIGH BLOOD PRESSURE)

Imperial College London. Free statins with fast food could neutralize heart risk, scientists say. *ScienceDaily,* August 12, 2010. www.sciencedaily.com/releases/2010/08/100812083608.htm.

Pal S, Khossousi A, Binns C, et al. The effect of a fibre supplement compared to a healthy diet on body composition, lipids, glucose, insulin and other metabolic syndrome risk factors in overweight and obese individuals. *British Journal of Nutrition* 2011; 105(1):90–100.

Giacosa A, Rondanelli M. The right fiber for the right disease: An update on the psyllium seed husk and the metabolic syndrome. *Journal of Clinical Gastroenterology* 2010; 44 Suppl 1:S58–S60.

Mori TA, Bao DQ, Burke V, et al. Docosahexaenoic acid but not eicosapentaenoic acid lowers ambulatory blood pressure and heart rate in humans. *Hypertension* 1999; 34(2):253–260.

Nelin LD, Hoffman GM. L-arginine infusion lowers blood pressure in children. *Journal of Pediatrics* 2001; 139(5):747–749.

### (2) HIGH CHOLESTEROL

American Heart Association. *Cholesterol and atherosclerosis in children.* n.d. www.americanheart.org/presenter.jhtml?identifier=4499.

Linke A, Sonnabend M, Fasshauer M, et al. Effects of extended-release niacin on lipid profile and adipocyte biology in patients with impaired glucose tolerance. *Atherosclerosis* 2009; 205(1):207–213.

de Jongh S, Vissers MN, Rol P, et al. Plant sterols lower LDL cholesterol without improving endothelial function in prepubertal children with familial hypercholesterolaemia. *Journal of Inherited Metabolic Disease* 2003; 26(4):343–351.

Dennison BA, Levine DM. Randomized, double-blind, placebo-controlled, two-period crossover clinical trial of psyllium fiber in children with hypercholesterolemia. *Journal of Pediatrics* 1993; 123(1):24–29.

Kwiterovich PO. The role of fiber in the treatment of hypercholesterolemia in children and adolescents. *Pediatrics* 1995; 96(5):1005–1009.

Zibadi S, Rohdewald PJ, Park D, Watson RR. Reduction of cardiovascular risk factors in subjects with type 2 diabetes by Pycnogenol supplementation. *Nutrition Research* 2008; 28(5):315–320.

## (4) KAWASAKI SYNDROME

Takeshita S, Kobayashi I, Kawamura Y, et al. Characteristic profile of intestinal microflora in Kawasaki disease. *Acta Paediatrica* 2002; 91(7):783–788.

Deng YB, Li TL, Xiang HJ, et al. Impaired endothelial function in the brachial artery after Kawasaki disease and the effects of intravenous administration of vitamin C. *Pediatric Infectious Disease Journal* 2003; 22(1):34–39.

## (5) ANEMIC JAUNDICE (G6PD DEFICIENCY)

Wright RO, Woolf AD, Shannon MW, Magnani B. N-acetylcysteine reduces methemoglobin in an in-vitro model of glucose-6-phosphate dehydrogenase deficiency. *Academic Emergency Medicine* 1998; 5(3):225–229.

Corash L, Spielberg S, Bartsocas C, et al. Reduced chronic hemolysis during high-dose vitamin E administration in Mediterranean-type glucose-6-phosphate dehydrogenase deficiency. *New England Journal of Medicine* 1980; 303(8):416–420.

## (6) CONGENITAL HEART DEFECTS

Tanner K, Sabrine, N, Wren C. Cardiovascular malformations among preterm infants. *Pediatrics* 2005; 116(6):e833–e838.

Godwin KA, Sibbald B, Bedard T, et al. Changes in frequencies of select congenital anomalies since the onset of folic acid fortification in a Canadian birth defect registry. *Canadian Journal of Public Health* 2008; 99(4):271–275.

Olgar S, Ertugrul T, Nisli K, et al. Fish oil supplementation improves left ventricular function in children with idiopathic dilated cardiomyopathy. *Congestive Heart Failure* 2007; 13(6):308–312.

Aufricht C, Ties M, Wimmer M, et al. Iron supplementation in children after cardiopulmonary bypass for surgical repair of congenital heart disease. *Pediatric Cardiology* 1994; 15(4):167–169.

Liu D, Liu S, Huang Y, et al. Effect of selenium on human myocardial glutathione peroxidase gene expression. *Chinese Medical Journal* 2000; 113(9):771–775.

Huang Y, Han L, Guo J. [Protective effect of selenium on human erythrocyte rheology]. *Zhonghua Yi Xue Za Zhi* 1998; 78(2):101–104. [Chinese]

Gu J, Li J, Liu S. [Protective effect of *Salvia miltiorrhizae composita* on myocardium in patients undergoing open heart surgery]. *Zhongguo Zhong Xi Yi Jie He Za Zhi* 1998; 18(2):68–70. [Chinese]

## (7) MEGALOBLASTIC ANEMIA (GIANT RED BLOOD CELLS)

Khanduri U, Sharma A. Megaloblastic anaemia: Prevalence and causative factors. *National Medical Journal of India* 2007; 20(4):172–175.

Monfort-Gouraud M, Bongiorno A, Le Gall MA, Badoual J. [Severe megaloblastic anemia in child breast fed by a vegetarian mother]. *Annales de Pédiatrie* 1993; 40(1):28–31. [French]

Katar S, Nuri Ozbek M, Yaramis A, Ecer S. Nutritional megaloblastic anemia in young Turkish children is associated with vitamin B-12 deficiency and psychomotor retardation. *Journal of Pediatric Hematology/Oncology* 2006; 28(9):559–562.

Simsek OP, Gönç N, Gümrük F, Cetin M. A child with vitamin B12 deficiency presenting with pancytopenia and hyperpigmentation. *Journal of Pediatric Hematology/Oncology* 2004; 26(12):834–836.

## (10) CONJUNCTIVITIS (PINKEYE)

Stoss M, Michels C, Peter E, et al. Prospective cohort trial of *Euphrasia* single-dose eye drops in conjunctivitis. *Journal of Alternative and Complementary Medicine* 2000; 6(6):499–508.

Russo V, Stella A, Appezzati L, et al. Clinical efficacy of a *Ginkgo biloba* extract in the topical treatment of allergic conjunctivitis. *European Journal of Ophthalmology* 2009; 19(3):331–336.

## (12) PINGUECULA AND PTERYGIUM (YELLOW SPOT ON THE WHITE OF THE EYE)

Nakaishi H, Yamamoto M, Ishida M, et al. Pingueculae and pterygia in motorcycle policemen. *Industrial Health* 1997; 35(3):325–329.

Kaji Y, Oshika T, Amano S, et al. Immunohistochemical localization of advanced glycation end products in pinguecula. *Graefe's Archive for Clinical and Experimental Ophthalmology* 2006; 244(1):104–108.

## (13) OTITIS EXTERNA (SWIMMER'S EAR)

Nogueira JC, Diniz Mde F, Lima EO. In vitro antimicrobial activity of plants in acute otitis externa. *Brazilian Journal of Otorhinolaryngology* 2008; 74(1):118–124.

Farnan TB, McCallum J, Awa A, et al. Tea tree oil: In vitro efficacy in otitis externa. *Journal of Laryngology and Otology* 2005; 119(3):198–201.

Pai ST, Platt MW. Antifungal effects of *Allium sativum* (garlic) extract against the *Aspergillus* species involved in otomycosis. *Letters in Applied Microbiology* 1995; 20(1):14–18.


## (14) OTITIS MEDIA (MIDDLE EAR INFECTION)

Juntti H, Tikkanen S, Kokkonen J, et al. Cow's milk allergy is associated with recurrent otitis media during childhood. *Acta Oto-laryngologica* 1999; 119(8):867–873.

Linday LA, Shindledecker RD, Dolitsky JN, et al. Plasma 25-hydroxyvitamin D levels in young children undergoing placement of tympanostomy tubes. *Annals of Otology, Rhinology and Laryngology* 2008; 117(10):740–744.

Cameron C, Dallaire F, Vézina C, et al. Neonatal vitamin A deficiency and its impact on acute respiratory infections among preschool Inuit children. *Canadian Journal of Public Health* 2008; 99(2):102–106.

Aladag I, Guven M, Eyibilen A, et al. Efficacy of vitamin A in experimentally induced acute otitis media. *International Journal of Pediatric Otorhinolaryngology* 2007; 71(4):623–628.

Yilmaz T, Koçan EG, Besler HT, et al. The role of oxidants and antioxidants in otitis media with effusion in children. *Otolaryngology—Head and Neck Surgery* 2004; 131(6):797–803.

Sarrell EM, Mandelberg A, Cohen HA. Efficacy of naturopathic extracts in the management of ear pain associated with acute otitis media. *Archives of Pediatrics and Adolescent Medicine* 2001; 155(7):796–799.


## (17) BENIGN PAROXYSMAL POSITIONAL VERTIGO

Richard W, Bruintjes TD, Oostenbrink P, van Leeuwen RB. Efficacy of the Epley maneuver for posterior canal BPPV: A long-term, controlled study of 81 patients. *Ear, Nose, and Throat Journal* 2005; 84(1):22–25.

Teixeira LJ, Machado JN. Maneuvers for the treatment of benign positional paroxysmal vertigo: A systematic review. *Brazilian Journal of Otorhinolaryngology* 2006; 72(1):130–139.


## (19) EPISTAXIS (NOSEBLEED)

Galley P, Thiollet M. A double-blind, placebo-controlled trial of a new veno-active flavonoid fraction (S 5682) in the treatment of symptomatic capillary fragility. *International Angiology* 1993; 12(1):69–72.

## (20) RHINITIS (NASAL INFLAMMATION)

Kuitunen M, Kukkonen K, Juntunen-Backman K, et al. Probiotics prevent IgE-associated allergy until age 5 years in cesarean-delivered children but not in the total cohort. *Journal of Allergy and Clinical Immunology* 2009; 123(2):335–341.

Bucca C, Rolla G, Oliva A, Farina JC. Effect of vitamin C on histamine bronchial responsiveness of patients with allergic rhinitis. *Annals of Allergy* 1990; 65(4):311–314.

Roschek B, Fink RC, McMichael M, Alberte RS. Nettle extract (*Urtica dioica*) affects key receptors and enzymes associated with allergic rhinitis. *Phytotherapy Research* 2009; 23:920–926.


## (21) SINUSITIS

Shoseyov D, Bibi H, Shai P, et al. Treatment with hypertonic saline versus normal saline nasal wash of pediatric chronic sinusitis. *Journal of Allergy and Clinical Immunology* 1998; 101(5):602–605.

Freeman SR, Sivayoham ES, Jepson K, de Carpentier J. A preliminary randomised controlled trial evaluating the efficacy of saline douching following endoscopic sinus surgery. *Clinical Otolaryngology* 2008; 33(5):462–465.

Braun JM, Schneider B, Beuth HJ. Therapeutic use, efficiency and safety of the proteolytic pineapple enzyme Bromelain-POS in children with acute sinusitis in Germany. *In Vivo* 2005; 19(2):417–421.


## (23) PHARYNGITIS (SORE THROAT)

Hubbert M, Sievers H, Lehnfeld R, Kehrl W. Efficacy and tolerability of a spray with Salvia officinalis in the treatment of acute pharyngitis: A randomised, double-blind, placebo-controlled study with adaptive design and interim analysis. *European Journal of Medical Research* 2006; 11(1):20–26.


## (24) STREP THROAT

Groppo FC, Ramacciato JC, Motta RH, et al. Antimicrobial activity of garlic against oral streptococci. *International Journal of Dental Hygiene* 2007; 5(2):109–115.


## (25) POSTNASAL DRIP

Ratjen F, Wönne R, Posselt H-G, et al. A double-blind placebo controlled trial with oral ambroxol and N-acetylcysteine for mucolytic treatment in cystic fibrosis. *European Journal of Pediatrics* 1985; 144(4):374–378.

Boogaard R, de Jongste JC, Merkus PJ. Pharmacotherapy of impaired mucociliary clearance in non-CF pediatric lung disease: A review of the literature. *Pediatric Pulmonology* 2007; 42(11):989–1001.

## (26) TONSILLITIS

Onerci M, Kus S, Ogretmenoglu O. Trace elements in children with chronic and recurrent tonsillitis. *International Journal of Pediatric Otorhinolaryngology* 1997; 41(1):47–51.

Yang Y, Wang LD, Chen ZB. [Effects of *Astragalus membranaceus* on TH cell subset function in children with recurrent tonsillitis]. *Zhongguo Dang Dai Er Ke Za Zhi* 2006; 8(5):376–378. [Chinese]

Yilmaz T, Koçan EG, Besler HT. The role of oxidants and antioxidants in chronic tonsillitis and adenoid hypertrophy in children. *International Journal of Pediatric Otorhinolaryngology* 2004; 68(8):1053–1058.


## (27) ORAL CANDIDIASIS (THRUSH)

Sabitha P, Adhikari PM, Shenoy SM, et al. Efficacy of garlic paste in oral candidiasis. *Tropical Doctor* 2005; 35(2):99–100.

Nyst MJ, Perriens JH, Kimputu L, et al. Gentian violet, ketoconazole and nystatin in oropharyngeal and esophageal candidiasis in Zairian AIDS patients. *Annales de la Société Belge de Médecine Tropicale* 1992; 72(1):45–52.


## (30) CELIAC DISEASE

De Angelis M, Rizzello CG, Fasano A, et al. VSL#3 probiotic preparation has the capacity to hydrolyze gliadin polypeptides responsible for celiac sprue. *Biochimica et Biophysica Acta* 2006; 1762(1):80–93.

Stenman SM, Venäläinen JI, Lindfors K, et al. Enzymatic detoxification of gluten by germinating wheat proteases: Implications for new treatment of celiac disease. *Annals of Medicine* 2009; 41(5):390–400.


## (31) CONSTIPATION

Castillejo G, Bulló M, Anguera A, et al. A controlled, randomized, double-blind trial to evaluate the effect of a supplement of cocoa husk that is rich in dietary fiber on colonic transit in constipated pediatric patients. *Pediatrics* 2006; 118(3):e641–e648.

Bekkali NLH, Bongers MEJ, Van den Berg MM, et al. The role of a probiotics mixture in the treatment of childhood constipation: A pilot study. *Nutrition Journal* 2007; 6:17.


## (32) DIARRHEA

Scrimgeour AG, Lukaski HC. Zinc and diarrheal disease: Current status and future perspectives. *Current Opinion in Clinical Nutrition and Metabolic Care* 2008; 11(6):711–717.

Sazawal S, Black RE, Ramsan M, et al. Effect of zinc supplementation on mortality in children aged 1–48 months: A community-based randomised placebo-controlled trial. *Lancet* 2007; 369(9565):927–934.

Long KZ, Rosado JL, Montoya Y, et al. Effect of vitamin A and zinc supplementation on gastrointestinal parasitic infections among Mexican children. *Pediatrics* 2007; 120(4):e846–e855.

Ou-Yang WX, You JY, Duan BP, Chen CB. [Application of food allergens specific IgG antibody detection in chronic diarrhea in children]. *Zhongguo Dang Dai Er Ke Za Zhi* 2008; 10(1):21–24. [Chinese]

Kligler B, Hanaway P, Cohrssen A. Probiotics in children. *Pediatric Clinics of North America* 2007; 54(6):949–967.

### (33) COLIC

Savino F, Pelle E, Palumeri E, et al. Lactobacillus reuteri (American Type Culture Collection strain 55730) versus simethicone in the treatment of infantile colic: A prospective randomized study. *Pediatrics* 2007; 119(1):e124–e130.

Savino F, Cresi F, Castagno E, et al. A randomized double-blind placebo-controlled trial of a standardized extract of *Matricariae recutita, Foeniculum vulgare* and *Melissa officinalis* (ColiMil) in the treatment of breastfed colicky infants. *Phytotherapy Research* 2005; 19(4):335–340.

### (34) GERD/REFLUX/HEARTBURN

Higginbotham TW. Effectiveness and safety of proton pump inhibitors in infantile gastroesophageal reflux disease. *Annals of Pharmacotherapy* 2010; 44(3):572–576.

Romano C, Chiaro A, Comito D, et al. Proton pump inhibitors in pediatrics: Evaluation of efficacy in GERD therapy. *Current Clinical Pharmacology* 2011 Jan 11 PMID: 21235462. [epub ahead of print]

### (35) IRRITABLE BOWEL SYNDROME

Austin GL, Dalton CB, Hu Y, et al. A very low-carbohydrate diet improves symptoms and quality of life in diarrhea-predominant irritable bowel syndrome. *Clinical Gastroenterology and Hepatology* 2009; 7(6):706–708.

Atkinson W, Sheldon TA, Shaath N, Whorwell PJ. Food elimination based on IgG antibodies in irritable bowel syndrome: A randomised controlled trial. *Gut* 2004; 53(10):1459–1464.

Saha L, Malhotra S, Rana S, et al. A preliminary study of melatonin in irritable bowel syndrome. *Journal of Clinical Gastroenterology* 2007; 41(1):29–32.

Camilleri M. Probiotics and irritable bowel syndrome: Rationale, putative mechanisms, and evidence of clinical efficacy. *Journal of Clinical Gastroenterology* 2006; 40(3):264–269.

Kuttner L, Chambers CT, Hardial J, et al. A randomized trial of yoga for adolescents with irritable bowel syndrome. *Pain Research and Management* 2006; 11(4):217–223.

## (36) GASTROENTERITIS (STOMACH BUG)

Szymanski H, Pejcz J, Jawien M, et al. Treatment of acute infectious diarrhoea in infants and children with a mixture of three Lactobacillus rhamnosus strains: A randomized, double-blind, placebo-controlled trial. *Alimentary Pharmacology and Therapeutics* 2006; 23(2):247–253.

Sarker SA, Sultana S, Fuchs GJ, et al. *Lactobacillus paracasei* strain ST11 has no effect on rotavirus but ameliorates the outcome of nonrotavirus diarrhea in children from Bangladesh. *Pediatrics* 2005; 116(2):e221–e228.

Dubey AP, Rajeshwari K, Chakravarty A, Famularo G. Use of VSL#3 in the treatment of rotavirus diarrhea in children: Preliminary results. *Journal of Clinical Gastroenterology* 2008; 42 Suppl 3 Pt 1:S126–S129.

## (37) GASTROINTESTINAL CANDIDIASIS

Pereira AP, Ferreira ICFR, Marcelino F, et al. Phenolic compounds and antimicrobial activity of olive (Olea europaea L. Cv. Cobrançosa) leaves. *Molecules* 2007; 12(5):1153–1162.

## (38) ACUTE PANCREATITIS

Xiong J, Zhu S, Zhou Y, et al. Regulation of omega-3 fish oil emulsion on the SIRS during the initial stage of severe acute pancreatitis. *Journal of Huazhong University of Science and Technology: Medical Sciences* 2009; 29(1):35–38.

Yang SQ, Xu JG. [Effect of glutamine on serum interleukin-8 and tumor necrosis factor-alpha levels in patients with severe pancreatitis]. *Nan Fang Yi Ke Da Xue Xue Bao* 2008; 28(1):129–131. [Chinese]

## (39) PEPTIC ULCER

Okabe S, Takeuchi K, Honda K, Takagi K. Effects of acetylsalicylic acid (ASA), ASA plus L-glutamine and L-glutamine on healing of chronic gastric ulcer in the rat. *Digestion* 1976; 14(1):85–88.

## (40) CROHN'S DISEASE

Onken JE, Greer PK, Calingaert B, Hale LP. Bromelain treatment decreases secretion of pro-inflammatory cytokines and chemokines by colon biopsies in vitro. *Clinical Immunology* 2008; 126(3):345–352.

Gupta P, Andrew H, Kirschner BS, Guandalini S. Is Lactobacillus GG helpful in children with Crohn's disease? Results of a preliminary, open-label study. *Journal of Pediatric Gastroenterology and Nutrition* 2000; 31(4):453–457.

## (41) ULCERATIVE COLITIS

Vernia P, Annese V, Bresci G, et al. Topical butyrate improves efficacy of 5-ASA in refractory distal ulcerative colitis: Results of a multicentre trial. *European Journal of Clinical Investigation* 2003; 33(3):244–248.

Hanai H, Iida T, Takeuchi K, et al. Curcumin maintenance therapy for ulcerative colitis: Randomized, multicenter, double-blind, placebo-controlled trial. *Clinical Gastroenterology and Hepatology* 2006; 4(12):1502–1506.

Miele E, Pascarella F, Giannetti E, et al. Effect of a probiotic preparation (VSL#3) on induction and maintenance of remission in children with ulcerative colitis. *American Journal of Gastroenterology* 2009; 104(2):437–443.


## (42) HERNIA

Botto LD, Mulinare J, Erickson JD. Occurrence of omphalocele in relation to maternal multivitamin use: A population-based study. *Pediatrics* 2002; 109(5):904–908.


## (43) ATTENTION DEFICIT HYPERACTIVITY DISORDER

Johnson M, Ostlund S, Fransson G, et al. Omega-3/omega-6 fatty acids for attention deficit hyperactivity disorder: A randomized placebo-controlled trial in children and adolescents. *Journal of Attention Disorders* 2009; 12(5):394–401.

Mousain-Bosc M, Roche M, Polge A, et al. Improvement of neurobehavioral disorders in children supplemented with magnesium-vitamin $B_6$. I. Attention deficit hyperactivity disorders. *Magnesium Research* 2006; 19(1): 46–52.

Lyon MR, Cline JC, Totosy de Zepetnek J, et al. Effect of the herbal extract combination *Panax quinquefolium* and *Ginkgo biloba* on attention-deficit hyperactivity disorder: A pilot study. *Journal of Psychiatry and Neuroscience* 2001; 26(3):221–228.


## (44) AUTISM

Cohly HH, Panja A. Immunological findings in autism. *International Review of Neurobiology* 2005; 71:317–341.

Enstrom A, Krakowiak P, Onore C, et al. Increased IgG4 levels in children with autism disorder. *Brain, Behavior, and Immunity* 2009; 23(3):389–395.

Mousain-Bosc M, Roche M, Polge A, et al. Improvement of neurobehavioral disorders in children supplemented with magnesium-vitamin $B_6$. II. Pervasive developmental disorder-autism. *Magnesium Research* 2006; 19(1):53–62.

Chez MG, Buchanan CP, Aimonovitch MC, et al. Double-blind, placebo-controlled study of L-carnosine supplementation in children with autistic spectrum disorders. *Journal of Child Neurology* 2002; 17(11):833–837.

## (45) DEPRESSION

Murakami K, Miyake Y, Sasaki S, et al. Fish and n-3 polyunsaturated fatty acid intake and depressive symptoms: Ryukyus Child Health Study. *Pediatrics* 2010; 126(3):e623–e630.

Murakami K, Miyake Y, Sasaki S, et al. Dietary folate, riboflavin, vitamin B-6, and vitamin B-12 and depressive symptoms in early adolescence: The Ryukyus Child Health Study. *Psychosomatic Medicine* 2010; 72(8):763–768.

## (46) HEADACHE

Hershey AD, Powers SW, Vockell AL, et al. Coenzyme Q10 deficiency and response to supplementation in pediatric and adolescent migraine. *Headache* 2007; 47(1):73–80.

Miano S, Parisi P, Pelliccia A, et al. Melatonin to prevent migraine or tension-type headache in children. *Neurological Sciences* 2008; 29(4):285–287.

Peres MF, Zukerman E, da Cunha Tanuri F, et al. Melatonin, 3 mg, is effective for migraine prevention. *Neurology* 2004; 63(4):757.

## (49) STRESS AND ANXIETY

Samarkandi A, Naguib M, Riad W, et al. Melatonin vs. midazolam premedication in children: A double-blind, placebo-controlled study. *European Journal of Anaesthesiology* 2005; 22(3):189–196.

## (50) INSOMNIA

Bendz LM, Scates AC. Melatonin treatment for insomnia in pediatric patients with attention-deficit/hyperactivity disorder. *Annals of Pharmacotherapy* 2010; 44(1):185–191.

## (52) HYPOTHYROIDISM

Patrick L. Iodine: Deficiency and therapeutic considerations. *Alternative Medicine Review* 2008; 13(2):116–127.

## (53) TYPE 1 DIABETES MELLITUS

Stene LC, Joner G. Use of cod liver oil during the first year of life is associated with lower risk of childhood-onset type 1 diabetes: A large, population-based, case-control study. *American Journal of Clinical Nutrition* 2003; 78(6):1128–1134.

Hyppönen E, Läärä E, Reunanen A, et al. Intake of vitamin D and risk of type 1 diabetes: A birth-cohort study. *Lancet* 2001; 358(9292):1500–1503.

Matsuda T, Ferreri K, Todorov I, et al. Silymarin protects pancreatic ß-cells against cytokine-mediated toxicity: Implications of c-Jun NH$_2$-terminal kinase and Janus kinase/signal transducer and activator of transcription pathways. *Endocrinology* 2005; 146(1):175–185.

## (54) TYPE 2 DIABETES MELLITUS

Anderson RA. Chromium and polyphenols from cinnamon improve insulin sensitivity. *Proceedings of the Nutrition Society* 2008; 67(1):48–53.

Huerta MG, Roemmich JN, Kington ML, et al. Magnesium deficiency is associated with insulin resistance in obese children. *Diabetes Care* 2005; 28(5):1175–1181.

## (55) MEASLES

Fawzi WW, Herrera MG, Willett WC, et al. Dietary vitamin A intake and the incidence of diarrhea and respiratory infection among Sudanese children. *Journal of Nutrition* 1995; 125(5):1211–1221.

Yalçin SS, Yurdakök K, Ozalp I, Coskun T. The effect of live measles vaccines on serum vitamin A levels in healthy children. *Acta Paediatrica Japonica* 1998; 40(4):345–349.

## (60) CHICKEN POX

Thomas SL, Wheeler JG, Hall AJ. Micronutrient intake and the risk of herpes zoster: A case-control study. *International Journal of Epidemiology* 2006; 35(2):307–314.

## (62) HERPES SIMPLEX (COLD SORE)

Koytchev R, Alken RG, Dundarov S. Balm mint extract (Lo-701) for topical treatment of recurring herpes labialis. *Phytomedicine* 1999; 6(4):225–230.

Vynograd N, Vynograd I, Sosnowski Z. A comparative multi-centre study of the efficacy of propolis, acyclovir and placebo in the treatment of genital herpes (HSV). *Phytomedicine* 2000; 7(1):1–6.

## (64) PERTUSSIS (WHOOPING COUGH)

Vidakovics MLP, Paba J, Lamberti Y, et al. Profiling the *Bordetella pertussis* proteome during iron starvation. *Journal of Proteome Research* 2007; 6(7):2518–2528.

## (65) FEVER

Section on Clinical Pharmacology and Therapeutics and Committee on Drugs, American Academy of Pediatrics. Fever and antipyretic use in children. *Pediatrics* 2011; 127(3):580–587.

## (66) BRUXISM (TEETH GRINDING)

Lobbezoo F, Lavigne GJ, Tanguay R, Montplaisir JY. The effect of catecholamine precursor L-dopa on sleep bruxism: A controlled clinical trial. *Movement Disorders* 1997; 12(1):73–78.

## (67) BRUISES

Seeley BM, Denton AB, Ahn MS, Maas CS. Effect of homeopathic Arnica montana on bruising in face-lifts: Results of a randomized, double-blind, placebo-controlled clinical trial. *Archives of Facial Plastic Surgery* 2006; 8(1):54–59.

## (68) FIBROMYALGIA

Lister RE. An open, pilot study to evaluate the potential benefits of coenzyme Q10 combined with Ginkgo biloba extract in fibromyalgia syndrome. *Journal of International Medical Research* 2002; 30(2):195–199.

## (69) JUVENILE RHEUMATOID ARTHRITIS

Vargová V, Vesely R, Sasinka M, Török C. [Will administration of omega-3 unsaturated fatty acids reduce the use of nonsteroidal antirheumatic agents in children with chronic juvenile arthritis?]. *Casopís Lékaru Ceskych* 1998; 137(21):651–653. [Slovak]

Alpigiani MG, Ravera G, Buzzanca C, et al. [The use of n-3 fatty acids in chronic juvenile arthritis.] *Pediatria Medica e Chirurgica* 1996; 18(4):387–390. [Italian]

## (73) BROKEN BONE

Ryan LM, Brandoli C, Freishtat RJ, et al. Prevalence of vitamin D insufficiency in African American children with forearm fractures: A preliminary study. *Journal of Pediatric Orthopedics* 2010; 30(2):106–109.

## (75) ASTHMA

Camargo CA, Rifas-Shiman SL, Litonjua AA, et al. Maternal intake of vitamin D during pregnancy and risk of recurrent wheeze in children at 3 y of age. *American Journal of Clinical Nutrition* 2007; 85(3):788–795.

Brehm JM, Celedón JC, Soto-Quiros ME, et al. Serum vitamin D levels and markers of severity of childhood asthma in Costa Rica. *American Journal of Respiratory and Critical Care Medicine* 2009; 179(9):765–771.

Olsen SF, Østerdal ML, Salvig JD, et al. Fish oil intake compared with olive oil intake in late pregnancy and asthma in the offspring: 16 y of registry-based follow-up from a randomized controlled trial. *American Journal of Clinical Nutrition* 2008; 88(1):167–175.

Harik-Khan RI, Muller DC, Wise RA. Serum vitamin levels and the risk of asthma in children. *American Journal of Epidemiology* 2004; 159(4):351–357.

## (76) BRONCHIOLITIS (INFANT BRONCHITIS)

Marzian O. [Treatment of acute bronchitis in children and adolescents. Non-interventional postmarketing surveillance study confirms the benefit and safety of a syrup made of extracts from thyme and ivy leaves]. *MMW Fortschritte der Medizin* 2007; 149(27–28 Suppl):69 74. [German]

Shenai JP, Chytil F, Stahlman MT. Vitamin A status of neonates with bronchopulmonary dysplasia. *Pediatric Research* 1985; 19(2):185–188.

## (78) CYSTIC FIBROSIS

Stafanger G, Koch C. N-acetylcysteine in cystic fibrosis and Pseudomonas aeruginosa infection: Clinical score, spirometry and ciliary motility. *European Respiratory Journal* 1989; 2(3):234–237.

## (79) INFLUENZA (SEASONAL AND H1N1)

Zakay-Rones Z, Thom E, Wollan T, Wadstein J. Randomized study of the efficacy and safety of oral elderberry extract in the treatment of influenza A and B virus infections. *Journal of International Medical Research* 2004; 32(2):132–140.

Predy GN, Goel V, Lovlin R, et al. Efficacy of an extract of North American ginseng containing poly-furanosyl-pyranosyl-saccharides for preventing upper respiratory tract infections: A randomized controlled trial. *CMAJ: Canadian Medical Association Journal* 2005; 173(9):1043–1048.

## (80) PNEUMONIA

Bhandari N, Bahl R, Taneja S, et al. Effect of routine zinc supplementation on pneumonia in children aged 6 months to 3 years: Randomised controlled trial in an urban slum. *British Medical Journal* 2002; 324(7350):1358–1361.

## (82) ACNE

Adebamowo CA, Spiegelman D, Berkey CS, et al. Milk consumption and acne in teenaged boys. *Journal of the American Academy of Dermatology* 2008; 58(5):787–793.

Adebamowo CA, Spiegelman D, Danby FW, et al. High school dietary dairy intake and teenage acne. *Journal of the American Academy of Dermatology* 2005; 52(2):207–214.

Shalita AR, Smith JG, Parish LC, et al. Topical nicotinamide compared with clindamycin gel in the treatment of inflammatory acne vulgaris. *International Journal of Dermatology* 1995; 34(6):434–437.

## (85) CONTACT DERMATITIS (DIAPER RASH)

Wolff HH, Kieser M. Hamamelis in children with skin disorders and skin injuries: Results of an observational study. *European Journal of Pediatrics* 2007; 166(9):943–948.

## (86) ATOPIC DERMATITIS (ECZEMA)

Wickens K, Black PN, Stanley TV, et al. A differential effect of 2 probiotics in the prevention of eczema and atopy: A double-blind, randomized, placebo-controlled trial. *Journal of Allergy and Clinical Immunology* 2008; 122(4):788–794.

Sausenthaler S, Koletzko S, Schaaf B, et al. Maternal diet during pregnancy in relation to eczema and allergic sensitization in the offspring at 2 y of age. *American Journal of Clinical Nutrition* 2007; 85(2):530–537.

## (87) IMPETIGO

Cutler RR, Wilson P. Antibacterial activity of a new, stable, aqueous extract of allicin against methicillin-resistant Staphylococcus aureus. *British Journal of Biomedical Science* 2004; 61(2):71–74.

## (88) HEAD LICE

Mumcuoglu KY, Miller J, Zamir C, et al. The in vivo pediculicidal efficacy of a natural remedy. *Israel Medical Association Journal* 2002; 4(10):790–793.

## (89) PSORIASIS

Syed TA, Ahmad SA, Holt AH, et al. Management of psoriasis with Aloe vera extract in a hydrophilic cream: A placebo-controlled, double-blind study. *Tropical Medicine and International Health* 1996; 1(4):505–509.

## (91) TINEA (RINGWORM, ATHLETE'S FOOT, JOCK ITCH)

Satchell AC, Saurajen A, Bell C, Barnetson RS. Treatment of interdigital tinea pedis with 25% and 50% tea tree oil solution: A randomized, placebo-controlled, blinded study. *Australasian Journal of Dermatology* 2002; 43(3):175–178.

Al-Waili NS. An alternative treatment for pityriasis versicolor, tinea cruris, tinea corporis and tinea faciei with topical application of honey, olive oil and beeswax mixture: An open pilot study. *Complementary Therapies in Medicine* 2004; 12(1):45–47.

## (92) WARTS

Focht DR, Spicer C, Fairchok MP. The efficacy of duct tape vs cryotherapy in the treatment of verruca vulgaris (the common wart). *Archives of Pediatrics and Adolescent Medicine* 2002; 156(10):971–974.

## (94) ENURESIS (BED-WETTING)

Egger J, Carter CH, Soothill JF, Wilson J. Effect of diet treatment on enuresis in children with migraine or hyperkinetic behavior. *Clinical Pediatrics* (Philadelphia) 1992; 31(5):302–307.

Ferrara P, Marrone G, Emmanuele V, et al. Homotoxicological remedies versus desmopressin versus placebo in the treatment of enuresis: A randomised, double-blind, controlled trial. *Pediatric Nephrology* 2008; 23(2):269–274.


## (95) PREMENSTRUAL SYNDROME

Walker AF, De Souza MC, Vickers MF, et al. Magnesium supplementation alleviates premenstrual symptoms of fluid retention. *Journal of Women's Health* 1998; 7(9):1157–1165.

Agha-Hosseini M, Kashani L, Aleyaseen A, et al. *Crocus sativus* L. (saffron) in the treatment of premenstrual syndrome: A double-blind, randomised and placebo-controlled trial. *BJOG: An International Journal of Obstetrics and Gynaecology* 2008; 115(4):515–519.


## (96) MENORRHAGIA (ABNORMAL PERIODS)

Massart F, Parrino R, Seppia P, et al. How do environmental estrogen disruptors induce precocious puberty? *Minerva Pediatrica* 2006; 58(3):247–254.

Ziaei S, Zakeri M, Kazemnejad A. A randomised controlled trial of vitamin E in the treatment of primary dysmenorrhoea. *BJOG: An International Journal of Obstetrics and Gynaecology* 2005; 112(4):466–469.


## (97) URINARY TRACT INFECTION

Hess MJ, Hess PE, Sullivan MR, et al. Evaluation of cranberry tablets for the prevention of urinary tract infections in spinal cord injured patients with neurogenic bladder. *Spinal Cord* 2008; 46(9):622–626.


## (99) OBESITY

Matsuyama T, Tanaka Y, Kamimaki I, et al. Catechin safely improved higher levels of fatness, blood pressure, and cholesterol in children. *Obesity* (Silver Spring) 2008; 16(6):1338–1348.


## (100) FAILURE TO THRIVE

Saran S, Gopalan S, Krishna TP. Use of fermented foods to combat stunting and failure to thrive. *Nutrition* 2002; 18(5):393–396.


## PART III: BODY SYSTEM REMEDIES

## CHAPTER 5

Kogan MD, Blumberg SJ, Schieve LA, et al. Prevalence of parent-reported diagnosis of austism spectrum disorder among children in the US, 2007. *Pediatrics* 2009; 124(5):1395–1403.

# — ABOUT THE AUTHOR —

**DR. JARED M. SKOWRON IS A NATIONAL EXPERT** in natural medicine for children. Author of *Fundamentals of Naturopathic Pediatrics,* his life's work is dedicated to the optimal health of children, using natural therapies. Faculty at University of Bridgeport, and founder of their Pediatric & Autism Clinic, he has helped thousands of children fulfill their optimal potential. Dr. Skowron is vice-president of the Pediatric Association of Naturopathic Physicians and can help your child feel their best, www.100NaturalRemedies.com.

# — INDEX —

Underscored references indicate boxed text and charts.